ANALYZING WITHIN-SUBJECTS EXPERIMENTS

ANALYZING WITHIN-SUBJECTS EXPERIMENTS

John W. Cotton
UNIVERSITY OF CALIFORNIA,

SANTA BARBARA

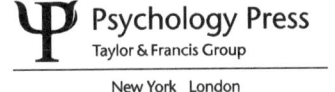

Psychology Press
Taylor & Francis Group

New York   London

Lawrence Erlbaum Associates, Inc., Publishers
10 Industrial Avenue
Mahwah, New Jersey 07430-2262

Cover design by Kathryn Houghtaling Lacey

Library of Congress Cataloging-in-Publication Data

Cotton, John Whealdon, 1925-
Analyzing within-subjects experiments / John W. Cotton
    p.   cm.
Includes bibliographical references and index.
ISBN 0-8058-2804-4 (alk. paper)
1. Crossover trials. I. Title
R653.C76C87 1997
615.5'07'2--DC21   97-8624
                                                      CIP

First Published by Lawrence Erlbaum Associates, Inc., Publishers
10 Industrial Avenue
Mahwah, New Jersey 07430

Reprinted 2010 by Psychology Press

The final camera copy for this work was prepared by the author, and therefore the publisher takes no responsibility for consistency or correctness of typographical style. However, this arrangement helps to make publication of this kind of scholarship possible.

To Corliss

Contents

Preface

This book is intended to fill an empty niche in the statistical toolbox of behavior scientists. Most of us know how to analyze continuous data from randomly assigned treatment groups of subjects. We also know how to assess practice effects for a single group of subjects given a constant treatment on each of several stages of practice. However, except in the case of the repeated measures Latin square design, we are not facile in analyzing data from different subjects receiving different treatments at different times in an experiment (i.e., in a so-called crossover design). As chapter 1 states, and later chapters elaborate, randomization of treatment sequences for different subjects may lead to unbiased conventional estimates of treatment effects and of time-related effects. However, the standard errors of such estimates may be unduly large because the error sums of squares include contributions from nuisance variables (such as stage-of-practice effects when treatment effects are of interest).

Because this text is an introductory one, we give minimal attention to two topics of importance with crossover designs: (a) modification of significance tests when error scores have complicated covariance structures and (b) analysis of crossover design data when many observations have been made on each organism serving as an experimental subject. The former problem may be treated by such devices as empirical generalized least squares estimation and ante dependence analysis (Jones & Kenward, 1989). The latter problem may require use of regression analysis with autoregressive errors (De Carlo, 1994) or of more advanced techniques rarely used with crossover design data to date, such as Kalman filtering procedures (Chatfield, 1989; Jones, 1993; Smith, 1996).

ACKNOWLEDGMENTS

Although I bear sole responsibility for the contents of this text, I express special appreciation to three experts on crossover designs who have provided me information, inspiration, and stimulation with their writings, correspondence, and face-to-face discussions: Byron Jones, Mike Kenward, and David Ratkowsky. Lynne Edwards made direct and indirect contributions to chapter 6, for which I thank her sincerely. I also thank Frank and Kam Rust for introducing me to Ventura Publisher and for many other kindnesses. This permitted me to prepare camera-ready copy for the present book. I am very grateful to Carol B. DeCanio for doing the correspondence necessary to obtain permission for reproduction of certain previously printed materials and for helping with related bibliographic matters as well as making helpful suggestions about book design.

I thank Larry Erlbaum and Bob Kidd for their support of this book and other Erlbaum personnel (Kathleen Dolan, Editorial Associate; Kate Graetzer, Editorial Assistant; Art Lizza, Vice President of Production, and Kathryn Houghtaling-Lacey, Graphic Designer) for copy editing, editorial, typesetting advice, and cover design. I will always admire my book production editors from Lawrence Erlbaum Associates, Marcy Pruiksma and Nicole Bush, for their technical expertise, teaching ability, and patience as they guided me through the intricacies of book preparation and "typesetting by computer." I especially thank my daughter, Carolyn Fishel, for volunteering to prepare the subject and author indexes; which she did in a thoughtful, principled manner. Most of all, I thank my wife Corliss, to whom this book is affectionately dedicated, for her help with proofreading, her sustained encouragement of this project, and for our life together during the past 50 years.

—John W. Cotton

1

An Orientation to Within-Subjects Designs

INTRODUCTION

What Is a Within-Subjects Design?

A *within-subjects design* is one in which every subject receives two or more trials on which the response is to be measured. The treatment may or may not change from trial to trial or from subject to subject on a given trial.

What Is a Crossover Design?

A *crossover design* is a within-subjects experimental design in which each subject receives two or more different tasks or treatments, crossing over from one to another and possibly back again in later stages. (This book uses the term *Stage* in many places where *Trial* might be expected by some readers. For behavior scientists, a *trial* is a unit of experimentation such as a warning signal followed by a test stimulus and a response to it. However, for biologists and medical statisticians, a *trial* is an experiment or at least a subexperiment, often labeled a "clinical trial," for example, when one is evaluating different drugs or other therapeutic treatments for effectiveness.)

Several within-subjects designs (most of them crossover designs as well) are briefly described later, together with reference to them elsewhere, as in chapters of this book. A major purpose of this book is to illustrate appropriate data analysis methods for use with a variety of such within-subjects and crossover designs. Because normally distributed data are assumed, analysis of variance techniques receive primary attention here.

TYPES OF WITHIN-SUBJECTS DESIGNS

Table 1.1 summarizes relevant features of some within-subjects designs that are important to behavior scientists. This table characterizes their experimental plans as well as indicating the purposes, such as assessing within-subjects treatment effects, for which they have been employed in behavioral research. Table 1.1 also tells where each design is discussed in this book.

TABLE 1.1

A Historical Classification of Within-Subjects Designs

VARIETY OF WITHIN-SUBJECTS DESIGN	MAIN PLACES DISCUSSED
Constant Treatment Within-Subjects Designs	
One-Group Split-Plot Designs	Chapter 2
Multigroup Split-Plot Designs	Marginally relevant material in chapters 3, 5, and 10
Historically Focused on Within-Subjects Treatment Effects	
Randomized Block Designs	Chapters 2, 3, and 13
Factorial Within-Subject Designs	Chapters 5 and 13
Historically Focused on Stage and Treatment Effects	
Latin Square Repeated Measurements Designs	Lightly in chapters 5, 6, and 13
Block Randomization Designs	Chapters 11 and 13
Historically Focused on the Point at Which Treatment Change Is Introduced	
Pretest-Posttest Control Group Designs	Chapters 6 and 13
Switching Treatments in Blocks (e.g., Balaam Designs)	Chapters 7 and 13
Alternating Treatment Designs	Chapters 8 and 13
Multiple Baseline Designs	Chapters 9, 10, and 13
Counterbalanced Designs	Chapters 12 and 13

Which Kinds of These Designs Have Psychologists Used to Assess Stage (or Trial) Effects?

The two experimental designs listed here are typical of designs focusing on effects of stages:

1. *Simplest Within-Subjects Design (One-Group Split-Plot Repeated Measurements Design).* Uses a single group with some number *n* of different subjects and some number *p* of stages under a constant treatment. This design is employed to look for differential effects of treatments varying within subjects and to assess differences in performance by different subjects. This design is treated in chapter 2.

2. *Multigroup Split-Plot Design.* Some number *G* of groups with a different treatment for each group, *n* subjects per group with *p* stages under a constant treatment. This design is somewhat related to material in chapters 3, 5, and 10. It is treated fully in such sources as Milliken and Johnson (1984) and Kirk (1995). The multigroup split-plot design permits assessment of group, effects, stage effects, group by stage effects, and subject effects.

Which Within-Subjects Designs Have Psychologists Used Primarily to Assess Treatment Effects?

1. *Randomized Block Design.* Uses some number *n* of subjects with $p = T$ treatments, each on a different stage. Order of treatment is randomized separately for each subject. Part of Bethell-Fox and Shepard's (1988) Experiment 2 on mental rotation approximates a 6-treatment randomized block design. This design receives traditional discussion in chapter 2 (primarily assessing differential effects of treatments varying within subjects) and a more thorough analysis in chapter 3 (also assessing stage effects and carryover effects, i.e., effects of prior treatments on performance on the current stage).

2. *Two-Way Factorial Within-Subjects Design.* One example of a two-way factorial design has each of *n* subjects receive all possible combinations of two treatment factors. If there are *J* levels of Treatment Factor 1 and *K* levels of Treatment Factor 2, this means that there will be *JK* different stages of testing, one for each possible combination of the two factors. For example, Treatment Factor 1 in an attitude manipulation experiment could be the context (lecture or discussion) in which arguments on a topic are presented and Treatment Factor 2 could be the type of argument (emotional or factual) that is presented.

Multi-way within-subjects factorial designs with more than two treatment factors are also possible. These designs can be used to test for main effects and interactions of the within-subject treatment factors and also for stage effects and carryover effects. More than two levels of one or more treatment factors can also be employed. See chapter 5 for a discussion of factorial within-subjects designs.

Which Designs Have Psychologists Used to Assess Both Stage and Treatment Effects?

1. *Latin Square Repeated Measurements Designs*. There are $n = p = T$ subjects each receiving p stages, one on each of the T treatments with every stage involving each treatment exactly once. This kind of design is treated only as a secondary topic in chapters 5 and 6. However, it is well suited to the assessment of subject effects, within-subjects treatment effects, stage effects, and carryover effects.

2. *Block Randomized Designs*. Each of n subjects receives B blocks of $p = T$ stages. In each block each of T treatments is presented to each subject once in some random order. This design may be used for the assessment of treatment, stage, and carryover effects. In a more complicated example, what Bethell-Fox and Shepard (1988) call the final two blocks of their Experiment 2 is a block randomized experiment with a 2 by 3 factorial appearing in each block. There are $B = 6$ blocks of 6 stages. See chapter 11 for a discussion of block randomized designs.

Which Designs Are Used to Assess Effects of the Point at Which Treatment Change Is Introduced?

1. *Switching Treatments in Blocks*. For example, $A^m A^m$ versus $A^m B^m$ versus $B^m A^m$ versus $B^m B^m$ groups of n subjects each, with Treatments A and B in blocks of $p \geq 1$ stages. When $m = 1$, this is the so-called Balaam design of chapter 7. This general class of design may also be used for the assessment of treatment and carryover effects and also for stage effects if $m \geq 2$.

2. *Alternating Treatment Designs*. $A^m B^m A^m B^m$ and $B^m A^m B^m A^m$ patterns for separate groups of n subjects each, $m \geq 1$, as in chapter 8. This category of design also can be employed for the assessment of treatment, stage, and carryover effects. It is especially popular in clinical psychology or similar research areas in which the reversibility of therapeutic effects is of interest.

3. *Multiple Baseline Designs.* For example, AAA versus AAB versus ABB groups of *n* subjects each, as in chapter 9. As usual, it is possible to employ this design for the assessment of treatment, stage, and carryover effects. It has the advantage of checking for changed effects of introducing a treatment change at different stages of an experiment or at different chronological points.

4. *Counterbalanced Designs.* For example, ABBA versus BAAB groups of *n* subjects each, as in chapter 12. Or ABCCBA versus ACBBCA versus BACCAB versus BCAACB versus CABBAC versus CBAABC groups of *n* subjects each. Again, these designs may be used for checking on treatment, stage, and carryover effects. Counterbalanced designs have the same average stage of presentation for each treatment, giving a symmetry to their designs. An early use of them in psychology was to produce constant average performance under different treatments if no differential effects appeared. However, this required an assumption of linear stage effects (Gottsdanker, 1978), which is not necessary in the statistical analysis methods presented here. Appropriate methods of significance testing specific to counterbalanced designs probably do not appear yet in the psychological literature.

BACKGROUND ON ANALYSIS
OF WITHIN-SUBJECTS DESIGNS

What Are Traditional Sources of Data Analysis Methods for These Designs?

The split-plot, randomized block, two-way factorial within-subject, and Latin square repeated measurements designs tend to be discussed in most advanced behavioral science texts on statistics and experimental design (e.g., Girden, 1992; Keppel, 1982; Kirk, 1995; Maxwell & Delaney, 1990; Myers, 1979). These and similar sources are excellent for the designs just mentioned, provided that there is no need to separate carryover effects (also called residual effects) from treatment effects. Note that carryover effects can also be viewed as transfer effects due to prior treatment or to treatment change. Except in Latin square designs, traditional analysis methods also have difficulty in separating stage effects from treatment effects. It should be noted that several of the sources just cited do mention the need to use analysis techniques adequate to separate time-related effects from within-subjects treatment effects. However, they do not indicate how such analyses should proceed. This leaves the investigator knowing that data analysis really should perform this separation but not knowing how to do so.

For block randomized designs, Shaughnessy and Zechmeister (1990) recommended one analysis of variance separating subject and treatment effects from error and a second one-way analysis of variance of the same data to separate trial effects from error.

Some other designs, such as switching treatments within blocks designs, alternating treatment designs, and multiple baseline designs tend to be discussed nonstatistically in experimental psychology texts and statistically in the operant journal literature. See also Barlow and Hersen (1984), Kratochwill (1978), and Kratochwill and Levin (1992).

Are There Better Sources Permitting Simultaneous Assessment of Time-Related Effects?

We recommend that, for data from most within subjects designs, modern analysis methods be used. These are crossover design methods that can simultaneously test for treatment, trial, and carryover effects in all of the previously mentioned designs and others for which those effects are technically estimable. The least mathematically challenging modern sources may be Ratkowsky, Evans, and Alldredge (1993) and Senn (1993). The former details sophisticated analyses of all designs previously mentioned, except for block randomized designs, variants of the Balaam design for which $n > 1$, alternating treatment designs, and multiple baseline designs.

The most statistically sophisticated crossover designs book is Jones and Kenward (1989). It treats the same designs as Ratkowsky et al., plus others. A special strength of this book is further analysis methods in which unusual multivariate methods are applied to crossover designs (e.g., the analysis of data from what we would call a *randomized block design*, Jones and Kenward).

Crossover theory data analysis methods for all of the designs mentioned above appear in current versions of Cotton (1993, 1994) or the present volume. Other recommended sources are Crowder and Hand (1990), Lunneborg (1994), Milliken and Johnson (1984, especially chap. 32), and Searle (1987). Lunneborg introduced crossover designs in the context of statistical modeling for biological and behavioral scientists; Searle was very strong on analysis of variance but had little or nothing to say about within-subject designs.

GOOD NEWS: As mentioned earlier, most recommended sources make it plain that it is not necessary to assume linear trend of stage effects in order to use and interpret data from within-subject counterbalanced designs.

Why Not Simply Focus on Multivariate Statistics As a Source of Analysis Methods for Within-Subjects Designs?

Multivariate statistical methods are directly applicable in repeated measurements studies with single- and multiple-group split-plot designs because those designs involve comparable response vectors for each subject, the first response coming from Stage 1, the second from Stage 2, and so on. So techniques such as MANOVA (multivariate analysis of variance) are easily applied there. Unfortunately, most other within-subject designs involve different treatments at different stages of a subject's service in an experiment. Therefore, an inappropriate analysis method will fail to separate time-related effects from the effects of those different treatments.

In the multivariate statistical literature, the models for crossover designs of primary interest in the present book are called Multiple Design Models (MDMs; Seber, 1984). The multivariate analysis of data involving such models seems not to be nearly as well developed as that for data from other within-subject designs; we cannot really speak of MANOVA as an option for crossover designs (MDMs). However, we have mentioned that Jones and Kenward (1989) were strong in adapting multivariate techniques to crossover designs. Especially in chapters 3 and 8, we discuss some applications of multivariate techniques, using conservative procedures as necessary to compensate for failures to meet assumptions for application of univariate methods. However, our treatment of this topic is very brief. The reader should rely on other sources, such as Jones and Kenward, for serious treatments of this topic. There one will find special techniques such as ante-dependence analysis and empirical generalized least squares that can be useful in the behavioral science despite not having been used frequently in psychology or related disciplines in past research.

TOOLS OF THE PRESENT BOOK: ANOVA
AND THE SAS® GLM STATISTICAL PACKAGE

This book is intended to focus as much as possible on computational techniques appropriate to the analysis of data from within-subjects and, especially crossover within-subjects, designs. Therefore, it is largely a collection of examples of hypothetical data from the designs listed in Table 1.1, together with illustrative data analyses for them. Theoretical background is presented only as it proves needed. Much of the interpretation of SAS® GLM output is explained in chapter 4, which does not cover any new designs.

All response measures examined here are assumed to be continuous variables, partially justifying use of analysis of variance (often abbreviated ANOVA). For an introduction to the analysis of crossover design data that are categorical rather than continuous, see Jones and Kenward (1989).

For computation, the present book primarily uses the SAS® statistical system, giving special attention to its GLM (General Linear Model) procedure. Relevant manuals are available both for personal computers (SAS Institute Inc., 1985, 1988a, 1988b) and for larger computers such as those with the UNIX operating system as a base (SAS Institute Inc., 1989a, 1989b, 1989c, 1989d, 1990). Because the use of SAS® is quite similar for both kinds of computers, we cite only the latter hereafter. The meaning of GLM, a unified way of modeling data to be used in analysis of variance, covariance, and regression analysis, is explained next. It is a statistical concept that is not tied to any single statistical package. However, SAS® GLM is particularly well suited to analyzing data describable by the GLM.

Chapter 6 tells how to use BMDP™ (Dixon, Brown, Engelman, Hill, & Jennrich, 1990), SPSS® (Norusis, 1990a, 1990b), or SYSTAT™ (Wilkinson, 1989) for data analysis problems like those illustrated here with SAS® GLM. However, there are enough difficulties or ambiguities involved in using those other programs with crossover design data to make us feel that you need to master chapters 1 through 5 before attempting to use an alternate statistical package with such data.

Beginning in chapter 3, there are occasional references to mathematical programming languages such as GAUSS (Aptech Systems, 1993).

Such systems have the advantage of allowing the user to write out the General Linear Model for a specific design and see exactly what it implies about a related data set rather than obtaining results more indirectly via a conventional statistical package. Near the end of the book (chapter 12 and appendix 2), we go so far as to explain the use of specific GAUSS programs in situations where their use is much more feasible than that of SAS®. However, in chapter 8 we spare the reader the study of this new language even where it would be desirable, choosing instead to use SAS® GLM in a somewhat unnatural way. Finally, chapter 13 asks what makes a good experimental design from a statistical standpoint. This chapter relates the efficiency and variance of estimators information from earlier chapters to the topics of optimality and practical optimality. It goes on to compare current designs with others in non-psychological sources and to consider topics such as the use of *baseline observations* (observations in the absence of special treatment) or *wash-out observations* (baseline types of observations made between observations under special treatment).

THE IDEA OF THE GENERAL LINEAR MODEL

Now we present a preliminary topic central to the remainder of this text. The General Linear Model is a model for any regression analysis or analysis of variance data set based on continuous (ordinarily also normally distributed) scores and linear equations. What makes this kind of model general is the breadth of application of equations like 1.3 and 1.4 below to regression analysis, analysis of covariance, and analysis of variance. Although a General Linear Model can be written without matrices (i.e., in so-called *scalar* form), we will be most interested in its representation in matrix form. If you are not acquainted with simple concepts of matrix algebra, you should use appendix 1 as a reference from now on.

In this introductory section we deal with an example so simple that we could not do a useful data analysis on it. We have two groups of subjects but only one subject per group with one observation per subject. This would prevent performing a two-group *t*- or *F*-test with data from it. However, some parameter estimation and other central ideas about the General Linear Model will be present even in this simple case. We deal both with simple algebraic (scalar) and more complicated (matrix) notation.

The General Linear Model in Scalar Form

Let $Y_1 = 21 + 15 + 1.3$ and $Y_2 = 21 + 7 + (-1.2)$ be predictions for two persons, the first coming from Group 1 and the second coming from Group 2. We could say that 21 is a population intercept (much like a population mean) applying to members of each group. Also, 15 is a treatment effect for members of Group 1, and 7 is a treatment effect for members of Group 2. Finally, 1.3 is an error component or score for the one person known to fall in Group 1, and -1.2 is an error component for the one person known to fall in Group 2. If we let the intercept be represented by μ, the treatment effect for any member of Group 1 be α_1, the treatment effect for any member of Group 2 be α_2, the error for the one subject in Group 1 be e_1, and the error for the one subject in Group 2 be e_2, we can write:

$$Y_1 = \mu + \alpha_1 + e_1 \tag{1.1a}$$

and $\qquad Y_2 = \mu + \alpha_2 + e_2 \tag{1.1b}$

Sophisticated readers who expected $\sum_{g=1}^{2} \alpha_g = 0$ should read chapter 5 to see why the most general models and the SAS® GLM statistical system in particular do not include this constraint in their initial statement.)

There is some advantage in asking that every parameter (non-error component) of the model under examination be included in each of the predictive equations employed. Therefore, we rewrite each of our predictive equations to include both treatment effects, α_1 and α_2:

$$Y_1 = (1)\mu + (1)\alpha_1 + (0)\alpha_2 + e_1 \tag{1.2a}$$

and $\qquad Y_2 = (1)\mu + (0)\alpha_1 + (1)\alpha_2 + e_2 \tag{1.2b}$

Because every parameter is included in the predictive equation for each observation, this form is specially suited to representing a General Linear Model (GLM). Also, there are coefficients for each parameter: 1 1 0 for μ, α_1, and α_2 in Equation 1.2a and 1 0 1 for them in Equation 1.2b.

The General Linear Model in Matrix Form

The entries in these two equations turn out to be consistent with a matrix multiplication example in appendix 1: The coefficients just listed form a matrix, $X = \begin{pmatrix} 1 & 1 & 0 \\ 1 & 0 & 1 \end{pmatrix}$, which we call the *design matrix* because it reflects the experimental design employed in this experiment. Also, the parameters form a so-called *parameter vector*, $\beta = \begin{pmatrix} \mu \\ \alpha_1 \\ \alpha_2 \end{pmatrix}$. Then $X\beta = \begin{pmatrix} \mu + \alpha_1 \\ \mu + \alpha_2 \end{pmatrix}$.

Suppose that we also have a vector $E = \begin{pmatrix} e_1 \\ e_2 \end{pmatrix}$. We can then write a new matrix equation:

$$Y = X\beta + E \tag{1.3}$$

$$Y = \begin{pmatrix} \mu + \alpha_1 + e_1 \\ \mu + \alpha_2 + e_2 \end{pmatrix} = \begin{pmatrix} \mu + \alpha_1 \\ \mu + \alpha_2 \end{pmatrix} + \begin{pmatrix} e_1 \\ e_2 \end{pmatrix} \tag{1.4}$$

These equations implicitly define a vector $Y = \begin{pmatrix} Y_1 \\ Y_2 \end{pmatrix}$ called the *observation vector* or *vector of observed scores*, and the error vector E is the vector of error scores according to this model. The matrix Equations 1.3 and 1.4 are each shorthand for the scalar Equations 1.1a and 1.1b or 1.2a and 1.2b. In either scalar or matrix form, they form the model for a two-group study with one subject per group. If we had several subjects per group, Equation 1.3 would still hold but with a modified Y, X, and E. Equation 1.4 would have as many rows as the number of scalar equations required with several subjects. This illustrates the fact that a matrix equation can be used as a specially compact way to write a single equation instead of a set of equations.

In later chapters of this book we will see that our statistical packages are built around matrix equations such as (1.3) or (1.4). Using the terminology of the General Linear Model, we can say that a statistical analysis has two purposes beyond low-level description of a data set: (a) Estimation of parameters in the parameter vector β or functions of those parameters if not all of them can be directly estimated, and (b) testing hypotheses about those parameters. Let us turn now to chapter 2 to see how to satisfy those purposes.

2

Two-Way Experimental Plans: Split-Plot and Randomized Block Designs

INTRODUCTION TO MODELS WITH PRACTICE OR TREATMENT EFFECTS, BUT NOT BOTH

Now we are ready to use the General Linear Model with a pair of superficially parallel within-subjects designs. Each uses a rectangular array of data. We can arbitrarily label subjects as the row variable and stages of practice (first design) or treatments (second design) as the column variable, depending on which design is involved. Statistically identical analysis methods will be illustrated for both designs. However, chapter 3 will show that the second (subjects by treatments) design is better analyzed with techniques in that chapter.

ANALYZING ONE-GROUP SPLIT-PLOT DATA

Suppose that there are six subjects in this experiment, each being measured on three stages of a task in which scores may change with time, possibly due to practice or to fatigue. This is an example of what is called a *one-group repeated measurements design* or a *one-group split-plot design.*

Two Models for Data From This Design

We might suppose that some subjects would have high scores and others would have low scores in this experiment. Also, scores might tend to go up from stage to stage (if high scores mean good performance). Furthermore, there may be some fluctuation in performance that seems random rather than a consequence of known factors in the experiment.

Finally, maybe there is some fixed starting place or intercept, regardless of which subject or stage is involved.

Although we do not often discuss sampling assumptions in this book, you should presume that, unless otherwise stated, each data analysis presented is built on the assumptions of random sampling of subjects from an identifiable population of potential subjects and of random sampling of error scores of the sort described in the model equation. A reasonable equation (part of the basic set of assumptions or model) for data from such a design might be:

$$Y_{ij} = \mu + s_i + \pi_j + e_{ij} \tag{2.1}$$

where i and j refer to Subject i and Stage j. Then the score Y_{ij} for Subject i on Stage j becomes an additive constant (intercept or starting place), μ, plus a random subject effect, s_i, for Subject i plus an effect π_j for Stage j and an error component, e_{ij}, specific to Subject i on Stage j. We assume that subject effects are independently and identically distributed (i.i.d.) with normal distributions having a mean of zero and a variance of σ_s^2. A compact representation of this assumption is that the s_i are i.i.d. $N(0, \sigma_s^2)$. Error components (e_{ij}) for each subject are assumed to be normally distributed with a mean of 0 and the further property that the variance of the difference in error components for the same subject on different stages, $Var(e_{ij} - e_{ij'})$, is constant for all pairs of different stages. Error components for different subjects are assumed independent, implying $Cov(e_{ij}, e_{i'j'}) = 0$ for different subjects, regardless of whether different stages are involved. Also, we assume $Cov(s_i, e_{i'j'}) = 0$ regardless of whether $i = i'$.

The former assumptions also imply that the Y_{ij} have a sphericity property: *Sphericity* is defined as present if and only if there is equality of variances for all differences of scores for pairs of stages on the same stages, such as the variance of $Y_{i1} - Y_{i2}$ (Stage 1 score minus Stage 2 score) compared to the variance of $Y_{i1} - Y_{i3}$, of $Y_{i2} - Y_{i3}$, etc. Sphericity holds because Equation 2.1 and its associated assumptions imply that $Var(Y_{ij} - Y_{ij'}) = Var(\pi_j + e_{ij} - \pi_{j'} - e_{ij'}) = Var(e_{ij} - e_{ij'})$, which has already been assumed constant for all pairs of different stages. Note that exclusion of subject effects, s_i, from (2.1) would not change the variances of our difference scores.

Digression on Alternate Definitions of Sphericity. The cited definition is equivalent to saying that sphericity holds when the so-called Huynh-Feldt (Huynh & Feldt, 1970) or Type H covariance structure to be discussed in chapter 3 is present. Sphericity was originally defined (e.g., Mauchly, 1940) as being what is now called *compound symmetry* or *uniform covariance structure*, specifically that the variances of Y are constant for all stages and that Y values for any pair of stages have the same correlation regardless of which pair was correlated. However, many authors (e.g., Kirk, 1995; Morrison, 1990) point out that the F-distribution holds in the presence of conventional assumptions plus the Type H covariance matrix or, equivalently, the equal variances of difference scores just invoked to define sphericity. It happens that the original Mauchly test is also a test of the newer sphericity assumption (Morrison, 1990).

If we want to be more specific about the nature of the effects of stages, we may recall that complicated trends can be composed of elements such as linear, quadratic, and cubic terms. Therefore, a second reasonable equation is:

$$Y_{ij} = \beta_0 + s_i + j\,\beta_1 + j^2\beta_2 + e_{ij} \qquad (2.2)$$

Then the score Y_{ij} for Subject i on Stage j becomes an additive constant, β_0; plus a random subject effect, s_i; plus a linear effect of the stage, $j\,\beta_1$; plus a quadratic effect of the stage, $j^2\beta_2$; plus an error compontent, e_{ij}, specific to Subject i on Stage j. The same assumptions about subject effects and error components apply here as in Equation 2.1.

One advantage of Equation 2.2 is that it includes linear and quadratic terms, permitting tests of the kind of trend in stage effects, rather than merely allowing a test of the presence of stage effects, as with Equation 2.1. Because only three stages are involved for any one subject in the current example, all data could be fitted perfectly with a separate quadratic equation for each subject. Therefore, no cubic or more complicated term is included in Equation 2.2. Either a linear trend, quadratic trend, or both would be consistent with nonzero stage effect differences in Equation 2.1.

A Hypothetical Repeated Measurements Study

Table 2.1 displays a hypothetical set of data for the specific design just mentioned. We want to analyze them with a computer statistical program, the SAS® package (SAS Institute Inc., 1989c). This program will employ the SAS® General Linear Model (GLM) procedure, called PROC GLM.

TABLE 2.1

Hypothetical Data for a One-Group Repeated Measurements Experiment

(Responses are number of t's crossed per minute in a proofreading task)

Subject	Stage 1	Stage 2	Stage 3	Mean
1	95.9	117.9	136.6	116.80
2	109.6	130.2	152.1	130.63
3	98.4	119.1	139.8	119.10
4	107.9	129.3	151.0	129.40
5	114.5	132.0	153.6	133.37
6	106.4	128.1	145.2	126.57
Mean	105.45	126.10	146.38	125.98

Method A: Two-Way ANOVA Test for Subject and Stage Effects Using SAS® GLM

A Relevant Computer Program

Here is one way to analyze the data of Table 2.1 based on the model in Equation 2.1. Think of the data as conforming to a two-way design with subjects as rows and stages as columns. Then it is natural to treat row effects as random and column effects as fixed. Our program will first evaluate these two kinds of effects.

The program will then compute the power of the test of subject (random) effects for a stated size of such effects, that size being a minimal size for detection: It is the smallest size that we would not want to lead to a nonsignificant F-test. Next the power of the test for stage effects (fixed effects) will be computed. Again there will be a stated size of such effects, that size being the smallest size that we would not want to miss in our analysis, judging stage effects to be nonsignificant when they indeed do exist in the population. Table 2.2 displays our SAS® GLM program for analyzing our hypothetical data in the way just outlined.

TABLE 2.2

A Two-Way ANOVA Program for Analyzing the Data
of Table 2.1

```
* PROGRAM GLM1GRP.SAS;
DATA A; INPUT SUBJ STAGE Y @@; CARDS;
1 1   95.9      1 2 117.9      1 3 136.6
2 1 109.6      2 2 130.2      2 3 152.1
3 1   98.4      3 2 119.1      3 3 139.8
4 1 107.9      4 2 129.3      4 3 151.0
5 1 114.5      5 2 132.0      5 3 153.6
6 1 106.4      6 2 128.1      6 3 145.2
RUN;
PROC GLM;  CLASS SUBJ STAGE;
MODEL Y = SUBJ STAGE/INVERSE; RANDOM SUBJ;
MEANS SUBJ;  MEANS STAGE;
DATA B;  VAR1 = 'RANDOM SUBJECTS';
F5PCNT_R = FINV(.95,5,10,0);  MULT_R = .1429;
POWER_R = 1 - PROBF(MULT_R*F5PCNT_R,5,10,0);
PROC PRINT DATA = B;
DATA  C; VAR2 = 'FIXED STAGES';
F5PCNT_F=FINV(.95,2,10,0);  LAMBDA = 19.0;
POWER_F = 1 – PROBF(F5PCNT_F,2,10,LAMBDA);
PROC PRINT DATA = C;
TITLE 'GLM1GRP — Analyzing Table 2.1 data by testing for subject
and stage effects.'; RUN;
```

The bold-faced section would not be typed differently than other parts of the program. It can be run as given, but the truth is that a reasonable value of LAMBDA for that section was generated by running the program once without it and again with it, using the initial results, as shown next, to help decide the value for LAMBDA. Because it uses data obtained in the present experiment, this is called a post hoc estimate of the size of stage effects and thus yields a post hoc estimate of power.

It is preferable, however, to quantify one's expectations about the size of population differences among different stage means and to compute LAMBDA before running the program the first time. A disadvantage of the post hoc method is that one is computing the probability of finding significance if certain sample mean differences were population values. But, if they were correct as assumed, we would not need to know the power value!

Some Rules About Symbols Used in a SAS® GLM Program

Let us try to understand how a program like this one is constructed and what it is saying. You should learn that each SAS® GLM command is ended by a semi-colon. It is permissible to include more than one command on a single line or to have a command continue to a new line so long as its semi-colon is at the end of the full command. A line beginning with an asterisk in the leftmost position begins a comment — it is infomation for the user, not instructions to the computer. Therefore, any comments are optional; omit them unless they may be useful to remind you what the program means or is about.

The main data unit (called *data step* in SAS® manuals) includes an arbitrary name for the data ("A" in this case) plus an input statement naming the variables to be recorded, an atavistic command called "CARDS;" (stemming from ancient times when computers used IBM cards as input), and the actual values of the data variables. Because the input statement in this program begins: "INPUT SUBJ STAGE Y", each line below the cards statement has three successive categories as follows:

Category 1 is the subject number.
Category 2 is the stage value for that subject.
Category 3 is the Y score for that subject and stage.

Note that some categories contain more than one column of data (e.g., a Y of 95.9 uses four columns of numerals or decimals plus blank spaces around the overall number, 95.9). Also notice, that because of the "@@" symbols in the "INPUT" statement, it is possible to record more than one set of the three categories on each line. In fact, each line has all the data for a certain subject such as Subject 1.

A procedure step such as "PROC GLM" tells what kind of analysis to do next; here it must include a "CLASS" statement telling which variables fall into groups or classes such as Stage 1 or Subject 1. The "PROC GLM" step also includes such commands as the "MODEL" statement, implying a mathematical model to be fitted to the data: "MODEL Y = SUBJ STAGE;" is a quick way to say that the previous model is Equation 2.1: $Y_{ij} = \mu + s_i + \pi_j + e_{ij}$. Notice that SAS® does not need us to type μ or error into its model; they are taken for granted. Also "RANDOM SUBJ;" says to treat the subjects factor as random rather than fixed, and "MEANS SUBJ;" or "MEANS STAGE;" says to compute the means for the factor specified. This is not necessary but can be helpful in filling in a data table such as Table 2.1.

This program actually includes three data steps. The last two, beginning "DATA B;" and "DATA C;", are used to compute power values rather than to store conventional data. Ideally, they should be run with dummy data and prior estimates of parameter values, made before the real experiment. If power is too low (perhaps less than 0.80 for any important variable) by such computations, then the experiment should be redesigned by such measures as increasing the number of subjects used. Then a study with adequate power can be conducted. On the other hand, there are occasions when you may already have run an experiment before computing its power for a certain hypothesis test. It could be that power is only 0.50, say, whereas the test statistic, such as t or F, is significant. Consider yourself lucky. There is nothing wrong with saying there is evidence of an effect when power is low! But, if power is low and the test statistic is not significant, you have a reason to feel your experiment was inconclusive.

A line beginning "TITLE" and followed by a message inside single quotation marks, concluding with a semi-colon, tells SAS® what title to place at the top of each page of output. Title commands are optional. The command "RUN;" appears at the very end of a SAS® program, saying that the program should now be run.

There was also an earlier "RUN;" command that you will not find in most discussions of SAS® programs: At the beginning of the first line after all the data entries have appeared, SAS Institute, Inc. (1989d) uses a ";" and Ratkowsky, Evans, and Alldredge (1993) use a "RUN;" command to say that the data have been entered. We prefer the "RUN;" because it is easier to see. If a line begins solely with ";", one may not notice it and eventually delete the semi-colon completely. At one time, omission of such an ending for a set of data would cause the requested statistical analysis to be aborted. Now, however, this is not true except in unusual cases. At least one author (Stevens, 1996, p. 28) omits these commands from his sample programs.

Be careful not to foul up your data entry by including any semi-colon(s) after the "CARDS;" statement and before the "RUN;" statement just discussed! Fortunately, SAS® is pretty patient with us in terms of spacing. Just don't run two words together or split a word into two partial words.

A Matrix Form of Equation 2.1

We already know the model in Equation 2.1 for observations from an experiment with a possibly different random effect for each subject and a possibly different fixed effect for each stage. Now let us write a matrix form of that equation:

$$Y = X\beta + E \tag{2.3}$$

With our six subjects and three stages, we can write the transpose Y' of the observation vector for Equation 2.3 as:

$$Y' = \left(Y_{11}\ Y_{12}\ Y_{13}\ Y_{21}\ Y_{22}\ Y_{23}\ Y_{31}\ Y_{32}\ Y_{33}\ Y_{41}\ Y_{42}\ Y_{43} \right.$$

$$Y_{51}\ Y_{52}\ Y_{53}\ Y_{61}\ Y_{62}\ Y_{63}),$$

and the design matrix as: $X = \begin{pmatrix} 1\ 100000\ 100 \\ 1\ 100000\ 010 \\ 1\ 100000\ 001 \\ 1\ 010000\ 100 \\ 1\ 010000\ 010 \\ 1\ 010000\ 001 \\ 1\ 001000\ 100 \\ 1\ 001000\ 010 \\ 1\ 001000\ 001 \\ 1\ 000100\ 100 \\ 1\ 000100\ 010 \\ 1\ 000100\ 001 \\ 1\ 000010\ 100 \\ 1\ 000010\ 010 \\ 1\ 000010\ 001 \\ 1\ 000001\ 100 \\ 1\ 000001\ 010 \\ 1\ 000001\ 001 \end{pmatrix}$ Also the transpose of the parameter vector is: $\beta' = \left(\mu\ s_1\ s_2\ s_3\ s_4\ s_5\ s_6\ \pi_1\ \pi_2\ \pi_3\right)$ and the transpose of the error vector is:

$$E' = \left(e_{11}\ e_{12}\ e_{13}\ e_{21}\ e_{22}\ e_{23}\ e_{31}\ e_{32}\ e_{33}\ e_{41}\ e_{42}\ e_{43}\right.$$

$$\left. e_{51}\ e_{52}\ e_{53}\ e_{61}\ e_{62}\ e_{63}\right).$$

The most important things to remember about these matrices are: (1) The rows of the design matrix correspond to the rows of the observation vector, organized with the three observations for Subject 1 preceding the three observations for Subject 2, etc. (2) The columns of the design matrix correspond to the rows of the parameter vector. Extra spacing in X emphasizes these points, with the first column being a 1 implying that μ applies to each observation. The next group, with six columns, is relevant to subject effects, s_i, with ones for the first three observations in the first column of such effects, followed by zeroes for all other observations; the next column applies to Subject 2, and so on. The final group, with three columns, applies to period effects, π_j, with ones in Positions 1, 4, 7, . . ., of the first column of such effects and zeros elsewhere, etc. (3) We state without proof that $(X'X)^{-1}$, the inverse of the matrix product, $(X'X)$, does not exist.

Method and Meaning of the Power Calculations in an SAS® Program

You probably know from earlier statistics courses that a power value is the probability of rejecting the null hypothesis when a certain size of effect is present. SAS® is able to compute power values both for fixed and for random effects once the size is specified for which power is to be found. See SAS Institute Inc. (1990) for a listing of SAS® statistical functions such as those used in our own power calculations. Using SAS® GLM to find power for random effects is relatively easy. However, using it to compute power for fixed effects is more difficult; the method for fixed effects illustrated next will include some matrix calculations.

Finding a Relevant Power Value for a Variable Having Random Effects. In the "DATA B;" section of the Table 2.2 program, power is calculated for subjects, a random effect. As noted in many sources (e.g., Hays, 1994), the power function for a random effect is calculated using the ordinary (central) F-distribution. The command "VAR1 = 'SUBJECT';" defines subject as the variable for which power is to be calculated. The next command "F5PCNT_R = FINV(.95,5,10,0);" has entries (socalled arguments) in four slots inside the parentheses of the SAS® function FINV. The first entry, .95, is used to specify the $1 - .95 = .05$ significance level of F for an experiment. The second entry, 5, specifies 5 degrees of freedom for the numerator (subjects). The third, 10, specifies 10 degrees of freedom for the denominator (error), as is true for the current example. The fourth entry, 0, follows from the fact that the ordinary (central) F-distribution just mentioned has what is known as a noncentrality parameter of zero. Using MULT_R to represent a measure of random effects, a further command, "MULT_R = .1429;", says that the critical effect size index for random effects discussed shortly below is equal to .1429. The next command, "POWER_R = 1 – PROBF(MULT_R*F5PCNT_R,5,10,0);" says to compute this power with the SAS® function PROBF for an F = MULT_R times F5PCNT_R with 5 and 10 degrees of freedom and 0 as the value of the noncentrality parameter.

Selecting an Appropriate Effect Size for a Variable Having Random Effects. To decide on an appropriate value of MULT_R, we needed first to know (or by running most of the program above an extra time to find out) that $E(MS_{Subjects}) = \sigma^2 + p\sigma_s^2 = \sigma^2 + 3\sigma_s^2$ (where the number of fixed conditions, p, is 3 stages in this example) and $E(MS_{Error}) = \sigma^2$ for this design with three observations per subject. If there are subject effects, then σ_s^2 is positive rather than zero. In that case there is a quantity F_1 which has the central F-distribution, but it is

$$F_1 = \frac{\sigma^2}{\sigma^2 + p\sigma_s^2}F = \frac{\sigma^2}{\sigma^2 + 3\sigma_s^2}F \qquad (2.4)$$

where the F is computed for subjects by SAS® GLM. The ratio used as a multiplier of F in 2.4 is what we call MULT_R in our aforementioned computer program. A very small true value of MULT_R means that there is (compared to σ^2 and taking p into account also) a very large value of σ_s^2 in the population from which we are sampling. When we calculate power for a significance test of this kind, we are selecting a MULT_R value that represents the largest ratio and the smallest effect we feel would be very important not to infer as statistically significant.

This judgment is somewhat arbitrary, as is the judgment about how much power is desired with a given study and MULT_R value. Here is one kind of reasoning that could be made: Unless the variance for subjects, σ_s^2, is at least twice as large as the variance for error, σ^2, it may not be serious if we conclude there are no significant subject effects. But when this condition holds exactly, our ratio, $\dfrac{\sigma^2}{\sigma^2 + 3\sigma_s^2}$, is equal to $1/7 = .1429$. This is why we set MULT_R = .1429 in the program of Table 2.2.

Finding a Relevant Power Value for a Variable Having Fixed Effects. In the "DATA C;" section of our program, power is calculated for the fixed effects associated with stages. As noted by Hays (1994), the power function for a set of fixed effects is calculated using the noncentral F-distribution. Accordingly, this section of the program uses the SAS® function "PROBF" with a nonzero value in its last argument to reflect that kind of distribution.

In Table 2.2 the command "VAR2 = 'FIXED STAGES';" is used to specific stages as the fixed variable for which power is to be calculated. The next command "F5PCNT_F = FINV(.95,2,10,0);" uses the SAS® function FINV to find the $1 - .95 = .05$ significance level of the central F distribution for an experiment with 2 degrees of freedom for the numerator (stages) and 10 degrees of freedom for the denominator (error) in this case. A further command, "LAMBDA = 19.0;", says that the effect size parameter, λ, for fixed effects discussed next is equal to 19. The next command, "POWER_F = 1 – PROBF(F5PCNT_F,2,10, LAMBDA);" says to compute this power with the SAS® function PROBF for a noncentral F5PCNT_F with 2 and 10 degrees of freedom and LAMBDA = 19 as the noncentrality parameter.

BEWARE: When you define a new "DATA" step, the most recent one operates for anything below it until a new one or an even older one is invoked again. So once you have run the existing program in Table 2.2, you will have gone through "DATA A;", "DATA B;", and "DATA C;" with C for fixed stages power still being operative even if you add a new "PROC" without specifying a new data step. This means that you must be very careful in your use of "DATA" steps.

Suppose that now you want to use "DATA A" again with a new "MODEL" statement. You will not have to type the "DATA A" step again; what you must do is to type "PROC GLM DATA = A;" and follow with your new model statement and related material.

Selecting an Appropriate Effect Size for a Variable Having Fixed Effects. When we specify a value of LAMBDA in our computer program, we are giving a minimum value for fixed effects, the smallest amount of effects that have to be identified if present. If λ is really smaller than LAMBDA, we believe it not to be necessary that our test for this kind of fixed effects should prove to be significant. But, if λ is really as large or larger than LAMBDA, we do want a high probability of significance (and thus a large value of power). If the computed probability, POWER_F, is larger than .80, for example, we may decide that it is adequate.

This judgment is somewhat arbitrary, as is the judgment about how much power is desired with a given study and LAMBDA value. Here is a reasonable method for setting its value: When we test hypotheses of no fixed effects of a certain kind within the General Linear Model, we are also testing the hypothesis that a matrix equation of a certain form holds:

$$H: K'\beta = 0 \tag{2.5}$$

In testing for stage of practice effects based on Equation 2.1 or Equation 2.3, the matrix $K' = \begin{pmatrix} 0\,0\,0\,0\,0\,0\,0\,1\,0\,-1 \\ 0\,0\,0\,0\,0\,0\,0\,0\,1\,-1 \end{pmatrix}$ is the transpose of a matrix that does not need to be shown here. The rows of K' refer to the first and second components of estimators of stage effects, and the columns correspond to all 10 parameters of β. When we perform the matrix multiplication implied by the hypothesis above, we obtain the desired result: $H: K'\beta = \begin{pmatrix} \pi_1 - \pi_3 \\ \pi_2 - \pi_3 \end{pmatrix} = \begin{pmatrix} 0 \\ 0 \end{pmatrix} = 0$. Because, as noted earlier, $(X'X)^{-1}$ does not exist, we usually must assess differences between parameters rather than individual parameters themselves. So our hypothesis is that the differences between Stage 1 and Stage 3 effects and between Stage 2 and Stage 3 effects are both equal to zero. Searle's (1971) Equation 70 can be applied to this example to show that $F = \dfrac{MS_{Stages}}{MS_{Error}}$ has the central F-distribution with 2 and 10 degrees of freedom when this H is true. However, if it is not true, F will have the noncentral F-distribution with 2 and 10 degrees of freedom and noncentrality parameter:

$$\lambda = \frac{1}{\sigma^2} (K'\beta)'(K'GK)^{-1}(K'\beta) \tag{2.6}$$

holds, where a generalized inverse with properties defined in appendix A1 is $G = (X'X)^{-}$ based on our design matrix. (Because a generalized inverse rather than a standard inverse is used here, the − superscript does not need a "1" beside it.) To set a value of LAMBDA to a reasonable minimum value in our power calculation plan, we need three building blocks: a value of σ^2, an appropriate value of $K'\beta$, and a value of $(K'GK)^{-1}$.

The one building block for stage effects that is fully determined by the time we conduct our experiment is the calculation of $(K'GK)^{-1}$, which can be shown algebraically to be equal to $\begin{pmatrix} g_{88} & g_{89} \\ g_{89} & g_{99} \end{pmatrix}^{-1}$. For ex-

ample, G is computed when we invoke the INVERSE option in the MODEL command of our program in Table 2.2. The g values come from the portion of computer output for G labeled Stage 1 and Stage 2 on its rows and columns. The inverse required proves to be:

$(K'GK)^{-1} = \begin{pmatrix} \dfrac{1}{3} & \dfrac{1}{6} \\ \dfrac{1}{6} & \dfrac{1}{3} \end{pmatrix}^{-1} = \begin{pmatrix} 4 & -2 \\ -2 & 4 \end{pmatrix}$. But, what should we do about our other

building blocks? The usual advice is to try to find independent information about the size of σ^2. Lacking that information here, we note that $MS_{Error} = 1.597$. To be conservative, we make a guess that σ^2 is no larger than 2. To find an appropriate value of $K'\beta$, we arbitrarily say that $\pi_1 - \pi_3 = -3.5355$ and $\pi_2 - \pi_3 = -1.4142$ represent a minimimally sized combination of effects to identify. This makes $K'\beta = \begin{pmatrix} \pi_1 - \pi_3 \\ \pi_2 - \pi_3 \end{pmatrix} = \begin{pmatrix} -3.5355 \\ -1.4142 \end{pmatrix}$.

Combining all three building blocks (a vector of hypothesized parameter differences, a related inverse of a function of the generalized inverse, and a hypothesized value for the variance) lets us write an equation for LAMBDA , our best judgment of the true λ:

$$LAMBDA = \frac{1}{\sigma^2} (K'\beta)' (K'GK)^{-1}(K'\beta) \qquad (2.7)$$

$$= \frac{1}{2} (-3.5355 \ -1.4142) \begin{pmatrix} 4 & -2 \\ -2 & 4 \end{pmatrix} \begin{pmatrix} -3.5355 \\ -1.4142 \end{pmatrix} = 19$$

This value is employed in the "DATA C" section of our program in Table 2.2 after obtaining its value by using the output just mentioned from an earlier run of the program.

Results of Analyzing Table 2.1 Data With a SAS® GLM Program

When the program of Table 2.2 is run, we obtain the following results:

TABLE 2.3
ANOVA for Table 2.1 Data, Based on the Program in Table 2.2

Source	Sum of Squares	df	Mean Square	F
Subjects	659.59	5	131.92	82.59****
Stages	5,026.75	2	2,513.37	1,573.59****
Error	15.97	10	1.60	—

Note. **** $p < 0.0001$.

As stated in this table, there are highly significant subject effects and stage effects.

Elsewhere in the output from this program, we find that the power of the test for subject effects was 0.79 for the random effect size (for subjects) being considered. Also the power of the test for stage effects was 0.92 for the fixed effect size (for stages) considered. This suggests adequate power for the stages effects of most interest in this experiment. Power for testing the subject effects is lower than the 0.80 we might desire, but close enough in view of the fact that we have no great need to establish presence or absence of subject effects in this case.

We have already mentioned that power calculations after a study is conducted should be viewed with caution. This point is illustrated by noting that, once we know that subject effects are significant in Table 2.3, it is not important to know that the power of that test is slightly lower than we would like: at least our result fell into the 79% of experiments in which significance should occur. A second reason for caution, of course, is that our estimate of σ^2 may have been quite wrong.

Other Helpful Approaches to Computer-Based Power Calculations. O'Brien and Muller (1993) discuss statistical power at length, also providing information on currently no-cost SAS® programs for computing power values. Their programs and theoretical presentation are extremely useful; research workers interested in power calculations are strongly encouraged to read their material and follow O'Brien and Muller's (1993) instructions for obtaining these free programs, somewhat updated in the files now obtained with those instructions. Using their programs, we have confirmed the two fixed effects power calculations reported in the present chapter. This required use of their section 8.3 approach and writing analogues of their program listings 8.4.1 and 8.4.3 appropriate to the current design. One advantage of their technique is the calculation of power for as many different significance levels and different possible effects sizes as desired.

Interpretation of the noncentrality parameter λ or its specified value LAMBDA in our programs is simplified by O'Brien and Muller's emphasis on relationships between λ and "exemplary" data sets, sums of squares, and F-values based on hypothesized parameter values rather than observed data. For example, our use of their approach to calculate power for our six-subject, three-stage example led to 18 "exemplary data points" reflecting hypothesized intercept, subject, and stage parameters but no error components. Careful application of O'Brien and Muller's Eq. 8.39 yields an intuitively pleasing alternate to (2.6):

$$\lambda = \frac{SS_{Stages\ with\ assumed\ parameter\ values\ but\ no\ error}}{\sigma^2} \tag{2.8}$$

This equation is closely related to definitions of the noncentrality parameter for F by Maxwell and Delaney (1990) and others. The present book omits a corrective procedure in O'Brien and Muller's UnifyPow program, called F-TRAP because it checks arguments to the PROBF function in SAS® to be sure they will not improperly generate a near zero probability due to a bug in SAS®. Research users of this book may well choose to use UnifyPow.sas or to make comparable lengthy corrections of power calculation procedures such as those in Table 2.2. A new commercially produced package for computing required sample sizes in order to gain stated power values, nQuery Advisor® (Elashoff, 1997) appears to be user-friendly and quite broad in its capabilities.

Method B: A Repeated Measurements Test of Stage Effects and Their Polynomial Components

Computer Program

Suppose that we want to use Equation 2.2 as our model in testing whether the trend from stage to stage in our data from Table 2.1 is linear or quadratic, the only two possibilities when there are significant differences in performance on three stages. Table 2.4 is a SAS® GLM program for a method that tests separately for these effects. This analysis uses sets of so-called orthogonal polynomials in the estimation and hypothesis testing procedure.

TABLE 2.4

A Program for Performing a Test of Polynomial Trend of the
Hypothetical Repeated Measurements Data of Table 2.1

```
* PROGRAM IS REP_MEAS.SAS;  DATA DEMO;
INPUT SUBJ Y1 Y2 Y3; CARDS;
 1   95.9  117.9  136.6
 2  109.6  130.2  152.1
 3   98.4  119.1  139.8
 4  107.9  129.3  151.0
 5  114.5  132.0  153.6
 6  106.4  128.1  145.2
RUN; PROC GLM; MODEL Y1-Y3 = / NOUNI;REPEATED STAGE
3 (1 2 3) POLYNOMIAL / PRINTE SUMMARY; TITLE 'REP_
MEAS.SAS-Polynomial trend analysis for Table 2.1 data.'; RUN;
```

Interpreting What This SAS® Program Has to Say

We already know what the data step in Table 2.4 means. The "PROC GLM" step defines a model for predicting scores for Stages 1 through 3, beginning with "MODEL Y1-Y3;". A "REPEATED" statement reading "REPEATED STAGE 3 (1 2 3) POLYNOMIAL / PRINTE SUMMARY;" tells the computer to use the stage variable to indicate three repeated measures for each subject, to test differences between stage performance on the three measures, to assess separate polynomial components of scores as a function of stages, and to display that output in summary form. By a polynomial component of a score, we mean that each Y_{ij} is split in this instance into three component scores: $(Y0)_{ij}$ for the zero-order or mean component, $(Ylin)_{ij}$ for the linear component, and $(Yquad)_{ij}$ for the quadratic component. This is analogous (but different!) to doing one data analysis for Stage 1 data, another for Stage 2 data, and still another for Stage 3 data; it splits the data into three sets of six data points, leading to 5 df for error in each case rather than a single estimate of error with 15 df. This model is more or less the model of Eq. 2.2, but it looks quite different from our earlier model statement because we are using the "REPEATED" command in our present analysis. An important difference is that we do not test for subject effects; they actually are included in the mean square for error in the present analysis.

The parenthesized (1 2 3) could be omitted because 1, 2, and 3 are evenly spaced. However, it does not hurt anything to include it; we become conscious of this kind of symbol pattern, needed in any application of "POLYNOMIAL" where the effects are not evenly spaced. The slash, /, means that one or more options are to be used.

Here the option "PRINTE" means, among other things, that a so-called E matrix of sums of squares and cross-products (discussed in chapt. 3) will be printed out and that a so-called sphericity test (discussed shortly) will be performed. In this example, the option "NOUNI" (short for "No Univariate Statistics") in the "MODEL" command causes the computer to omit tests specific to each stage of the experiment, such as tests of the hypothesis that the mean response on Stage 1 is zero. The "REPEATED" statement and related expressions permit us to perform several tests: the sphericity test just mentioned, a test for polynomial effects to be defined, and multivariate tests to be ignored here for the most part.

Difficulties of Parameter Estimation and Power Computation in Orthogonal Polynomial Analysis

Because no way of estimating the precise size of polynomial effects appears to be associated with the use of the "REPEATED" command in SAS® GLM, we defer discussion of power for tests of polynomial effects until chapter 3. We state without proof, however, that the power of the overall test of stage effects is unchanged from that for the analysis in Table 2.3.

Analyzing Table 2.1 Data With a Repeated Measures Command

Results of testing for any stage effects. Table 2.5 is based on the output from the SAS® GLM program of Table 2.4. Our first information about stage effects does not refer to polynomial trend:

TABLE 2.5
Part of Repeated Measurements Polynomial Trend ANOVA
Results for Table 2.1 Data

Source	Sum of Squares	df	Mean Square	F
Stages	5,026.75	2	2,513.37	1,573.59****
Error	15.97	10	1.60	—

Note.   **** $p < 0.0001$.

Notice that no test for subject effects is conducted by SAS® GLM when it uses the "REPEATED" command. It was possible to obtain such a test with our first SAS® GLM program (see Tables 2.2 and 2.3), but much important output of the current program, presented next, was missing then. Notice that the same numbers for stages and error appear as in Table 2.3. The stage effect is highly significant just as before, with all numbers in the current table being the same as corresponding ones in Table 2.4

Interpretation of Results of Assessing Sphericity. If sphericity holds in a repeated measurements design in addition to the other assumptions of analysis of variance, then the Table 2.4 program and Table 2.5 analysis are somewhat justified. One by-product of using the "REPEATED" statement in a SAS® GLM program is that adjustments are reported in the significance level of each time-related test. The purpose of these adjustments is to correct for any possible failure of the sphericity assumption. The original test for stage effects in Table 2.5 is reported to yield a significance level of 0.0001, but what happens when the G-G or Geisser-Greenhouse (Geisser & Greenhouse, 1958) and H-F or Huynh-Feldt (Huynh & Feldt, 1970) epsilon (ε) corrections are employed?

First we (or our computer package, in this case) multiply original numerator and denominators *df* values by the ε reported in the program output for G-G or a different ε for H-F (neither is shown here). This gives corrected degree of freedom values, which may even be fractional. Then we either enter an appropriate *F*-table with corrected *df*'s, invoke our SAS® FINV function with fractional *df*'s, or (as here) let our computer program tell us the corrected significance values. For the present data analysis, the G-G and H-F corrections give exactly the same significance level ($p = 0.0001$) to four decimal places as the uncorrected *F*. See statistics textbooks such as Kirk (1995) or Maxwell and Delaney (1990) for a fuller treatment of these corrections and associated epsilon values.

Earlier we also mentioned that the "PRINTE" option in the "REPEATED" command of the program activates a Mauchly test of whether an assumption of sphericity is acceptable. Simulation studies by Cornell, Young, Seaman, and Kirk (1992), and predecessors whose work they discuss suggest that this test has problems: It will falsely reject the null hypothesis with probability greater than $\alpha = 0.05$ (for example) with certain kinds of nonnormal data but falsely reject with probability less than α with kinds. In addition its power for detecting certain kinds of failure of sphericity in small-sample normal data with larger ratios of numbers of stages to numbers of subjects is usually lower than an alternate test by John (1971, 1972). Cornell (1992) et al. also cite evidence favoring alternate tests in place of performing G-G or H-F adjustments of significance levels from the original *F*-test. Nonetheless this book focuses on such adjustments as reasonably powerful procedures with accurate conservative statements about the true value of α when the assumption of normality holds. Readers are encouraged to adapt the present examples by using more advanced techniques such as those just mentioned and others cited in Kirk (1995) when they would be specially helpful.

Partly because of its computational convenience in SAS® GLM, we report the results of the Mauchly test for the present example, showing that here the Mauchly and ε-correction approaches yield the same conclusions: The output of the program of Table 2.4 reports a test of sphericity saying that Mauchly's criterion was used and that the resulting χ^2 of 0.18 with two degrees of freedom did not even approach statistical significance. This is consistent with the G-G and H-F adjustments in telling us that our use of the analysis of variance of repeated measurements here seems to meet the assumption of sphericity. Notice that SAS® ordinarily does not test for sphericity unless the "REPEATED" command in GLM is used.

Results of Testing for Different Degrees of Polynomial Trend in Stage Effects. The line of our program of Table 2.4 reading "REPEATED 3 (1 2 3) POLYNOMIAL/PRINTE SUMMARY;" ensures that this repeated measurements analysis will break down the two degrees of freedom for stages into one degree of freedom each for linear and quadratic components of trend, testing each for significance. Somewhat arbitrary power calculations (not part of Table 2.4) suggest a power of 0.51 for linear trend (β_1) and 0.140 for quadratic trend (β_2). The test for STAGE.1 (linear trend) is summarized in Table 2.6:

TABLE 2.6

Test for Linear Trend from Polynomial Analysis
for Repeated Measurements Study

Source	Sum of Squares	df	Mean Square	F
Linear (Stages)	5,026.61	1	5,026.61	3,278.23****
Error	7.67	5	1.53	—

Note. **** $p < 0.0001$.

Clearly there is a highly significant linear trend (called *Mean* in this part of the SAS® output). Notice that the sum of squares for Mean in Table 2.6 is almost as large as that for stages in Table 2.5. This suggests that the quadratic component for these data will not be significant. In fact the output for that test (not displayed here) confirms that inference. One handy feature of this breakdown of the test of treatment effects into separate tests of polynomial components is that it may lead to a simple description of overall effects, just as it does in this case. A further convenience is that, because only one degree of freedom is needed in the numerator of any F-test for a single polynomial component (or any other contrast we might assess), the sphericity assumption need not be made nor tested.

You may have noticed that the degrees of freedom for error in Table 2.6 are only 5 instead of the 10 in Table 2.3, with related changes in error sums of squares and mean squares. This is because the polynomial analysis converts observed scores into polynomial scores for each subject. The six subjects of this experiment each have one linear score and one quadratic score (not ordinarily shown in SAS® GLM output), with the analysis of linear scores testing the hypothesis that their population mean is zero. Understandably there are only five df for the linear analysis. The quadratic analysis is comparable.

ANALYZING MULTIGROUP DATA
WITHOUT TIME-RELATED EFFECTS

The two programs presented in Tables 2.2 and 2.4 will now be adapted for the analysis of data from *randomized block designs* using subjects as blocks in which treatments are to be randomly arranged. Simply ignoring the fact that time is varying in such an experiment, one could substitute "treatments" for "stages" throughout the previous analyses.

Warning

This kind of randomized block design analysis is presented here because it is discussed in most books on experimental design in statistics, is applicable to much agricultural research, and also is often proposed in behavioral science texts. In any case where both time-related and within-subject treatment effects might be present, users are strongly advised to choose other methods instead, such as those of chapter 3. This permits finding such effects if present and also permits reducing the estimate of error variance by taking out contributions from time-related effects. Another potential problem is that subjects may not have been selected randomly from some population, making it difficult to justify traditional significance testing procedures even if time-related effects are absent. See the end of this chapter for a discussion of randomization tests that can alleviate this problem in some cases.

Example

Specific Design

We illustrate this randomized block design analysis with hypothetical data for a familiar example from cognitive psychology: Shepard and Metzler (1971) wanted to know how well people could decide whether two perspective drawings of three-dimensional objects represented the same object or not. The drawings might be different, or they might be the same and oriented the same way, or they might be the same except that one was rotated a certain number of degrees (e.g., 30° in the picture plane) from the way the other was oriented. Here is a characterization of these three types of stimulus pairs:

Pair Type 1	Pair Type 2	Pair Type 3
Two different figures	The same figure twice with constant orientation	The same figure, but with 30° rotation
(nonmatching pair)	(matching, unrotated pair)	(matching, rotated pair)

Subjects tested with these kinds of stimuli made very few errors in deciding whether the same basic stimulus appeared in any given pair. However, the time they required to respond was greatly affected by the amount of rotation of a figure compared to its matching example. If the number of degrees of rotation was large (up to 180°), it took longer for a subject to respond "Same" than if there were a smaller rotation or no rotation (0°) at all.

Why did this effect occur? One possibility suggested by Shepard and Metzler is that subjects needed to "mentally rotate" one figure (i.e., move it around in one's head to see if it matched the other). With a large angle of physical rotation, the corresponding mental rotation would take longer than with a smaller rotational angle.

Let us over-simplify Shepard and Metzler's experiment by assuming that every subject received exactly one test of a matching stimulus pair at 0° rotation, one at 30° rotation, one at 90° rotation, and one at 180° rotation, plus several tests with nonmatching pairs. We will ignore nonmatching pairs and look only at hypothetical data for matching pairs.

Suppose that there were ten subjects in this experiment and that the four matching pairs for each subject were presented in a random order selected separately for each subject. For example, Subject 1 might have received a 0°, 180°, 90°, and 30° order of test trials. Subject 2 might have received a 30°, 0°, 180°, and 90° order of test trials. Other randomly selected orders would occur for the other eight subjects. The reason we have called this a *randomized block design* is that subjects are one kind of "block" used in experimentation, and treatments are randomized within each subject or block. The usual analysis of a randomized block experiment in psychology is pretty much the same as the analysis in a two-way ANOVA or repeated measurements ANOVA by methods shown next.

Hypothetical Data

Table 2.7 displays a hypothetical set of data showing response times for the four types of rotated figures for our ten subjects. This table can be used in developing two SAS® GLM programs for a traditional random blocks analysis of variance, with and without explicit repeated measurements options. Specific treatment orders are presented in chapter 3.

TABLE 2.7
Hypothetical Data for a Mental Rotation Experiment
(Responses in .01 sec units)

Subject	Treatment (Angle of Rotation in Degrees)				Mean
	0°	30°	90°	180°	
1	62.0	41.7	170.1	407.1	170.22
2	72.3	109.1	132.9	306.2	155.12
3	61.5	45.6	274.6	346.8	182.12
4	99.4	123.9	207.6	363.3	198.55
5	21.5	96.6	96.3	254.4	117.20
6	1.5	97.0	176.7	250.2	131.35
7	1.0	38.1	94.1	154.1	71.82
8	95.2	90.9	203.5	491.2	220.20
9	60.3	51.0	292.8	383.3	196.85
10	62.3	96.7	93.8	138.1	97.72
Mean	53.70	79.06	174.24	309.47	154.12

Method A Revisited: A Two-Way SAS® PROC GLM Test for Treatment and Subject Effects

Model and Computer Program

Let us first consider a two-way design with subjects as rows. However, we use treatments rather than trials as columns. Much as for Equation 2.1 earlier, we see that a reasonable equation for data from such a design might be:

$$Y_{ik} = \mu + s_i + \tau_k + e_{ik} \tag{2.9}$$

where i and k now refer to Subject i and Treatment k. Then the score Y_{ik} for Subject i on Treatment k becomes an additive constant, μ, plus a random subject effect, s_i, for Subject i plus an effect τ_k for Treatment k and an error component, e_{ik}, specific to Subject i on Treatment k. We make the same assumptions about s_i and e_{ij} as with Equation 2.1. Table 2.8 uses the PROC GLM method of Table 2.2 with the change that subjects and treatments are used in the new model in place of subjects and stages.

TABLE 2.8

A Program for Performing a Randomized Block Design Analysis
(Two-Way ANOVA) of the Hypothetical Mental Rotation Data
of Table 2.7

```
* Program RANBLOC.SAS
Treatments are labeled A, B, C, and D for 0, 30, 90, and 180 degrees
rotation. $ after treat says that letters, not numbers, are used.  ;
data rotate; input subj treat $ y @@; cards;
 1 A 62.0   1 B   41.7   1 C 170.1   1 D 407.1
 2 A 72.3   2 B 109.1   2 C 132.9   2 D 306.2
 3 A 61.5   3 B   45.6   3 C 274.6   3 D 346.8
 4 A 99.4   4 B 123.9   4 C 207.6   4 D 363.3
 5 A 21.5   5 B   96.6   5 C   96.3   5 D 254.4
 6 A   1.5   6 B   97.0   6 C 176.7   6 D 250.2
 7 A   1.0   7 B   38.1   7 C   94.1   7 D 154.1
 8 A 95.2   8 B   90.9   8 C 203.5   8 D 491.2
 9 A 60.3   9 B   51.0   9 C 292.8   9 D 383.3
10 A 62.3  10 B   96.7  10 C   93.8  10 D 138.1
run; proc glm; class subj treat; model y = subj treat;
```

(Contiuued)

TABLE 2.8
(Continued)

```
random subj/test;  means subj; means treat;
data power_r;  var1 = 'random subjects'; f5pcnt_r = finv(.95,9,27,0);
mult_r = .1111;  power_r = 1 - probf(mult_r*f5pcnt_r,9,27,0);
proc print data = power_r;
data power_f; var2 = 'Fixed treatments'; f5pcnt_f=finv(.95,3,27,0);
lambda = 5.0;  power_f = 1 - probf(f5pcnt_f,3,27,lambda);
proc print data = power_f;
title 'Mental rotation data.  RANBLOC.SAS.'; run;
```

Interpreting What This SAS® Program Has to Say

Notice that most of this program is written in lower case symbols rather than the upper case symbols of Table 2.2. This is not important. SAS® accepts both kinds of symbols in all cases of interest to us. Some information about the interpretation of Table 2.8 appears in the comment lines at the very beginning of it.   A series of comment lines typically begins with an asterisk on its first line and closes with a semicolon at the end of its last line.   Notice that the "data rotate;" statement assigns the name "rotate" to our dataset.

A "PROC GLM" step always includes a "CLASS" statement such as the present one, "class subj treat;" saying that the predictor variables listed in that statement are qualitative, not quantitative. So, subjects and treatments are qualitative or class variables in this analysis. The "model y = subj treat;" statement here tells us that the predicted y or Y_{ik} is equal to an additive constant (not shown in Table 2.8 but present as μ in Eq. 2.8), plus a subject effect plus a treatment effect. So the MODEL statement in this program is a shorthand way of stating the model equation we want to use for this data set. The statements "means subj;" and "means treat;" after a model command involving subjects and treatments tell SAS® GLM to find the means for each subject and for each treatment, needed in data tables such as Table 2.7.   The "/test" option in the "random subjects" statement instructs SAS GLM® to use F-tests consistent with this random effect.

More Rules About Symbols Used in a SAS® Program

The input statement in this program is interpreted in a similar way to that for Table 2.2: Because it says "input subj treat $ y @@;", each line below the cards statement begins with three categories: Category 1 is the subject number; category 2 is the treatment, labeled with a letter (as indicated by $ after "treat" in the input statement); and category 3 is the value of the observation, y, or Y_{ik} in the notation of Equation 2.8.

As before, the "@@" symbols tell us that more than one set of these categories appears on any line. The order in which these other values are presented is the same as for the first three columns. Notice that, after each Y_{ik} score, there are extra blank spaces left to help the reader tell that a new set of input information is being provided. You may use this sort of extra spacing when it is convenient for you; SAS® does not require it, however.

Computing Power of Subject Effects and Treatment Effects Tests Here

Selecting an Appropriate Effect Size for Random Subject Effects. Because there are $T = 4$ treatments corresponding to the three stages of our previous example, our previous Equation 2.4 for the distribution of an F for subject effects is modified to read:

$$F_1 = \frac{\sigma^2}{\sigma^2 + 4\sigma_s^2} F$$

where 4 is the number of observations per subjects (= the number of treatments in this case) and the F is computed for subjects by SAS® GLM. The ratio used as a multiplier of F in this equation is again called MULT_R in our computer program. As before, when we calculate power for the significance test of subject effects, we are selecting a MULT_R value that represents the largest ratio and the smallest effect we feel would be very important not to infer as statistically significant. Again we set our value of MULT_R at a value based on the relation $\sigma_s^2 = 2\sigma^2$, implying MULT_R = 1/9 = 0.1111. Table 2.8 uses this MULT_R value in its "DATA POWER_R:" step for random subject effects. Otherwise, the power calculation for random subject effects is just as it was in our earlier example, Table 2.2.

MULT_R can be given a different value if we have more information available, such as evidence that we need to protect only against subject effects of $\sigma_s^2 = 3\sigma^2$ or larger, making MULT_R = 1/13. In many cases, even this $\sigma_s^2 = 3\sigma^2$ value might be an underestimate, making a larger value of σ_s^2 and a smaller value of MULT_R appropriate.   The power value will increase accordingly as MULT_R declines in value.

Finding a Relevant Power Value for a Variable Having Fixed Effects.   The transpose of the parameter vector for this experiment is given as:

$$\beta' = (\mu \; s_1 \; s_2 \; s_3 \; \ldots \; s_{10} \; \tau_1 \; \tau_2 \; \tau_3 \; \tau_4)$$

and the design matrix is given as:

$$X = \begin{pmatrix}
1 & 1 & 0 & 0 & \ldots & 0 & 1 & 0 & 0 & 0 \\
1 & 1 & 0 & 0 & \ldots & 0 & 0 & 1 & 0 & 0 \\
1 & 1 & 0 & 0 & \ldots & 0 & 0 & 0 & 1 & 0 \\
1 & 1 & 0 & 0 & \ldots & 0 & 0 & 0 & 0 & 1 \\
1 & 0 & 1 & 0 & \ldots & 0 & 1 & 0 & 0 & 0 \\
1 & 0 & 1 & 0 & \ldots & 0 & 0 & 1 & 0 & 0 \\
1 & 0 & 1 & 0 & \ldots & 0 & 0 & 0 & 1 & 0 \\
1 & 0 & 1 & 0 & \ldots & 0 & 0 & 0 & 0 & 1 \\
1 & 0 & 0 & 1 & \ldots & 0 & 1 & 0 & 0 & 0 \\
1 & 0 & 0 & 1 & \ldots & 0 & 0 & 1 & 0 & 0 \\
1 & 0 & 0 & 1 & \ldots & 0 & 0 & 0 & 1 & 0 \\
1 & 0 & 0 & 1 & \ldots & 0 & 0 & 0 & 0 & 1 \\
\ldots & \ldots & \ldots & \ldots & & \ldots & & \ldots & \ldots & \ldots \\
1 & 0 & 0 & 0 & \ldots & 1 & 1 & 0 & 0 & 0 \\
1 & 0 & 0 & 0 & \ldots & 1 & 0 & 1 & 0 & 0 \\
1 & 0 & 0 & 0 & \ldots & 1 & 0 & 0 & 1 & 0 \\
1 & 0 & 0 & 0 & \ldots & 1 & 0 & 0 & 0 & 1
\end{pmatrix}$$

where . . . entries reflect obviously defined missing rows or columns. The first column refers to μ, the next set of columns to subject effects, and the last group of columns to treatment effects. The hypothesis about any fixed effects to be tested is our earlier equation

$$H: K'\beta = 0 \tag{2.5}$$

In testing for treatment effects based on Equation 2.8, the matrix K' is the transpose of the following matrix: $K = \begin{pmatrix} 0 & 0 & 0 \\ 0 & 0 & 0 \\ 0 & 0 & 0 \\ 0 & 0 & 0 \\ \dots\dots \\ 1 & 0 & 0 \\ 0 & 1 & 0 \\ 0 & 0 & 1 \\ -1 & -1 & -1 \end{pmatrix}$. Here the rows

correspond to all 15 parameters of β (missing entries being zeroes), and the columns refer to the first through third components of estimators and thus also of sum of squares of treatment effects. When we perform the matrix multiplication implied by the previously mentioned hypothesis, we obtain: $H: K'\beta = \begin{pmatrix} \tau_A - \tau_D \\ \tau_B - \tau_D \\ \tau_C - \tau_D \end{pmatrix} = \begin{pmatrix} 0 \\ 0 \\ 0 \end{pmatrix} = 0.$ As in our earlier example,

$(X'X)^{-1}$ does not exist; we must use the generalized inverse, G, with a value $(X'X)^-$ instead. Therefore, we are working with differences between parameters rather than individual parameters themselves. So our hypothesis is that the differences between effects for Treatments A and D, B and D, and C and D are all zero.

Next we make a guess that σ^2 is no larger than 4000. To find an appropriate value of $K'\beta$, we arbitrarily say that $\tau_A - \tau_D = -60.00$, $\tau_B - \tau_D = -40.00$, and $\tau_C - \tau_D = -20.00$ represent a minimimally sized combination of effects to identify. This makes

$$K'\beta = \begin{pmatrix} \tau_A - \tau_D \\ \tau_B - \tau_D \\ \tau_C - \tau_D \end{pmatrix} = \begin{pmatrix} -60.00 \\ -40.00 \\ -20.00 \end{pmatrix}.$$

We can now substitute in an early general equation for LAMBDA:

$$\text{LAMBDA} = \frac{1}{\sigma^2} (K'\beta)' (K'GK)^{-1} (K'\beta) \tag{2.7}$$

Next we calculate $(K'GK)^{-1}$, finding it to be equal to:

$$\begin{pmatrix} g_{12,12} & g_{12,13} & g_{12,14} \\ g_{13,12} & g_{13,13} & g_{13,14} \\ g_{14,12} & g_{14,13} & g_{14,14} \end{pmatrix}^{-1}.$$ Having invoked the INVERSE option in the

MODEL command of our program in Table 2.8, we know that the g values come from the portion of computer output for **G** labeled Treatments A through C on its rows and columns. Thus we use part of the generalized inverse **G** of $(\mathbf{X'X})$, to obtain:

$$(\mathbf{K'GK})^{-1} = \begin{pmatrix} .2 & .1 & .1 \\ .1 & .2 & .1 \\ .1 & .1 & .2 \end{pmatrix}^{-1} = \begin{pmatrix} 7.5 & -2.5 & -2.5 \\ -2.5 & 7.5 & -2.5 \\ -2.5 & -2.5 & 7.5 \end{pmatrix}.$$ Given these results,

Equation 2.7 implies that

$$\mathrm{LAMBDA} = \frac{1}{4000} (-60.00 \ -40.00 \ -20.00) \begin{pmatrix} 7.5 & -2.5 & -2.5 \\ -2.5 & 7.5 & -2.5 \\ -2.5 & -2.5 & 7.5 \end{pmatrix} \begin{pmatrix} -60.00 \\ -40.00 \\ -20.00 \end{pmatrix},$$

which is equal to 5.0   This value is employed in the "DATA POWER_F;" section of our program in Table 2.8.

Results of Analyzing Table 2.7 Data
With a Two-Way ANOVA Method

When the program in Table 2.8 is run, one obtains the makings of the following analysis of variance table:

TABLE 2.9
Randomized Block ANOVA Results for Mental Rotation Data

Source	Sum of Squares	df	Mean Square	F
Subjects	84,182.11	9	9,353.57	2.66*
Treatments (Rotation Angles)	402,566.17	3	134,188.72	38.18****
Error	94,895.92	27	3,514.66	—

Note. * $p < 0.05$. **** $p < 0.0001$.

Table 2.9 shows significant ($p < 0.05$) differences among mean reaction times of different subjects and highly significant ($p < 0.0001$) differences among mean reaction times with different treatments. Power values are 0.983 for subject effects and 0.386 for treatment effects.

Method B Revisited: Repeated Measurements Tests for Treatment Effects and Their Polynomial Components

Computer Program

We now re-analyze the present data set using a program much like that of Table 2.4, a SAS® GLM program with a "repeated" command needed to test for polynomial components of trend. An analogue of Equation 2.2 related to Equation 2.9 for randomized block designs, but with cubic as well as linear and quadratic terms, is implicitly invoked here. Table 2.10 presents the program for the new analyses. Notice that the four scores for any one subject are now called y_1, y_2, y_3, and y_4 to tie them together rather than recording each as a separate y value. No test for subject effects is conducted; as before, the "repeated" statement for SAS® GLM does not lead to such tests.

TABLE 2.10

A Program for Performing a Test of Polynomial Trend
of Rotation Angle Effects in the Hypothetical Data of Table 2.7

```
*Program RANBLOCP.SAS for testing mental rotation data;
data rotate;
input subj y1 y2 y3 y4 @@; cards;
1 62.0 41.7 170.1 407.1    2 72.3 109.1 132.9 306.2
3 61.5 45.6 274.6 346.8    4 99.4 123.9 207.6 363.3
5 21.5 96.6  96.3 254.4    6  1.5  97.0 176.7 250.2
7  1.0 38.1  94.1 154.1    8 95.2  90.9 203.5 491.2
9 60.3 51.0 292.8 383.3   10 62.3  96.7  93.8 138.1
run; proc glm; model y1--y4 = / nouni;
repeated treat 4 (0 30 90 180) polynomial / printe printm summary;
title 'RANBLOCP.SAS.  Mental rotation data.  Polynomial trend fitted.'; run;
```

Difficulties of Parameter Estimation and Power Computation in This Orthogonal Polynomial Analysis

The power of the overall test of stage effects is unchanged from that for the analysis using Table 2.8. However, the same difficulties of estimation and power calculation appear for our linear, quadratic, and cubic trends here as in the polynomial analysis of stage effects in Table 2.4. We defer discussion of the "printm" option of the "repeated" command in Table 2.10 until chapter 3. The "summary" option of the same command is used to generate ANOVA tables for each contrast among within-subject factors.

Results of Testing Again for Treatment Effects

Before testing the significance of one or more specific polynomial trend components of data in this study, we need an overall test of treatment (rotation angle) effects. Table 2.11 shows the results of such an overall analysis of variance for the data of this hypothetical experiment. This table is based on material from the output obtained by running the SAS® program of Table 2.10.

TABLE 2.11
Part of Polynomial Trend ANOVA Results for Table 2.7 Data

Source	Sum of Squares	df	Mean Square	F
Treatments (Rotation Angles)	402,566.17	3	134,188.72	38.18****
Error	94,895.92	27	3,514.66	—

Note. **** $p < 0.0001$.

Except for the absence of a test for subject effects, Tables 2.9 and 2.11 are completely consistent with each other, yielding exactly the same numerical entries as before. Mean reaction times for different rotation angles again differ in a highly significant fashion.

Testing Sphericity and Correcting for Its Absence

For this data set a Mauchly test yields $\chi^2(5) = 13.45$, $p < 0.0195$. Despite previous concerns about the value of this test, we may wonder if an alternative is needed for the F-test. So we examine adjusted significance levels based on the so-called Geisser-Greenhouse and Huynh-Feldt epsilon (ε) corrections, reported in computer output as 0.5678 and 0.6868, respectively. In this case the adjusted significance levels are both 0.0001, just as was the originally reported level. So the significant treatment effect of Table 2.11 holds, even after correction for possible failure of the sphericity assumption.

Results of Testing for Different Degrees of Trend in Treatment Effects

We already know that Shepard and Metzler concluded that mean reaction time increases as angle of rotation of one picture compared to its matching picture increases. They went farther and concluded that this trend is a straight line trend (i.e., that mean reaction time increases linearly as angle of rotation increases). The line of our program of Table 2.10 reading "repeated treat 4 (0 30 90 180) polynomial / printe printm summary;" ensures that this repeated measurements analysis will break down the three degrees of freedom for treatments into one degree of freedom each for linear, quadratic, and cubic trends, testing each for significance. Accordingly, the present method applied to Shepard and Metzler's data could test for linearity while also taking into account any effects associated with the stage of practice at which each observation was taken.

Notice that 0, 30, 90, and 180 are not equally spaced; listing them here is required if the computer analysis is to be accurate. Often a user may omit "printe printm" above because s(he) has minimal interest in the error sum of squares and cross-products matrix or sphericity test provided by "printe" or the transformation matrices for contrasts provided by "printm". The "summary" option is more important because it provides for display of the separate ANOVA tests for different polynomial components or other contrasts.

The very last part of the SAS® output for this program reports these three tests, saying, "TREAT.N represents the nth degree polynomial for TREAT". Tests for linear, quadratic, and cubic effects were conducted with this program. However, because the other polynomial effects are not significant, only the test for TREAT.1 (linear trend) is summarized in Table 2.12:

TABLE 2.12

Test for Linear Trend From Polynomial Analysis
for Mental Rotation Experiment

Source	Sum of Squares	df	Mean Square	F
Linear (Treatments)	400,794.59	1	400,794.59	59.79****
Error	60,333.83	9	6,703.76	—

Note. **** $p < 0.0001$.

Clearly there is a highly significant linear trend (called *Mean* for this part of the SAS® output). Notice that the sum of squares for Mean in Table 2.12 is almost as large as that for treatments in Table 2.11.

This suggests that the quadratic and cubic treatment components for these data will not be significant., which we previously noted to be true. One handy feature of the breakdown of the test of treatment effects into separate tests of linear, quadratic, and cubic effects is that it may lead to a simple description of overall effects, just as it does in this case.

METHOD C: RANDOMIZATION TESTS APPROPRIATE IN RANDOMIZED BLOCK DESIGNS WITHOUT RANDOM SELECTION OF SUBJECTS

Objections to the model for Y_{ik} in Equation 2.9 when subjects are not randomly sampled can be finessed by moving to a randomization test model: Following Kempthorne (1952), we do not assume normally distributed subject and error components, and we do not assume random sampling. Rather, we assume random assignment of the sequence of four treatments for each subject. This is likely to lead to selection of several of the 24 possible sequences such as (0°, 30°, 90°, and 180°) or (0°, 180°, 90°, and 30°). What we want to know is whether the differences in response means for the four rotational angles could have occurred because the random assignment of sequences happened by chance to put high scores with certain angles and low scores with other angles.

Kempthorne (1952) showed that the conventional F-test for treatment effects in a randomized block design is fairly satisfactory for the randomization assignment assumptions just made. It may also be useful in cases in which data are randomly sampled, but the assumptions of normality and equal variances are not met (Collier, Baker, & Mandeville, 1967). Jones and Kenward (1989) emphasized the importance of randomization of treatment sequences for different subjects.

Even more precise application of randomization theory to the randomized block design are possible using general methods discussed by Edgington (1995) and Manly (1991). If one can properly ignore the possibility of "nuisance effects" such as stage effects and carryover effects, then the randomization test approaches are worth exploring. Because of the focus of this book on such effects, we have no option henceforth but to treat subjects as randomly selected. Note, however, that an alternative is to treat subjects as having fixed effects, an approach that is mathematically equivalent to assuming sequence effects but no subject effects (Jones & Kenward, 1989).

THINGS TO REMEMBER

Major Analysis Options

1. With a one-group repeated measurements design, use a conventional two-way ANOVA analysis to assess subject effects and stage effects with F-tests dividing the mean square for a given effect by the mean square for error.

2. Or with a one-group repeated measurements design, employ a polynomial trend model and test which, if any, degrees of the fitted orthogonal polynomial equation are significant, as well as testing for overall differences among stages. Subject effects are not analyzed with this model.

3. In order to justify use of tests such as that in #2, we can test sphericity of data from repeated measurements designs (i.e., the assumption of equality of variances from all differences of scores for pairs as stages such as $Y_1 - Y_2$ for Stages 1 and 2). Sphericity is not assumed for data used in testing single degree of freedom effects such as linear-

ity, but sphericity is a theoretical requirement for effects such as stages with more than one *df*.

4. With a randomized block design, if it is known that no time-related effects are present, use a model involving subject effects and treatment effects but no others beyond error. The analysis method is similar (and could be identical!) to that in #1 for one-group repeated measurements designs except that treatment effects replace stage effects. If stage and/or carryover effects may be present, methods of chapter 3 should be considered.

5. Or with a randomized block design and no time-related effects, employ a polynomial trend model and test which, if any, degrees of the fitted orthogonal polynomial equation are significant.

6. With any of the aforementioned methods, compute power of random or fixed effects. Elementary methods are illustrated here; more sophisticated procedures have been programmed by O'Brien and Muller (1993). Power calculations for polynomial coefficients are not described.

Interpreting Results of Computational Methods Not Previously Discussed

1. Know that randomization tests, which can be used for analyzing data from some experimental designs even when the assumption of random sampling from a defined population is not reasonable, exist.

EXERCISES

1. Run the programs in Tables 2.2, 2.4, 2.8, and 2.10 to see if they work properly with the SAS® facilities on your computer.

2. Modify one of the previously mentioned programs by making up four scores for a fifth subject and analyzing the expanded data set.

3. Modify one of the aforementioned programs so that it will compute power values for the tests of random and fixed effects when a significance level of 0.01 is used instead of 0.05. Tell how the power values change with this modification in significance level.

3

Analyzing Data From
a Randomized Block Design
Experiment That May Exhibit
Time-Related Effects

INTRODUCTION

As in chapter 2, we deal with hypothetical data related to Shepard and Metzler's (1971) test of people deciding whether two drawings of three-dimensional geometrical objects were the same except for rotation. Again the principal experimental variable is the number of degrees (e.g., 90°) one stimulus is rotated from the way the other was oriented.

We now assume that we know the order in which each subject sees the four pairs of stimuli with different degrees of rotation. This permits us to employ methods of data analysis appropriate to cross-over designs (Jones & Kenward, 1989; Ratkowsky, Evans, & Alldredge, 1993) in order to test for stage effects and carryover effects as well as the treatment effects of primary interest in studies like the present one.

CROSSOVER DESIGN APPROACH
TO MENTAL ROTATION DATA

Again, we assume that there were 10 subjects in the mental rotation experiment and that the four matching pairs for each subject were presented in a random order selected separately for each subject. But we also assume, for example, that Subject 1 received a 0°, 180°, 90°, and 30° order of test trials. Table 3.1 displays the chapter 2 hypothetical set of data showing response times for the four types of rotated figures for our 10 subjects. But now it also includes information about the time order in which the stimuli were presented.

TABLE 3.1
Hypothetical Data for a Mental Rotation Experiment
(Responses in .01 second units)

Temporal Position of the Rotations (Angles in Degrees)

	1		2		3		4
(0°)	62.0	(180°)	407.1	(90°)	170.1	(30°)	41.7
(30°)	109.1	(0°)	72.3	(180°)	306.2	(90°)	132.9
(0°)	61.5	(90°)	274.6	(180°)	346.8	(30°)	45.6
(30°)	123.9	(0°)	99.4	(90°)	207.6	(180°)	363.3
(180°)	254.4	(30°)	96.6	(0°)	21.5	(90°)	96.3
(90°)	176.7	(30°)	97.0	(180°)	250.2	(0°)	1.5
(180°)	154.1	(90°)	94.1	(30°)	38.1	(0°)	1.0
(180°)	491.2	(0°)	95.2	(30°)	90.9	(90°)	203.5
(0°)	60.3	(90°)	292.8	(180°)	383.3	(30°)	51.0
(0°)	62.3	(30°)	96.7	(90°)	93.8	(180°)	138.1
	155.55		162.58		190.85		107.49
	53.70		79.06		174.24		309.47

Method A: Basic Analysis of Mental Rotation Data

Basic Approach

Now we need a model for data from this experiment that combines aspects of Equation 2.1 in chapter 2 for repeated measurements without treatment variation, and Equation 2.9 for treatment variation without stage effects. Such a model will include both four stage effects (let $p = 4$) and four treatment effects (let $T = 4$) in addition to the components common to both the original equations. Furthermore, there should be parameters for carryover effects, reflecting the effects of immediately prior treatments. Carryover effects sometimes have other names such as *residual effects* or *delayed treatment effects*. We do not have a hypothesis about their direction or magnitude in the present experiment, but want to be able to recognize them if they are present.

In view of the previous paragraph, a reasonable model for an observed score Y_{ijk} from Table 3.1 for Subject i on Stage j with Rotation Angle k (Treatment k) following Treatment k' on the previous stage is:

$$Y_{ijk} = \mu + s_i + \pi_j + \tau_k + \lambda_{k'} + e_{ijk} \tag{3.1}$$

Here μ is an additive constant, and the s_i are random subject effects for subjects identified with i; they are i.i.d. $N(0,\sigma_s^2)$. Also π_j is the effect of Stage j, τ_k is the effect of Treatment k, and $\lambda_{k'}$ is a carryover effect from Treatment k' on the previous stage of the experiment. The subject effects are independent of each other. We assume that error components e_{ijk} are normally distributed with mean zero and that the following variance-covariance matrix (or, more briefly labeled, covariance matrix) between different stages is assumed to hold for each subject:

$$\Sigma_e = \begin{pmatrix} \lambda + 2\gamma_1^* & \gamma_1^* + \gamma_2^* & \cdots & \gamma_1^* + \gamma_p^* \\ \gamma_1^* + \gamma_2^* & \lambda + 2\gamma_2^* & \cdots & \gamma_2^* + \gamma_p^* \\ \cdots & \cdots & \cdots & \cdots \\ \gamma_1^* + \gamma_p^* & \gamma_2^* + \gamma_p^* & \cdots & \lambda + 2\gamma_p^* \end{pmatrix}$$

Next we add assumptions of independence of error scores for different subjects, implying $Cov(e_{ijk}, e_{i'j'k'}) = 0$ for $i \neq i'$ regardless of whether different stages or treatments are involved. Also we assume

$Cov(s_i, e_{i'j'k'}) = 0$ regardless of whether $i = i'$. Given these assumptions, we can obtain the following covariance matrix for all observations Y_{ijk} in any single treatment-sequence group:

$$\Sigma = \begin{pmatrix} \lambda + 2\gamma_1 & \gamma_1 + \gamma_2 & .... & \gamma_1 + \gamma_p \\ \gamma_1 + \gamma_2 & \lambda + 2\gamma_2 & .... & \gamma_2 + \gamma_p \\ .... & .... & .... & .... \\ \gamma_1 + \gamma_p & \gamma_2 + \gamma_p & .... & \lambda + 2\gamma_p \end{pmatrix} \text{ where } \gamma_j = \gamma_j^* + 0.5\sigma_s^2.$$

The current definition of Σ is a representation of Type H structure obtained from Ratkowsky, Evans, and Alldredge (1993) by adding our specification of γ_j. in terms of γ_j^*.[1] Presence of a Type H structure for Σ is a necessary and sufficient condition of sphericity. This is equivalent to the definition of sphericity as holding if and only if the variances of difference scores from pairs of stages of the experiment are constant. Although the assumption of sphericity is an assumption about observed scores, our assumptions associated with Equation 3.1, including the covariance matrix Σ_e, show a close relation between covariance structures for errors and for observed scores.

Note that, with p stages, there are $p + 1$ different parameters in Σ, rather than the $p(p + 1)/2$ in a completely general covariance matrix. This yields a difference of $[p(p - 1)/2] - 1$ as the number of degrees of freedom for a test of this assumption about covariance structure. Because the covariance matrix of observed scores is modified by inclusion of subjects receiving different sequences of treatments, it is necessary to examine the covariance matrix of each treatment-sequence group separately before asking whether sphericity holds for all subjects in a crossover design experiment with different sequences of treatments.

Existing proofs are known to show that the F-distribution holds for

---

[1] It is necessary to mention that the λ and γ elements of a Type H structure are entirely different from a $\lambda_{k'}$ carryover effect and from any γ parameter in later equations predicting observations such as Y_{ijk}.

one-group and multi-group split-plot repeated measurements designs under conventional models that also include the sphericity assumption. In view of Crowder and Hand (1990) who started from a single group of subjects, each measured on p occasions, we presume that those proofs generalize to a wider class of crossover designs. However, note that in some crossover designs, Jones and Kenward (1989) made the somewhat stronger assumption that the distribution of errors e_{ijk} on different stages for the same subject have a uniform covariance structure (also called *compound symmetry*) with variance σ^2 for each stage and covariance $\rho\sigma^2$ for each pair of different stages.

A commonly used test for compound symmetry is different from the Mauchly test for sphericity (Ratkowsky et al., 1993). Jones and Kenward (1989) usually assumed uniform covariance structure and sometimes appeared to test it with the usual test for sphericity as Mauchly himself did. They also used a third procedure (a likelihood ratio test) in cases in which the covariance matrix was clearly being tested for uniformity. This procedure has the advantage that it can be performed even if lack of replication precludes presence of within-sequence information. We follow Ratkowsky et al. (1993), in using a sphericity assumption rather than a uniform covariance assumption for most of the crossover design experiments.

We now present a SAS® PROC GLM program for using the cross-over design model of Equation 3.1 to analyze the data just presented. In contrast to chapter 2, we are testing for any stage and carryover effects that may be present in these data. We also compute the power of tests of linear and quadratic components to be examined with commands to be added to this program later. This is addition to prior tests of subject and treatment effects.

Regrettably, common usage in power formulas gives one more meaning of lambda (λ) in Table 3.2 and elsewhere in this book. The reader is again warned to restrict the interpretation of any lambda to the context in which it appears. As in chapter 2, this lambda is simply an index of the smallest size of effect that we wish to be able to find with probability (power) having a stated value such as 0.80.

TABLE 3.2

A Program for Analyzing the Hypothetical Mental Rotation Data
of Table 3.1 to Take Into Account Possible Stage and Carryover Effects

---

* PROGRAM ROTATE.SAS;
data rotate; input subj stage treat carry y @ @ ;cards;

1	1	0	0	62.0	1	2	180	1	407.1	1	3	90	4	170.1	1	4	30	3	41.7
2	1	30	0	109.1	2	2	0	2	72.3	2	3	180	1	306.2	2	4	90	4	132.9
3	1	0	0	61.5	3	2	90	1	274.6	3	3	180	3	346.8	3	4	30	4	45.6
4	1	30	0	123.9	4	2	0	2	99.4	4	3	90	1	207.6	4	4	180	3	363.3
5	1	180	0	254.4	5	2	30	4	96.6	5	3	0	2	21.5	5	4	90	1	96.3
6	1	90	0	176.7	6	2	30	3	97.0	6	3	180	2	250.2	6	4	0	4	1.5
7	1	180	0	154.1	7	2	90	4	94.1	7	3	30	3	38.1	7	4	0	2	1.0
8	1	180	0	491.2	8	2	0	4	95.2	8	3	30	1	90.9	8	4	90	2	203.5
9	1	0	0	60.3	9	2	90	1	292.8	9	3	180	3	383.3	9	4	30	4	51.0
10	1	0	0	62.3	10	2	30	1	96.7	10	3	90	2	93.8	10	4	180	3	138.1

run ; proc glm; class subj stage carry treat;
model y = subj treat stage carry/solution e e1 e2 p; random subj;
data power_L; var1 = 'Orthogonal linear coefficient';
f5pcnt_L = finv(.95,1,21,0); lambda = 5;
power_L = 1-probf(f5pcnt_L,1,21,lambda); proc print data = power_L;
title 'Mental rotation data. ROTATE.SAS with all factors.'; run ;

Interpreting What This SAS® Program Has to Say

The most important new SAS® options in this program are "e e1 e2"
in the "model" command. In this chapter we tell their purpose and summarize some information about their results here. However, a detailed
description of their use is delayed until the next chapter. Basically, all
these options tell something about what can be estimated concerning the
data, given the current model and experimental design. Output from the
"e" option allows us to determine what could be estimated somehow; the
other options narrow that information down. Thus "e1" output lets us
know what can be estimated with what SAS® GLM calls a Type I analysis, and "e2" output lets us know what can be estimated with a Type II
analysis. We shall see many examples in which the sums of squares
and associated significance tests are not the same for all of the four
types of analysis performed with SAS® GLM. The three lines computing power ("data power_L . . . ") apply to testing for linear trend in
treatment effects; they are discussed in connection with Tables 3.7 and
3.8.

Findings From the Program of Table 3.2

Running this program yields the makings of Table 3.3:

TABLE 3.3

ANOVA Results for the Program in Table 3.2, Assessing Stage
and Carryover Effects in Addition to Traditional Randomized
Block Variables

		Type I		
Source	Sum of Squares	df	Mean Square	F
Subjects	84,182.11	9	9,353.57	3.49**
Treatments (Rotation Angles)	402,566.17	3	134,188.72	50.13****
Stages	34,250.45	3	11,416.82	4.27*
Carryovers	4,432.09	3	1,477.36	0.55
Error	56,213.38	21	2,676.83	—

		Type II		
Source	Sum of Squares	df	Mean Square	F
Subjects	79,623.80	9	8,847.09	3.31*
Treatments	326,274.69	3	108,758.23	40.63****
Stages	27,002.07	2	13,501.04	5.04*
Carryovers	4,432.09	3	1,477.36	0.55
Error	56,213.38	21	2,676.83	—

Note. $*p < 0.05.$ $** p < 0.01.$ $**** p < 0.0001.$

Before comparing Type I and II analyses in detail, we note two apparent inconsistencies between them:

(1) The total of Type I sums of squares is 581,644.20, but the total of Type II sums of squares is only 493,546.03. This is not a computational error. Rather, it reflects a difference in techniques. The total sum of squares for different types (I through IV) of GLM analyses will be constant if the designs are balanced, having equal numbers of observations in all possible cells. But many experimental designs and associated statistical models lack this property. In the simplest randomized block design that has stage and carryover effects modeled in addition to sub-

ject and treatment effects, meeting the assumption of balance proves to be impossible: One cannot always obtain each possible carryover an equal number of times with each stage and treatment combination. In such cases one may expect to find different total sums of squares for different analysis types using the same design, model, and dataset.

(2) The stages line for Type I shows three *df* whereas for Type II it shows only two. This phenomenon receives greater attention as we discuss expected mean squares and parameter estimation. Suffice it to say now that the degrees of freedom should be three if stage effects are assessed before carryovers and should be two if stages are assessed after carry-overs. A Type II analysis always assesses stage effects after carry-overs (actually after everything else except interaction), but a Type I analysis has the option of testing different effects in any conceivable order in which interaction tests follow main effect tests.

The Type I and II analyses in this table are consistent in showing significant ($p < 0.05$ or $p < 0.01$) differences among different subjects and stages. They also show highly significant ($p < 0.0001$) differences among mean reaction times with different rotation angles. So, in this example, the major conclusions do not change with changes from Type I to Type II analysis methods.

Because of the "e1 e2" options and the assumption of random effects (the "random subjects;" specification) in the program of Table 3.2, we are given the expected mean squares for this set of analyses (i.e., the average values of mean squares if a given experiment were performed an infinite number of times) under Types I and II analyses. Table 3.4 shows that these expected values each include a Var(Error) term, and most also include a so-called Q( ) expression showing what experimental variables affect its expected mean square. For example, with Type I the expected mean square for treatments includes Q(TREAT, STAGE, CARRY), telling us that treatment, stage, and carryover effects (if present) all contribute to that mean square. However, with Type II the expected mean square for treatments contains Q(TREAT), showing that any stage and carryover effects that may be present are not included in that expected mean square. Similarly, with Type I but not with Type II, there is possible contamination of stage effects by carryover effects. Because carryover effects are extracted last in both Types I and II analyses, each analysis has an expected mean square for carryovers with Q(CARRY) uncontaminated by other effects.

TABLE 3.4
Expected Mean Squares Obtained in the Analysis Associated
With Table 3.3

Type I

Source	Expected Mean Square
Subjects	Var(Error) + 4 Var(SUBJ) + Q(CARRY)
Treatments	Var(Error) + Q(TREAT,STAGE,CARRY)
Stages	Var (Error) + Q(STAGE, CARRY)
Carryovers	Var(Error) + Q(CARRY)
Error	Var(Error)

Type II

Source	Expected Mean Square
Subjects	Var(Error) + 3.8565 Var(SUBJ)
Treatments	Var(Error) + Q(TREAT)
Stages	Var (Error) + Q(STAGE)
Carryovers	Var(Error) + Q(CARRY)
Error	Var(Error)

Table 3.4 helps us to understand why we may prefer Type II to Type I or vice versa in a certain situation. We know from the philosophy of F-tests that a non-zero Q( ) makes it more likely than 0.05 (or some other significance level such as 0.01 or 0.001) that F will be significant. The reason we care what is included in Q( ) is that we want significance to result from the factor we are testing, not some other aspect of the experiment. If you want to obtain more specific information about the values within these Q( ) terms in an expected mean square value, see the Q option for the RANDOM command in the GLM section of the SAS® manual (SAS Institute Inc., 1989d).

Table 3.3 shows that Type I and Type II analyses lead to the same conclusions about significance with these data. However, because stage and treatment effects are both significant, Table 3.4 shows that the Type I expected mean square for treatments may be contaminated by stage effects even though it apparently is not contaminated by carryover effects, which are nonsignificant. Similar difficulties appear with tests of subject and stage effects. Accordingly, it looks as if the Type II analysis is a "safety-first" approach here.

The output of a Type I analysis depends on the order, such as subjects, treatments, stages, and carryovers. This current order makes the Type I analysis more like the traditional randomized block design analysis of chap. 2. The present $SS_{Treatments}$ value of 402,566.17 is exactly what would be obtained by the traditional method, but the SS_{Error} value is smaller with the present method because stage- and carryover sums of squares have now been extracted also.

Estimation of Effects. Table 3.5 displays some of the estimated parameters reported in response to the SOLUTION option in the MODEL command of our SAS® program. They are so-called ordinary least squares (OLS) estimates having desirable properties when the sphericity assumption and other model assumptions hold. These values do not change from one of the four types of analysis to another. As a consequence of Table 3.5 entries, predicted estimated reaction times (not shown here) increase with increased angle of rotation and change irregularly with stage of testing.

TABLE 3.5
Some Parameter Estimates Reported in the Analysis Associated
With Table 3.3

	Parameter	Estimate	
STAGE	2	77.22	B
	3	26.33	B
	4	0.00	B
TREAT	0	−255.65	B
	30	−228.64	B
	90	−129.85	B
	180	0.00	B

Output like this giving "Estimate" values, usually labeled "B" for Bias, may be interpreted once we know output from E, E1, E2, etc., options in the "model" statement. Except for random subject effects, when we use a constant model, the numerical estimates are the same with all four types of analysis, but what they really estimate may be different. The Type II Estimable Functions output (not shown here; see chapter 4 for an illustration of its use) based on the E2 command implies that a treatment parameter difference such as $\tau_0 - \tau_{180}$ or TREAT 0

– TREAT 180 is estimable. Output from the SOLUTION command can properly be used to estimate that parameter difference as the difference between Table 3.5's biased estimates of TREAT 0   (–255.65) and TREAT 180 (0.00).[2] This yields –255.65 as the difference between predicted response times under 0° and 180° rotation of figures. By the same basic method, $\tau_{30} - \tau_{180}$ is estimated as –228.64, and $\tau_{90} - \tau_{180}$ is estimated as –129.85.

This method also yields estimated values of $\pi_2 - \pi_4$ (STAGE 2 – STAGE 4) and $\pi_3 - \pi_4$ as 77.22 and 26.33, respectively, showing a decline in predicted response time with practice.   Unfortunately a STAGE 1 – STAGE 4 parameter difference is not estimable:

The Type II Estimable Functions output based on the E2 command plus the SOLUTION command implies that, despite a STAGE 1 B estimate (not shown in Table 3.5) appearing in computer output, we must ignore the possibility of estimating that difference because it is contaminated by carryover effects. Carryover parameter estimates are available in the computer output but also need not be shown since they are not statistically significant. In view of the Type II expected mean squares for subjects and for error values in Table 3.4, we can estimate Var(SUBJ) as [MS(Subjects) – MS(Error)/3.8565 = [8,847.09 – 2,676.83]/3.8565 = 1,599.96. The fixed subject effect estimates generated by the SOLUTION option need not be reported.

Examining Data to Check Adequacy of the Model Employed

Orientation. It is useful to employ graphs and further statistical analyses as means of checking whether our data are normally distributed and whether some data values are so extreme that they they should be rejected as so-called outliers, lying beyond the range of reasonable data for the present experiment. Some of the graphing or testing procedures are presented at this point. We focus on searches for consistency among subjects and upon evidence of nonnormality in the underlying data.

---

[2] The discussion of the ESTIMATE command in SAS® GLM (SAS Institute Inc., 1989d, p. 907) states that values of estimators for estimable linear functions of parameters are actually generated by matrix multiplication using the biased estimates now under discussion. This justifies the present computational advice.

   Plotting of Raw Data. First of all, we could display the raw scores, Y_{ijk}, values for each subject and stage of the experiment in a single graph. If a single treatment-sequence order were employed for all subjects, such a graph would help us to compare subjects under comparable conditions. The best we can do in the present situation is to show Fig. 3.1 below, plotting such data for Subjects 3 and 9, who received the treatment order of 0°, 90°, 180°, and 30°. We are happy to find that these two subjects exhibit very similar behavior at each point of the experiment.

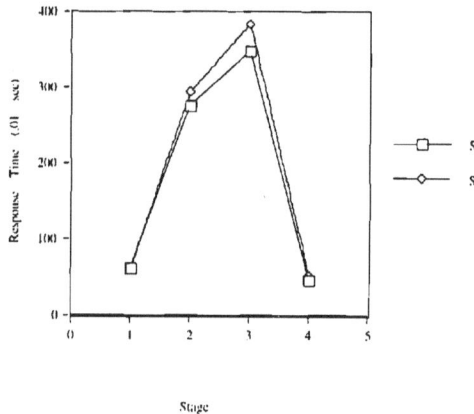

FIG. 3.1. Mean reaction times for two identically treated subjects.

   Testing Normality and Looking for Outliers With SAS®. Next we note that use of a "p" option in the program of Table 3.2 causes SAS® to report predicted Y_{ijk} values and residuals — discrepancies between observed and predicted values. We now display in Table 3.6 a SAS® program for testing for normality with a Shapiro-Wilks test statistic and providing a graphic display suggesting whether normality exists and whether any standardized residuals are unusually large. Such standardized residuals are defined as $\dfrac{(r - \bar{r})}{s_r}$, where $\bar{r}$ and s_r are the observed mean and standard deviation of the residuals, r. See Anscombe and Tukey (1963), Cook and Weisberg (1982), and Gentleman and Wilk (1975), for further orientation to tests of normality and searches for outliers. Chapter 5 also discusses this topic, using a robust method that requires replication of treatment sequences.

TABLE 3.6
Program for Checking Normality and Looking for Outliers

```
data rotate out trotate;  input obs_no resid  @ @;   tresid = resid/37.96536152;
cards;
 1  -14.08270803   2   31.97107257   3    9.31893847   4  -27.20730301
 5   17.47764380   6  -20.82818179   7   -6.57129418   8    9.92183217
 9  -26.48270803  10   17.41612410  11   11.01454650  12   -1.94796258
13   -2.83252109  14  -28.83834668  15  -10.43640754  16   42.10727531
17  -27.94141440  18   33.12291474  19   17.18565003  20  -22.36715037
21    9.96497660  22  -13.97508622  23  -24.00551829  24   28.01562790
25  -82.95507493  26  -22.88975246  27   37.53874560  28   68.30608179
29  105.85858560  30  -44.26863567  31  -58.30223598  32   -3.28771395
33  -42.40770803  34   20.89112410  35   32.78954650  36  -11.27296258
37   63.40092850  38   27.39876731  39   -8.53197112  40  -82.26772469
run; options ps 80; proc univariate data = rotate freq plot normal;
    var resid; id obs_no;
proc rank data = trotate normal = blom out = one; var tresid; ranks rtresid;
proc plot data = one;  title 'Program OUTLY.SAS';
title2 'NORMAL PROBABILITY PLOT OF STANDARDIZED
    RESIDUALS';
plot tresid*rtresid = '*';
proc print data = trotate; var tresid;
proc print data = one; var rtresid; run;
```

The first part of the program defines a data set called *rotate* including observation numbers and residuals from Table 3.2 output. That data step also computes standardized residuals labeled *tresid* in the program and outputted to a data file called *trotate* together with the original elements of *rotate*. Then a *proc univariate* procedure does a Shapiro-Wilks test of normality with the residuals as well as presenting a variety of frequency distributions, statistics, and plots. Because the normal probability plot with this procedure is not easy to interpret, we go on to use *proc rank* to normalize the scale of standardized residuals and *proc plot* to plot standardized residuals (*tresid*) and normalized ranks (called *rtresid* in the program). To the degree that such plots approximate straight lines, they suggest normality of underlying populations. Also to the extent that individual points fall far from the general trend of the graph, they suggest questionable data (outliers) that may need to be excluded from analysis. Two *proc print* commands are used to print numerical values of standardized residuals (tresid) and normalized ranks (rtresid). Finally, "options ps = 80;" sets page size to 80 lines.

Figure 3.2 shows the SAS® plot of standardized residuals against their normalized ranks. An advantage of plotting standardized residuals rather than residuals (there being no difference in the shapes of the two graphs) is that standardized residuals of more than about 2 in absolute size are quickly recongnized as quite high.

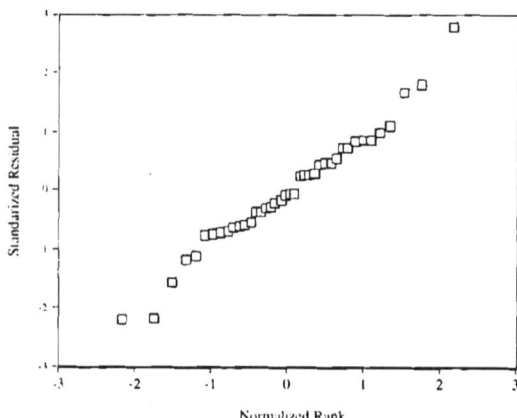

FIG. 3.2 Normal probability plot of standardized residuals against normalized ranks.

This graph shows some departure from a straight line trend. Also two data points lie below −2, and one lies above +2 on the standardized residual axis. If the theory of standard normal distributions applied exactly here, we would have expected our 40 residuals to include 5% or only 2 instead of 3 cases outside the range from −1.96 to +1.96. This suggests the possibility of an outlier but is not convincing evidence for one.

Now consider an earlier part of the output from the current SAS® program. The PROC UNIVARIATE subprogram yields a W statistic of 0.978733 with a probability of 0.7463 of obtaining as smaller or smaller a result when the underlying population is normal. A small W is taken as an indication of non-normality. This W-value gives us no reason to conclude that the deviations from a straight line in Fig. 3.2 reflect non-normality.

One reason for caution in interpreting existing tests of normality of residuals is to note the large difference between the number of degrees of freedom for error in the analysis of variance and the number of residuals to be compared by a test of normality. For example, the present experiment has 40 residuals but only 21 degrees of freedom for error in Table 3.3, rather than the 38 expected from a sample of 40 from which the population mean and standard deviation have been estimated. It may be fairly safe to follow common practice and assume that normality of error components implies normality of residuals. However, a more precise analyses might follow the lead of Wood (1978), who found the precise properties of residuals from data in a randomized block design. Similar new analyses might be appropriate for a variety of crossover designs. In fact, her technique would be appropriate for use with the current data if we were still considering the model in chapter 2 for mental rotation data, a randomized block model excluding time-related effects.

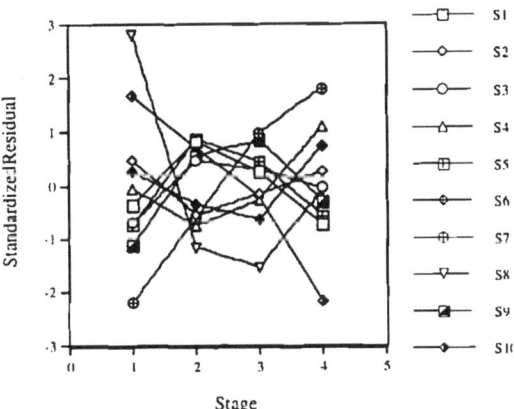

FIG. 3.3. Standardized residuals for each subject and stage number.

Figure 3.3 plots mean standardized residuals computed by the program of Table 3.6 for different subjects and stages. In view of the issue of larger numbers of standardized residuals than of df_{error} and because the mean standardized residual for any stage or for any subject is always zero, we may want to look primarily at Subjects 1 through 9 and Stages 1 through 3. This does not take into account constraints on the mean standardized residuals for different treatments or prior treatments, however. Looking at this smaller set leads us to identify Stage 1 as having the most questionable values, with Subject 7 being low and Subject 8 being high in standardized residuals. If this graph or Fig. 3.2 had shown more cases with extreme values or individual cases that were even more extreme, we might have gone on at this point to redo the program of Table 3.2 to omit questionable data points and see if new conclusions would be drawn from the new analysis of variance.

Variabilities of Estimates and Measures of Their Efficiency When a Carryover Is Used With a Randomized Block Design

This section discusses two closely related measures of how well a certain crossover design with a certain model can be used to estimate its effects. First, we consider the variance of estimating a given parameter or differences in parameters. Then we examine a measure of efficiency (on a scale from 0 to 100) for such an estimate. Each of these measures is controlled by the experimental design and associated model but not by the specific values of data obtained with the design.

The variance of an estimate of a parameter function is typically reported in $\frac{\sigma^2}{n}$ units so as to make it depend on the structure of the design and accompanying model rather than on the degree of variability in a specific experiment. Here n refers to the number of subjects per treatment sequence group, a factor controlling the variability of the sample mean for a group. We sometimes will call our variance measure in these units a *dimensionless variance*. For convenience, we imprecisely assume $n = 1$ and 10 sequences of this randomized block experiment.

To minimize the number of new methods in the present chapter, we delay description of a method of computing these variabilities of estimates of effects in $\frac{\sigma^2}{n}$ units until chapter 5. For now we simply report results to you so that you can see how the randomized block design studied here performs in this respect. We find that $\tau_0 - \tau_{180}$ or TREAT 0 – TREAT 180 is estimated with a dimensionless variance of 0.2908,

$\tau_{30} - \tau_{180}$ has a corresponding variance of 0.2237, and $\tau_{90} - \tau_{180}$ is estimated with a corresponding value of 0.2684. We also find such measures for $\pi_2 - \pi_4$ (STAGE 2 – STAGE 4) and $\pi_3 - \pi_4$ of 0.2273 and 0.2251, respectively. As noted earlier, it is impossible to estimate $\pi_1 - \pi_4$ in this example. The carryover parameter estimates for this design (not reported earlier because of their nonsignificance) have somewhat higher dimensionless variances (and, thus, lower sensitivities): 0.3154 for $\lambda_1 - \lambda_4$, 0.3557 for $\lambda_2 - \lambda_4$, and 0.3926 for $\lambda_3 - \lambda_4$. This decrease in sensitivity is to be expected in view of the fact that there are no carryovers in the model for Stage 1 of this experiment.

Now we examine an efficiency measure such as the one comparing the variance of a parameter or parameter difference such as TREAT 0 – TREAT 180 for that design to the corresponding variances for some more sensitive option such as the same experimental design but a model without carryover effects (Jones & Kenward, 1989; Ratkowsky, Evans, & Alldredge, 1993). Since the latter reference model yields a small variance of estimated quantities like TREAT 0 – TREAT 180, it can be used in the numerator of a ratio of variances for two models, reflecting their efficiency compared to each other. Once efficiency is defined as $E = 100 \dfrac{\text{Var}(\text{Estimator}_{\text{Reference Model}})}{\text{Var}(\text{Estimator}_{\text{Current Model}})}$, it is forced to have the desired range of possible values from 0 to 100 mentioned earlier.

A different efficiency measure may be obtained for each parameter function of interest. As with variances of estimators, we delay description of a method of computing efficiencies until chapter 5. For now we simply state that current variances and efficiencies are approximate — we report them to you so that you can see roughly how this design performs. We find that $\tau_0 - \tau_{180}$ or TREAT 0 – TREAT 180 is estimated with an efficiency $E = 68.78$, $\tau_{30} - \tau_{180}$ is estimated with an efficiency $E = 89.41$, and $\tau_{90} - \tau_{180}$ is estimated with an efficiency $E = 74.52$. We also find that $\pi_2 - \pi_4$ (STAGE 2 – STAGE 4) is estimated with an efficiency $E = 87.99$, and $\pi_3 - \pi_4$ is estimated with an efficiency $E = 88.85$. The carryover parameter estimates for this design (not reported earlier because of their nonsignificance) are also known to have high efficiencies: E for $\lambda_1 - \lambda_4 = 63.41$, E for $\lambda_2 - \lambda_4 = 56.23$, and E for $\lambda_3 - \lambda_4 = 50.94$. This set of efficiency values includes a few values quite near 100. However, most of them are of more moderate size.

It appears that the randomized block design may be used fairly efficiently with the model of Equation 3.1 even though the use of stage and carryover effects in the model tends to reduce the efficiency of estimation of the original parameters of interest, those for treatments. One is trading away some efficiency for the latter parameters in order to answer questions about the effects of practice (stages) and prior treatments (carryovers) on current behavior. Similarly, some designs are customarily associated with models having treatment and stage effects. Addition of carryover effects to those models may add information about carryovers while reducing the efficiency of estimation of the other effects of interest.

Method B: Using a Polynomial Model of Treatment Effects

Basic Approach

Just as Shepard and Metzler (1971) did (and chapter 2 explores without considering stage or carryover effects), we now want to check whether the basic trend of our mental rotation data is linear as a function of treatment (i.e., amount of rotation). We could therefore modify Equation 3.1 to include linear (β_1), quadratic (β_2), and/or cubic (β_3) components of treatment effects in that trend:

$$Y_{ijk} = \mu + s_i + \pi_j + \beta_1 k + \beta_2 k^2 + \beta_3 k^3 + \lambda_{k'} + e_{ijk} \tag{3.2}$$

Assumptions about other parameters would remain as they were for Equation 3.1 However, the actual analysis to be performed is the orthogonal polynomial analysis of a model parallel to Equation 3.2 and yielding conclusions reducible to conclusions about the parameters of that equation. The new model also invokes so-called $\psi_d(k)$ sets of d-order orthogonal polynomial coefficients for different orders d used in the equation:

$$Y_{ijk} = \mu + s_i + \pi_j + \alpha_1 \psi_1(k) + \alpha_2 \psi_2(k) + \alpha_3 \psi_3(k) + \lambda_{k'} + e_{ijk} \tag{3.3}$$

Why do we choose to use Equation 3.3 with its orthogonal polynomial parameters rather than Equation 3.2 with its more interesting parameters? Orthogonal polynomial analyses are performed for at least two reasons:

1. They define linear, quadratic, etc., effects in such a way that they are orthogonal to each other, permitting such strategies as testing for linear effects and then, without redoing the earlier analysis, testing for quadratic and/or cubic effects, and

2. Especially in the case of evenly spaced variables such as Stages 1, 2, 3, and 4, values of orthogonal polynomial coefficients of ψ_d for Order d are tabled or easy to compute; with four stages there are four coefficients for linear trend (Order 1), four for quadratic trend (Order 2), etc. The use of these coefficients in significance testing is simple enough to be performed with pocket calculators. Keppel (1982) is one of many sources of methods for computing such coefficients when spacing is unequal. One could do that kind of calculation explicitly here, but shortly we use a more convenient SAS® command instead, performing the Keppel calculations implicitly.

Unfortunately, some textbook discussions of orthogonal polynomial analysis describe significance testing but not estimation procedures. However, Kirk (1982) shows how to make numerical predictions of linear and quadratic trend for a four-level data set, writing a predictive equation in terms of what are called α values in Equation 3.3. For an eight-level data set, Draper and Smith (1981) go farther, also generating an unsimplified cubic equation in terms of the β values of equation but noting that there is little reason to perform that simplification. Note that in our context the orthogonal polynomial analysis may make α_1 for linear effects reflect an intercept as well; it may also make α_2 for quadratic effects reflect linear and lower-order effects as well, etc. However, no α_d estimate will reflect higher order effects ($\beta_{d'}$ for $d' > d$). So one simply needs to be careful in describing the meaning of an obtained value for a component such as α_1.

We could not find a way to perform estimation of polynomial constants, $\psi_d(k)$ values, for Equation 3.3 in SAS ® GLM when using the REPEATED command. However, use of that command plus a PRINTM option in the earlier program of Table 2.10 for the present data and a simpler model yielded the linear, quadratic, and cubic sets of four ψ_d coefficients each needed to progran computation of contrast tests and orthogonal polynomial estimates by the method of Table 3.7.

Again we use a SAS® PROC GLM program to produce analysis of variance results. The REPEATED command in SAS® GLM cannot be used with this model because both stage and treatment effects are included in the model. What is done instead is to find parameters α_d and t-statistics by performing ESTIMATE commands; equivalent F-testing of these parameters employs CONTRAST commands. Table 3.7 presents additions to our last program above, permitting the new analyses. Notice that the final CONTRAST command combines 1 df contrasts separated by commas in the program.

TABLE 3.7

A Partial Program for Analyzing Hypothetical Mental Rotation Data to Take Into Account Subject and Stage Effects While Looking for Orthogonal Polynomial Components of Treatment Effects

Add the following lines after "random subj;" in the middle of the existing program of Table 3.2:				
contrast 'linear' treat	−.5455447	−.3273268	.1091089	.7637626;
estimate 'linear' treat	−.5455447	−.3273268	.1091089	.7637626;
contrast 'quadratic' treat	.5128226	−.1709409	−.7407437	.3988620;
estimate 'quadratic' treat	.5128226	−.1709409	−.7407437	.3988620;
contrast 'cubic' treat	−.4351941	.7833495	−.4351941	.0870388;
estimate 'cubic' treat	−.4351941	.7833495	−.4351941	.0870388;
contrast 'treatments' treat	−.5455447	−.3273268	.1091089	.763726,
treat	.5128226	−.1709409	−.7407437	.3988620,
treat	−.4351941	.7833495	−.4351941	.0870388;

Hypothesis Testing and Estimation of Orthogonal Polynomial Effects

The results of the hypothesis tests just performed are shown in Table 3.8. This analysis shows a significant linear treatment component ($p < 0.0001$) and no significant quadratic or cubic treatment component. The estimated polynomial parameters are $\hat{\alpha}_1 = 200.14$, $\hat{\alpha}_2 = 4.16$, and $\hat{\alpha}_3 = 11.34$ in this case. There seems to be no need to convert these estimates to $\hat{\beta}$ values for Equation 3.2. As might be expected, the contrast command for treatments as a whole in Table 3.7 yields the same $SS_{Treatments}$ value and significance test results as shown for treatments in the Type II analysis of Table 3.3.

TABLE 3.8

Breakdown of Polynomial Components of Treatment Effects
for Hypothetical Mental Rotation Data

Source	Sum of Squares	df	Mean Square	F
Linear	309,487.88	1	309,487.88	115.62****
Quadratic	136.38	1	136.38	0.05
Cubic	973.05	1	973.05	0.36
Error	56,213.38	21	2,676.83	—

Note. **** $p < 0.0001$.

Power Calculations

Computation of power of random subject effects and overall fixed effects of stages, treatments, or carryovers is comparable to that performed in chapter 2. However, special attention needs to be paid to the computation of power for polynomial effects. Table 3.2 includes a data step called POWER_L for computing the power of the test for a linear effect. Because of our ignorance about the size of important linear effects for this data set, we simply set LAMBDA = 5, saying that the minimum detectable size of α_1^2 should be five times its variance, whatever that may be. Other parts of this data step set the significance level at 0.05 and the degrees of freedom at 1 and 21 as the rest of the analysis implies. The resulting power value is 0.569, which is smaller than one would like, despite the significant linear effect actually shown. The power of a quadratic or cubic effect test with LAMBDA = 5 is also 0.569, of course.

Method C: An Alternate Method for Use When Sphericity (Type H Covariance Structure) May Not Hold

Difficulties With Sphericity Testing in This Situation

Our original use of Mauchly's test of sphericity for these data in chapter 2 was improper if stage or carryover effects were also present. Assuming a proper model or new computational procedure, we wish to perform an overall test of sphericity for the covariance structure in our crossover design data. Ratkowsky, Evans, and Alldredge (1993) have provided helpful examples of performance of such a test. Our approach here must take into account the fact that only one treatment sequence (0°

90° 180° 30°) employs more than one subject, there being two subjects (Subjects 3 and 9) in this case. Because no covariance matrix can be estimated for the other sequences, we are not able to perform a better, 2-stage test (called a multisample sphericity test), to be illustrated in chapter 5. Nor do a more modern single sample 1-stage locally best invariant test or a 1-stage multisample sphericity test illustrated by Kirk (1995) seem appropriate here.

An Indirect Assessment of Nonsphericity in Table 2.1 Data

Approach. One option that will prove more useful than it first appears is to falsely apply the split-plot repeated measurements approach of Table 2.4 in chapter 2. Even though the split-plot model in Equation 3.4 is inappropriate to describe our data, it has the advantage of assigning the same number of parameters (36) as cells to the nine treatment sequence by four-stage segment of the data set, exactly predicting those cell means. This makes it what is called a *saturated model* (Jones & Kenward, 1989). By saturated, we mean that there can be no more complicated model that makes more accurate predictions of those cell means. A further advantage of using a saturated model is that a sophisticated estimation procedure, called *empirical GLS (Generalized Least Squares)* estimation gives the same parameter estimates regardless of whether the covariance matrix is estimated without refinement or under the assumption of uniform covariance or of Type H structure (Jones & Kenward, 1989; Ratkowsky, Evans, & Alldredge, 1993). This makes OLS and GLS estimators identical for the parameters of a saturated model.

Our general method will be to perform an analysis ignoring treatments but provisionally assessing effects of treatment sequences, stages, and interaction of sequences and stages in the process of attempting a Mauchly test and G-G or H-F corrections. This involves the multiple sequence group split-plot repeated measurements model:

$$Y_{gijk} = \mu + \gamma_g + s_i + \pi_j + \tau_k + (\gamma\pi)_{gj} + e_{gijk} \tag{3.4}$$

with g being a new index on sequence groups and γ_g and $(\gamma\pi)_{gj}$ being new parameters for sequence group and interaction of sequence group and stage effects, respectively. All other parameters have definitions given earlier. Because polynomial trends in time (stages) are not of interest now, we omit the POLYNOMIAL option from the REPEATED command in our program. Later, we ask the implications of this analysis for the earlier results in Table 3.3.

One point of possible controversy deserves attention here: Should the variance-covariance matrix Σ be indexed on stages or treatments? Because life proceeds along a time dimension, we choose to index Σ on stages, having successive rows be successive stages and also its columns. Table 3.9 is a program for the analysis just outlined.

TABLE 3.9

A Program for Assessing Sphericity of Hypothetical Mental Rotation Data
Under a Repeated Measurements Model

```
* PROGRAM ROTATEP.SAS;
data rotate; input subj seq y1 y2 y3 y4; cards;
 1 1   62.0 407.1 170.1   41.7
 2 2  109.1  72.3 306.2 132.9
 3 3   61.5 274.6 346.8   45.6
 4 4  123.9  99.4 207.6 363.3
 5 5  254.4  96.6  21.5  96.3
 6 6  176.7  97.0 250.2   1.5
 7 7  154.1  94.1  38.1   1.0
 8 8  491.2  95.2  90.9 203.5
 9 3   60.3 292.8 383.3  51.0
10 9   62.3  96.7  93.8 138.1
run ; proc glm; class seq; model y1—y4 = seq/nouni;
repeated stage 4/printe summary; title 'ROTATEP.SAS for assesing sphericity
in Table 3.1 data.'; run;
```

Results. Running this program yields a report in the LOG output of SAS® to the effect that multivariate tests could not be performed because of insufficient error degrees of freedom. The regular output reports that the Mauchly test could not be performed for the same reason. This is to be expected; the determinant of the sample covariance matrix $\hat{\Sigma}$ used in the Mauchly criterion will not exist unless the number of degrees of freedom for subjects within sequences is at least three rather than the present one.

Fortunately, there is a little bit of useful information available in the output from Table 3.9. The reported Geisser and Greenhouse (1958) G-G ε (epsilon) correction term is $\frac{1}{3}$ when rounded, indicating that a maximal correction for lack of sphericity is required (earlier work than

Geisser and Greenhouse's had shown a conservative correction of multiplying degrees of freedom in numerator and denominator by $\dfrac{1}{(J-1)}$ where J is the number of stages, or 4, in this case). A reported Huynh and Feldt (1976) H-F ε of $-69E11$ may be taken as an indication that this coefficient is undefined for the present analysis, causing an extraordinarily large negative result. Note that Huynh and Feldt did not state the upper and lower bounds on their coefficient. Whereas the G-G coefficient ranges from $\dfrac{1}{(J-1)}$ to 1, we know from the SAS® manual (SAS Institute Inc, 1989d) and other sources that the H-F ε can exceed 1, in which case no correction of F is performed; one simply treats that coefficient as if it were unity.

As mentioned earlier, this repeated measurements analysis uses a saturated model. Thus for 9 sequences and 4 stages there are 36 cells (not observations!), with 1 df for μ, 8 df for sequences, 3 df for stages, and 24 df for interaction, totalling 36 as desired. Given a total of 40 observations and 1 df for another non-error source, subjects within sequences, this leaves 3 for error.

Correcting for Nonsphericity in a Computationally Easy Way

Strategy. This section attempts to provide a testing procedure that does not require use of mathematical matrix programs like GAUSS (Aptech Systems, 1993) or multivariate techniques not easily employed with SAS® GLM or similar statistical packages. Let us now think back to the repeated measurements analysis method of Table 3.9, invoking the multigroup split-plot repeated measurements model of Equation 3.4. Despite the fact that nine different sequences were employed in the current experimental design, with only one sequence occurring twice, univariate tests of stage, sequence, and interaction effects were successfully performed. What can they tell us about performing a proper analysis based on a crossover model?

We know a G-G ε correction of $\frac{1}{3}$ for this data set and the model of (3.4). Because this model is saturated, the means for sequences and stages will be predicted exactly, as will all subject means not directly implied by sequence means. Any other saturated model will be equally accurate in prediction, even making the same, possibly inaccurate, predictions for individual scores and will therefore also yield the same estimated errors and $SS_{\text{Subj} \times \text{Stages}}$ value. Given Milliken and Johnson's

(1984) method of estimating the G-G ε value from estimated errors, this tells us that any other saturated model will also yield the same G-G ε value. This will be helpful in re-analyzing the data of Table 3.1 with a saturated carryover model.

$$Y_{gijk} = \mu + \gamma_g + s_{gi} + \pi_j + \tau_k + \lambda_{k'} + \lambda_{k''} + \lambda_{k'''}$$

$$+ (\pi\tau)_{jk} + (\tau\lambda)_{kk'} + (\gamma\pi)_{gj} + e_{gijk} \tag{3.5}$$

This equation uses elements of our original crossover model (3.1) and of our multi-group split-plot model (3.4) plus two new carryovers and two new interactions. A second-order carryover, $\lambda_{k''}$, is the carryover from a treatment two stages earlier; a third-order carryover, $\lambda_{k'''}$, has a corresponding definition. The new interactions are for stages by treatments, $(\pi\tau)_{jk}$, and for sequence groups by carryover, $(\gamma\pi)_{gj}$.

Tactics. We begin by performing a series of Type I analyses, each based on a different saturated crossover design model. If the original model of Equation 3.1 was correct except in assuming a spherical covariance structure, each of these analyses should show no significant effects after Type I extraction of the components of that equation. Significance will be assessed using the G-G coefficient of $\frac{1}{3}$ obtained in the saturated model split-plot analysis.

The next step will be to assess significance of the last component of Equation 3.1 to be entered into the model statement for a single Type I analysis based on Equation 3.5. Being conditional on extraction of all other non-error components of the original model and given nonsignificance of all new components in the current analysis, the G-G corrected test of this last component may be treated like a Type II analysis. Four such analyses will be conducted, one each for stage, treatment, carryover, and subject effects. The results of these analyses are intended to be conservative tests of the effects of interest in this experiment.

Justification of the application of G-G ε corrections to models other than standard models for 1-group or multi-group split-plot designs has appeared in Crowder and Hand (1990) who started from a single group of subjects, each measured on J occasions, with the covariance matrix of $J - 1$ orthonormal contrasts for the measures on those occasions being tested for sphericity and/or adjusted with the G-G ε coeficient. They

TABLE 3.10
A Conservative Crossover Design Program for Assessing
Treatment Effects in Hypothetical Mental Rotation Data

```
)T_SAT.SAS;

subj stage seq treat carry carry2 carry3 y @@;cards;
     62.0      1 2 1  180  1 0 0  407.1      1 3 1   90 4 1 0  170.1      1 4 1   30 3 ‹
    109.1      2 2 2    0  2 0 0   72.3      2 3 2  180 1 2 0  306.2      2 4 2   90 4 :
     61.5      3 2 3   90  1 0 0  274.6      3 3 3  180 3 1 0  346.8      3 4 3   30 4 :
    123.9      4 2 4    0  2 0 0   99.4      4 3 4   90 1 2 0  207.6      4 4 4  180 3 :
    254.4      5 2 5   30  4 0 0   96.6      5 3 5    0 2 4 0   21.5      5 4 5   90 1 :
    176.7      6 2 6   30  3 0 0   97.0      6 3 6  180 2 3 0  250.2      6 4 6    0 4 :
    154.1      7 2 7   90  4 0 0   94.1      7 3 7   30 3 4 0   38.1      7 4 7    0 2 :
    491.2      8 2 8    0  4 0 0   95.2      8 3 8   30 1 4 0   90.9      8 4 8   90 2 :
     60.3      9 2 3   90  1 0 0  292.8      9 3 3  180 3 1 0  383.3      9 4 3   30 4 :
     62.3     10 2 9   30  1 0 0   96.7     10 3 9   90 2 1 0   93.8     10 4 9  180 3 :
ss seq subj stage treat carry carry2 carry3;

)j(seq) stage carry treat carry2 carry3

:arry seq*stage/solution ss1 p; random subj(seq);

o saturate the model.  Tests treatment effects.'; run;
```

extend this approach to a 7-subject 2×4 within-subjects design, finding separate estimates of ε for the second main effect and its interaction. The first main effect, based on 1 *df* does not require a sphericity assumption.

Conservative Assessment of Treatment Effects. Table 3.10 shows the SAS® GLM program used for assessing treatment effects by the method just outlined. The results of Type I significance tests from Table 3.10 are given in Table 3.11. In this table *nr* indicates that an *F*, though available in computer output, is irrelevant to our basic analysis. In most cases this is because the expected mean square for the numerator reflects other effects beyond σ^2 and the source indicated for that line.

TABLE 3.11

Conservative Type I ANOVA Results Based on the Program in Table 3.10, Assessing Treatment Effects and Model in Equation 3.1 for Table 3.1 Data

Source	Sum of Squares	df	Mean Square	F
Sequences	83,748.56	8	10,468.56	*nr*
Subj(Seq)	433.65	1	433.65	*nr*
Stages	35,970.66	3	11,990.22	*nr*
Carryovers	79,003.35	3	26,334.45	*nr*
Treatments (Rotation Angles)	326,274.69	3 (-.>1)	108,758.23	789.26
Carry2	9,135.24	3 (-> 1)	3,045.08	22.10
Carry3	19,987.02	3 (-> 1)	6,662.34	48.35
Stage × Treat	25,330.39	9 (-> 3)	2,814.49	20.42
Treat × Carry	1,309.51	2 (-> $\frac{2}{3}$)	654.75	4.75
Stage × Seq	37.82	1 (-> $\frac{1}{3}$)	37.82	0.27
Error	413.39	3 (-> 1)	137.80	—

Consider the tests for Carry2 and Carry3, nominally involving 3 *df* for the numerator of the *F* involved, as well as 3 *df* for error. $F_{.05}(3,3)$ = 9.28, suggesting significance for each of these carryover effects if sphericity held. However, the -> signs for each indicate that, since ε =

.3333 for our Table 3.9 analysis, the ε-corrected numerator and denominator df's are 1 in each case. So a conservative test using these corrected values would be expected to reduce or abolish significance here. $F_{.05}(1,1) = 161$, much higher than the 22.10 and 48.35 for these two tests. Similarly for Stage × Treat, the corrected df values are 3 and 1, with $F_{.05}(3,1) = 216$, again well beyond the $F = 20.42$ reported above. Because the original design justified larger df's in the presence of sphericity, Draper and Joiner's (1984) warning against use of F-tests with 1 df for error may or may not be applicable here.

Two other F values, 4.75 for Treat × Carry with $\frac{2}{3}$ and 1 df, and 0.27 for Stage × Seq with $\frac{1}{3}$ and 1 df, cannot be assessed with conventional F tables because of their fractional df values. Use of our friend, the FINV command in SAS®, tells us that $F_{.05}(\frac{2}{3},1) = 134.80$ which is far higher than the observed value of 4.75. Alternatively, we find the total (55,799.98) of the five sums of squares for these final tests, as well as the total (6) of their corrected df values, yielding a corrected mean square for badness of fit of 9,300.00, a corrected mean square for error of $\frac{413.39}{1} = 413.39$, and an $F = 22.50$, compared to $F_{.05}(6,1) = 234$. Because there is no evidence of badness of fit, either with a composite test or with separate tests of several individual fixed effects in Equation 3.5, we conclude that the first part of the model may be adequate.

All that remains in the interpretation of Table 3.11 is to assess the effect of treatments. We have $F = 789.26$, compared to $F_{.05}(1,1) = 161$ or $F_{.01}(1,1) = 4,052$. So treatment effects are significant by a conservative test at the 0.05 level but not at the 0.01 level. In view of the nonsignificance of effects tested later in this table, we have done what we wanted to do, make a conservative Type II test of treatment effects.

Because our G-G correction, $\varepsilon = \frac{1}{3}$, is the most conservative possible, we have in effect performed a multivariate analysis for a crossover design, a class for which traditional multivariate procedures are rarely proposed. See Patel (1986) and Patel and Hearne (1980) for related work.

Conservative Assessment of Other Effects. The program of Table 3.10 needs to be run three more times with minor modifications each time. For testing stages, the only program change is to use the following MODEL statement in lieu of the current one and rerun:

MODEL Y = SEQ SUBJ(SEQ) TREAT CARRY STAGE CARRY2 CARRY3 TREAT*STAGE TREAT*CARRY SEQ*STAGE;

For testing 1st-order carryover, the corresponding statement is:

MODEL Y = SEQ SUBJ(SEQ) STAGE TREAT CARRY CARRY2 CARRY3 TREAT*STAGE TREAT*CARRY SEQ*STAGE;

For testing subject effects, pooled across sequences, we need the statement:

MODEL Y = TREAT CARRY STAGE SEQ SUBJ(SEQ) CARRY2 CARRY3 TREAT*STAGE TREAT*CARRY SEQ*STAGE;

and will add sums of squares for sequences and subjects in sequences before computing a mean square and an F for subjects (pooled across sequences).

OTHER TESTS OF EXPERIMENTAL EFFECTS
WHEN SPHERICITY DOES NOT HOLD

Conventional Crossover Design Methods

Here is a brief description of some other data analysis methods appropriate when sphericity does not hold. Ratkowsky, Evans, and Alldredge (1993) compare several approaches to the assessment of treatment, stage, and carryover effects when Type H structure does not hold. In each the basic method is to estimate parameters for an alternate variance-covariance matrix Σ, do any consequently required re-estimation of experimental effects, use the estimated matrix $\hat{\Sigma}$ in estimating standard errors for those effects, and compute significance tests based on those estimates. Ratkowsky et al. conclude that correction methods of this kind rarely make much difference in the conclusions from experiments; they believe that data analysis conducted under the sphericity assumption will ordinarily be satisfactory even if that assumption fails.

All of Ratkowsky et al.'s examples employ data with several replications of more than one treatment sequence. Persons with similar data will find those authors' methods easy to use because their illustrative examples are very complete. However, new computer packages or techniques, such as SAS® IML (SAS Institute Inc., 1985) or GAUSS (Aptech Systems, 1993), will be required.

Methods described by Jones and Kenward (1989) are available both for cases considered by Ratkowsky, Evans, and Alldredge and for data from experiments with inadequately replicated different sequences. The simplest method applies to replicated sequences such as ABAB versus BABA in our chapter 8 and ABBA versus BAAB in our chapter 12. This approach computes a single score (a so-called contrast) for each effect such as carryover and performs follow-up analysis on those scores (Jones & Kenward, 1989). This may be called a general approach of simplification by analyzing summary scores rather than all raw data directly.

A more complicated procedure employing ordinary least squares estimation with an unrestricted covariance structure (Jones & Kenward, 1989) is illustrated for one data set with replication within sequences and one with only one subject per sequence. This and other methods used by Jones and Kenward for dealing with minimally replicated sequences require more complicated computational effort or programs than are covered in the present book. However, the serious user of crossover designs needs to be able to apply these methods in addition to the methods illustrated here. Behavior scientists must increasingly deal with complicated techniques such as those just mentioned.

Ignoring Carryover Effects in a Design With Only One Treatment Order

Lorch and Myers (1990, Table 5) have used regression methods to analyze the times required for each of 10 subjects to read each of seven different sentences in the same order. Lorch and Myers evaluated effects of (a) serial position of a sentence, (b) number of words in a sentence, (c) number of new arguments in a sentence and (d) further but more or less unspecifiable variables affecting the reading of those sentences (regression sum of squares). Their serial position of a sentence corresponds to the current stage effects variable. Note that carryover effects were not assessed and that most variables were treated as quantitative variables with linear effects rather than as class variables.

THINGS TO REMEMBER

Major Analysis Options

1. Analyzing randomized block design data using a model involving subject effects, stage effects, treatment effects, and carryover effects in addition to an additive constant and error. Considering the possibility of using conservative tests when there is evidence that the sphericity assumption may not hold.

2. Analyzing randomized block design data using a model involving subject effects, stage effects, and linear, quadratic, and cubic treatment effects, in addition to an additive constant and error.

Interpreting Results of Computational Methods Not Previously Discussed

1. Understanding the Type I and Type II options in SAS® GLM.

2. Understanding expected mean squares from an analysis; using that information to indicate which type such as Type II may be most appropriate for a given analysis.

3. Understanding that information from E, E1 and E2 options can be used to tell what parameters or functions of parameters can be estimated in a given GLM data analysis.

4. Using SOLUTION command output plus estimability information to obtain desired parameter or parameter difference estimates.

5. Understanding predictive equations stated in terms of parameters from orthogonal polynomial analysis.

6. Understanding the computation of power of tests of orthogonal polynomial effects.

7. Understanding the interpretation of efficiency and variability (in $\frac{\sigma^2}{n}$ units) of estimates of specific functions of parameters in a given data analysis.

8. Remembering that any crossover design analysis method is built around a specific set of treatment sequences for the different subjects of the experiment. Also remembering that the dimensionless measures of variability of estimators and even the do-ability of a given hypothesis testing or estimability procedure may be impaired by certain other designs, such as having all subjects receive the same treatment sequence.

EXERCISES

1. Run the program combining Tables 3.2 and 3.7.

2. We could not use Table 2.4 in chapter 2 as a model to rewrite the ROTATE.SAS program in Table 3.2 to use the REPEATED option in measuring polynomial coefficients. However, we can go back to Table 2.4, and find the output resulting if you include PRINTM in the REPEATED command there.

(a) Now include that set of orthogonal polynomial coefficients in a modification of the program of Table 2.2 comparable to Table 3.7.

(b) Do you obtain the same sums of squares for polynomial coefficient and for error as originally obtained with Table 2.4? Discuss any discrepancies that you see. Hint: The revised Table 2.2 must assume sphericity *in all its tests*, but Table 2.4 does not.

4

Interpreting Estimability Information and Reported Estimates of Parameters in SAS® GLM Programs

INTRODUCTION

Most chapters of this book focus on the analysis of data from specific experimental designs. However, just as we needed theoretical background about matrices and the General Linear Model before dealing with the split-plot design of chapter 2, so we now need to think long and hard about SAS® GLM (SAS Institute Inc., 1989d) output from chapter 3 before we move to a new within-subjects design. Accordingly, the purpose of this chapter is to look at various ways to estimate parameters for within-subjects design models like the ones we have been considering thus far. Relevant information will come first from General Form of Estimable Functions (E) output generated by the E option in a SAS® GLM program and then from Type I, II, III, or IV Estimable Functions output generated by an E1, E2, E3, or E4 option in that program. Once we understand this estimability information, we are prepared to ask how to interpret both the (biased) estimates generated by the SOLUTION option of the MODEL command in a GLM program and the t-tests of significance for those estimates. In addition, we will discuss how to use estimability information to decide what functions can be estimated with the ESTIMATE command. Finally, we will relate these results to expected mean squares and any unusual degree of freedom values for specific significance tests.

INTERPRETING ESTIMABILITY TABLES
IN SAS® GLM OUTPUT

Interpretation of Output From the E Option of a MODEL Statement

To make this section very specific, let us consider the ROTATE.SAS program (Table 3.2) of the previous chapter, analyzing mental rotation data with a model testing for stage and carryover effects as well as traditional effects in randomized block design models. The output giving "Estimate values" must be interpreted in the light of what we are told about estimability because of output from the E and, for example, E2 options and of expected mean squares, especially those reported for TREAT, STAGE, and CARRY in the computer output. Because much of the information printed about subject effects refers to fixed effects and because we are assuming random effects, we discuss only the subject effect information relevant to that assumption.

Reading the General Form of Estimable Functions Output

What functions of fixed parameters can be estimated with this model, experimental design, and program? Table 4.1, the General Form of Estimable Functions (E) output generated by the E option in the SAS® GLM program just mentioned, can help to answer this question.

TABLE 4.1
General Linear Models Procedure
General Form of Estimable Functions

Effect		Coefficient	Effect		Coefficient
INTERCEPT		L1			
SUBJ	1	L2	SUBJ	6	L7
	2	L3		7	L8
	3	L4		8	L9
	4	L5		9	L10
	5	L6		10	L1-L2-L3-L4-L5-L6-L7-L8-L9-L10

(Continued)

TABLE 4.1
(Continued)

Effect		Coefficient	Effect		Coefficient
TREAT	0	L12	TREAT	90	L14
	30	L13		180	L1-L12-L13-L14
STAGE	1	L16	STAGE	3	L18
	2	L17		4	L1-L16-L17-L18
CARRY	0	L16	CARRY	3	L23
	1	L21		4	L1-L16-L21-L22-L23
	2	L22			

How do we use the information just given? Notice first that, for example, a term such as STAGE 1 refers to the parameter value for the first stage. Similarly, a term such as SUBJ 1 refers to the parameter value for the first subject. It can be shown that we can set a term or set of terms such as L16 or L17 to any desired numerical value or values and then develop an equation based on summing all effects multiplied by their coefficient values. Whatever that equation yields is an estimable function and a sample value can be computed, for example, with the ESTIMATE command discussed later in this chapter. A test of the hypothesis that this function is zero in the population is performed with a t-test also generated with that command.

Consider an example in which we set L17 = 1 and all other L values to 0. One way to see its consequences is to handwrite possible L-coefficient values and their consequences on your printed computer output. When the products of L values and parameters are summed, the result is a (possibly) weighted parameter or sum of parameters that can indeed be estimated within the current experimental design when the present model is assumed. Table 4.2 begins this process next (bold-face represents handwritten material).

Notice that the coefficient of every parameter except STAGE 2 and STAGE 4 becomes zero. So, adding up the products of each multiplier (L value) times parameter yields the fact that STAGE 2 – STAGE 4 = $\pi_2 - \pi_4$ is estimable with at least one type of analysis. To be more al-

TABLE 4.2

General Linear Models Procedure

General Form of Estimable Functions

Specialized for L17 = 0, All Else = 0

Effect	**Value**	**Coeff.**	**Effect**	**Value**		**Coeff.**
INTERCEPT	0	L1				
SUBJ	1	0	L2	SUBJ	6	0	L7
	2	0	L3		7	0	L8
	3	0	L4		8	0	L9
	4	0	L5		9	0	L10
	5	0	L6		10	0	L1-L2-L3-L4-L5-L6-L7-L8-L9-L10
TREAT	0	0	L12	TREAT	90	0	L14
	30	0	L13		180	0	L1-L12-L13-L14
STAGE	1	0	L16	STAGE	3	0	L18
	2	1	L17		4	1	L1-L16-L17-L18
CARRY	0	0	L16	CARRY	3	0	L23
	1	0	L21		4	0	L1-L16-L21-L22-L23
	2	0	L22				

gebraic (or more compulsive?) about this approach, we say that 0 INT +
0 SUBJ 1 + 0 SUBJ 2 + 0 SUBJ 3 + . . . + 0 SUBJ 16 + 0 TREAT 0
. . . + . . . 0 TREAT 180 + 0 STAGE 1 + 1 STAGE 2 + 0 STAGE 3 −
1 STAGE 4 + 0 CARRY 0 + 0 CARRY 1 + 0 CARRY 2 = STAGE 2
− STAGE 4 = $\pi_2 - \pi_4$ is estimable. A similar conclusion, that STAGE
3 − STAGE 4 is estimable, may be drawn by using this approach and
finding the consequences of setting L18 = 1 and all else equal to zero.

The case in which L16 = 1 and every other L coefficient = 0 is not
quite so pretty: The same summing of products of multipliers by parameters simplifies to the statement that STAGE 1 − STAGE 4 + CARRY 0
− CARRY 4 = $\pi_1 - \pi_4 + \lambda_0 - \lambda_4$ is estimable. Since no other combination of L values comes closer to telling us that STAGE 1 − STAGE 4 =
$\pi_1 - \pi_4$ is estimable, we see that we cannot estimate the difference between Stage 1 and Stage 4 effects no matter which type of analysis we
employ.

Our table showing the General Form of Estimable Functions can also be used to tell what can be estimated about pairs of treatment effects. Thus, setting L12 = 1 and all else equal to zero shows that TREAT 0 – TREAT 180 = $\tau_0 - \tau_{180}$ is estimable. We can also estimate carryover effect differences. However, because the F for carryover in the RO-TATE.SAS analysis was not significant, we do not explicitly check for estimability nor consider how to estimate such effects in this example.

The approach just discussed is intended to use the last effect in any group of parameters (family of parameters) as a reference point. Hence, we are subtracting STAGE 4 or TREAT 180 or CARRY 4 from some other level of STAGE or TREAT or CARRY. This is consistent with what is called the set-last-to-zero or set-to-zero approach in parameter estimation. That provides an intuitive explanation of the fact that our SOLUTION option output always yields a "0.0000 B" estimate for the last level of a given family of parameters. However, if an estimate of difference between some other pair of parameters is desired, the current table can tell us if it is estimable. For example, suppose that we set L12 = 1, L13 = –1, and all other L values equal to zero. Then Table 4.1 leads to a sum of products of multipliers and parameters equal to TREAT 0 – TREAT 30, showing that this specific difference is also estimable.

Interpretation of Estimability Information Relevant to a Specific ANOVA Type

Introduction

When a table of the General Form of Estimable Functions is examined, many different functions prove themselves estimable. In order to find out what we can estimate with a specific type of analysis, we need to use a command specific to that type. For example, to examine Type I Estimable Functions, we must invoke an E1 option for our MODEL statement. Because there are four types of analysis in SAS® GLM, we can invoke E1, E2, E3, or E4. Indeed we can use as many of these four options as we choose. However, because their output is quite long (and because we feel guilty about cutting down so many trees to make computer paper for our analyses!), we usually will not want to print results from more than one or two such options. Often we will get general information from the E option plus information based on the E2 option as well.

Interpreting Results of Using an E1, E2, E3, or E4 Option in a MODEL Statement

We illustrate this process by examining E2 output from the RO-TATE.SAS program. That output is special for Type II analysis, of course; what is estimable with Type II is often the same as for other types, but it is likely to be different from that for Type I when a cross-over design is employed.

Unlike output from the E option, the results of the current option yields several tables, one for each set of effects, such as stages, to be assessed. Table 4.3 shows part of that output for stages, based on the ROTATE.SAS program in Table 3.2:

TABLE 4.3
General Linear Models Procedure
Type II Estimable Functions for: STAGE

Effect		Coefficient
INTERCEPT	0	0
SUBJ	1	0
	2	0
	3	0
	. . .	0
	10	0
TREAT	. . .	0
STAGE	1	0
	2	L17
	3	L18
	4	–L17–L18
CARRY	. . .	0

All the Table 4.3 entries for TREAT and CARRY are zero and are not specifically shown here. Now we work very much as we did with output from the E option: Again, it can be shown that we can set any term or set of terms such as L17 or L17 and L18 to any desired numerical value or values and then develop an equation based on summing all effects multiplied by their coefficient values. For example, if we set L17 = 1 and L18 = 0, a quick look tells us that STAGE 2 – STAGE 4 = $\pi_2 - \pi_4$ is estimable in a Type II analysis. More algebraically, the table just shown implies that, for L17 =1 and L18 = 0, the quantity: 0 INT + 0 SUBJ 1 + 0 SUBJ 2 + 0 SUBJ 3 + . . . + 0 SUBJ 10 + 0 + . . . + 0 + 0 STAGE 1 + 1 STAGE 2 + 0 STAGE 3 – 1 STAGE 4 +   0 + . . .+ 0 = STAGE 2 – STAGE 4 is estimable within a Type II analysis.

The E2 information also tells us that, because the coefficient for STAGE 1 is 0, no function only of STAGE 1 and other stage parameters is estimable within a Type II analysis. Further, we can see from the E2 information that STAGE 3 – STAGE 4 (= $\pi_3 - \pi_4$) is estimable.

Comparable reasoning about treatment and carryover effects uses other little tables of the output, entitled "Type II Estimable Functions for: TREAT" or for "CARRY." It also helps in the recognition of the hypothesis tested by the F-tests for treatments and for carryover reported in the Type II analysis of variance based on the ROTATE.SAS program.

"SOLUTION" VERSUS "ESTIMATE" COMMANDS

The SOLUTION Option and (Biased) Parameter Estimation

Table 4.4 presents some of the more interesting results from the SOLUTION option of ROTATE.SAS.

TABLE 4.4

Parameter Estimates and t-Tests from the SOLUTION Option of ROTATE.SAS

Parameter		Estimate	t	p	Unbiased Estimate of
TREAT	0	–255.65 B	–9.16	0.0001	TREAT 0 – TREAT 180
	30	–228.64 B	–9.34	0.0001	TREAT 30 – TREAT 180
	90	–129.85 B	–4.84	0.0001	TREAT 90 – TREAT 180
					(Continued)

TABLE 4.4

(Continued)

Parameter		Estimate	t	p	Unbiased Estimate of
	180	0.00 B	.	.	
STAGE	1	67.44 B	2.34	0.0292	STAGE 1 – STAGE 4 + CARRY 0 – CARRY 4
	2	77.22 B	3.13	0.0050	STAGE 2 – STAGE 4
	3	26.33 B	1.07	0.2955	STAGE 3 – STAGE 4
	4	0.00 B	.	.	
CARRY	0	0.00 B	.	.	
	1	33.61 B	1.16	0.2603	CARRY 1 – CARRY 4
	2	18.73 B	0.61	0.5503	CARRY 2 – CARRY 4
	3	33.26 B	1.03	0.3166	CARRY 3 – CARRY 4
	4	0.00 B	.	.	

Output like this giving "Estimate" values, usually labeled "B" for Bias, is best interpreted once we know output from the E and E1 or E2, etc., options we have been discussing. The key to using the parameter estimates of Table 4.4 is to know that any estimable linear function of parameters may be generated as the corresponding linear combination of the (biased) parameter estimates produced by the SOLUTION option (inferrable from SAS Institute Inc., 1989d). Accordingly, TREAT 0 – TREAT 180 = $\tau_0 - \tau_{180}$ is estimated as $-255.65 - 0.00 = -255.65$ just as the final column of the table says. A more complex result is that STAGE 1 – STAGE 4 + CARRY 0 – CARRY 4 = $\pi_1 - \pi_4 + \lambda_0 - \lambda_4$ is estimated as $67.44 - 0.00 + 0.00 - 0.00 = 67.44$, just as the final column of the table says. Note that this column does not appear in SAS® output. Significance levels (p) for t are based on the 21 degrees of freedom for error reported in the ANOVA from ROTATE.SAS.

There is a sense in which the B for Bias is misleading. Indeed, 77.22 is biased as an estimate of the STAGE 2 effect. However, the results of running the commands in Table 4.2 tell us that 77.22 is unbiased as an estimate of the STAGE 2 – STAGE 4 effect difference. Similarly, the tabled t of 3.13 cannot be trusted to assess significance of the STAGE 2 effect, but it is perfectly acceptable for testing significance of the STAGE 2 – STAGE 4 effect difference. MORAL: The SOLUTION option output can be very useful if you take care to know what is really being assessed with it. Be especially careful not to misuse t and apply it to inadvertently test a hypothesis that does not interest you, such as that STAGE 1 − STAGE 4 + CARRY 0 − CARRY 4 = $\pi_1 - \pi_4 + \lambda_0 - \lambda_4$ is zero in the population from which your data was drawn.

The ESTIMATE Command As a Means of Parameter Estimation

Making Estimates Relevant to a Specific ANOVA Type

When we discuss a factorial within-subject design in chapter 5, we will find that SAS® GLM estimates main effects of a given factor quite differently with one technique than with another. It becomes especially important there to know the definition of a certain kind of treatment effects as a function of the type of analysis employed. For that reason we may use the ESTIMATE command to exhibit results associated with Estimable Functions for Type I, II, III, or IV, expecting to get different information from that obtained with the SOLUTION option of the MODEL command.

Estimating Parameters With the ESTIMATE Command

When needed, a SAS® ESTIMATE command must be included within a GLM procedure (PROC GLM) and after a MODEL statement. Its format begins with ESTIMATE, follows with a title included in single quotes, and ends with one or more parameter names each followed by weights for respective levels of the parameter. For example, we estimate STAGE 2 − STAGE 4 with the following command:

ESTIMATE 'STAGE2-STAGE4' 0 1 0 −1

We use minimal spacing inside these single quotes in order to be sure as much as possible of the title is actually printed out.

Notice that often we do not know which ESTIMATE commands to use until we have examined the output based on the E2 command. Similarly, without E or E2 information, we often do not know what linear combinations of biased estimates from the SOLUTION option to use in order to do estimation. It would be misleading to show ESTIMATE commands for this program without mentioning that the program was run at least once before in order to learn what was needed in it.

A tricky issue must be mentioned here: We can write an ESTIMATE command for any linear combination of parameters that proves estimable with the E command. The reason we let output from the E2 (or E1, E3, or E4 in other situations) option guide us in most of our selections for estimation is that we want to use the same estimated values as implicitly employed in the ANOVA routinely computed with the E2 option.

Because carryover effects were not significant in the analysis based on ROTATE.SAS, we do not bother to estimate them here. The following table shows estimation instructions to be included in the program of Table 3.2. A natural place to include them is right after the line ending "random subj;".

TABLE 4.5

Important ESTIMATE Commands for Inclusion in the Program of Table 3.2

ESTIMATE 'STAGE2-STAGE4' 0 1 0 –1;
ESTIMATE 'STAGE3-STAGE4' 0 0 1 –1;
ESTIMATE 'TREAT0-TREAT180' 1 0 0 –1;
ESTIMATE 'TREAT30-TREAT180' 0 1 0 –1;
ESTIMATE 'TREAT90-TREAT180' 0 0 1 –1;

When these commands are employed as recommended, they yield exactly the same results as are reported in Table 4.4 based on the SOLUTION command. However, the latter command routinely gives more estimates and significance tests than we may need to compute with the ESTIMATE command.

What happens if we try to estimate something that is not estimable? For example, we might try to estimate STAGE 1 – STAGE 4 with the command:

ESTIMATE 'STAGE1–STAGE4' 1 0 0 –1

Even if this command is placed in the proper part of the program we are using, no estimate of STAGE 1 – STAGE 4 will be printed out. The major clue to this failure appears in the LOG file or LOG window (not the OUTPUT) available after this SAS® run. There we are told that STAGE 1 – STAGE 4 cannot be estimated. On the other hand, once we know from the discussion of General Forms of Estimable Functions and of Table 4.1 output that STAGE 1 – STAGE 4 + CARRY 0 – CARRY 4 can be estimated, we know that the following command should work:

ESTIMATE 'ST1–ST4+CA0-CA4' STAGE 1 0 0 –1

CARRY 1 0 0 0 –1

It is not included in Table 4.5 because we have no special interest in estimating this quantity or testing it for significance.

Choosing Between the SOLUTION and ESTIMATE Commands

Careful linear combination of biased estimates from the SOLUTION command can be easier for estimation of linear functions of parameters than using the ESTIMATE command. However, there will often be cases in which the biased estimates from SOLUTION can be combined to yield unbiased estimates of parameter combinations of interest but SAS® cannot report an appropriate standard error or significance test for that combination without using the ESTIMATE command. A further advantage of using the ESTIMATE command is that it provides further verification that a given function of parameters is estimable when that estimation is attempted. If we know from the General Form of Estimable Functions (E command) that a certain function can be estimated, we can compute it from SOLUTION output. But, added confidence comes from use of the ESTIMATE command in addition.

MORE ABOUT EXPECTED MEAN SQUARES

From the preceding chapter, we know that the following expected mean squares apply to the Type II analysis of the ROTATE.SAS program:

Source	Type II Expected Mean Square
SUBJ	Var(Error) + 3.8565 Var(SUBJ)
TREAT	Var(Error) + Q(TREAT)
STAGE	Var(Error) + Q(STAGE)
CARRY	Var(Error) + Q(CARRY)
ERROR	Var(Error) (Not actually displayed in the EMS output of SAS®)

Because subjects are assumed random in our program, the best information about their effects comes from expected mean square values rather than the E2 information required with fixed effects. Comparing expected mean squares for subjects and for error suggests subtracting one from the other, yielding

$$E(MS_{subjects}) - E(MS_{error}) = 3.8565\ Var(Subjects).$$

If we take our observed mean squares from ROTATE.SAS output in the previous chapter as approximations of expected mean square values, we can say $MS_{subjects} - MS_{error} = 8{,}847.0892 - 2{,}676.8275 = 6{,}170.2617 \approx 3.8565\ Var(Subjects)$. In turn, this suggests that Var(Subjects) is about 1,599.9641 or that the standard deviation of subjects is about 40.00.

THINGS TO REMEMBER

1. The E option in a SAS® GLM MODEL statement yields output telling the General Form of Estimable Functions. From this output one can learn whether certain functions of model parameters can be estimated with some type of analysis (Type I through IV).

2. The E1 (or E2, E3, or E4) option in a SAS® GLM MODEL statement yields output telling the Type I Estimable Functions (or Type II, III, or IV) that are obtainable within a given family of parameters. There will be a separate table for each type of parameter, such as INTERCEPT, TREAT, or STAGE. One may find it possible to estimate a function of different stages in a Type II analysis, for example. How-

ever, for the Type II analysis of Table 3.2, no function of Stage 1 and other stages or other kinds of effects is estimable, causing loss of one degree of freedom in the numerator of an F-ratio for comparing the remaining stage effects.

3. We know that any estimable linear function of parameters may be generated as the corresponding linear combination of the (biased) parameter estimates produced by the SOLUTION option. Because information from the E option previously mentioned tells that such functions of parameters as TREAT 0 – TREAT 180 are estimable, one can estimate such functions as TREAT 0 – TREAT 180 from the biased estimates of their components.

4. Information from this E option can be also used to tell what functions of parameters can be estimated with an ESTIMATE command. Standard errors and significance tests for quantities estimated are also obtained thereby.

5. The expected mean square for a given family of effects within a given type of analysis can be used to determine whether there is a quadratic form Q for that effect uncontaminated with other effects, suggesting the possibility of a significance test for that family.

EXERCISES

1. Use output in Table 4.1 to estimate STAGE 2 – STAGE 3.

2. Use output in Table 4.2 to estimate TREAT 30 – TREAT 90.

3. Can you estimate STAGE 1 – STAGE 3? Explain.

4. Can you find out how to use a command related to the ESTIMATE command, the CONTRAST command, to test differences among the four treatment effects, comparable to performing the Type II F-test for treatment effects in Tables 3.2 and 3.3? Explain.

5

Analyzing Data From Within-Subject Factorial Designs, Taking Into Account Stage-of-Practice Effects

INTRODUCTION

The purpose of this chapter is to demonstrate an analysis method for 4-stage within-subject designs having two values for each of two factors, A and B. Much current analysis of data from this design follows recommendations by authors such as Girden (1992) and Kirk (1995) who considered the possibility of main effects of A and B plus their interactions, as well as interactions of subjects and those factors. (Winer, Brown, & Michels, 1991, made comparable suggestions for a more complicated design with one between-subjects factor in addition to the two within-subject factors just mentioned.) They do not assess time-related effects such as stage effects and carryover effects. However, when more than one of the 24 possible sequences of the 4 basic treatment combinations (pairs), A_1B_1 A_1B_2 A_2B_1 A_2B_2, are employed in an experiment, performance differences on a given treatment pair for subjects from different sequences might very well suggest that time-related effects are present. If three or more appropriate sequences are employed, it will be possible to disentangle treatment effects from the specific stage and carryover effects assumed in the model equation to be presented shortly.

The main example shown next (Young, McWeeny, Ellis, & Hay, 1986) concerns recognition of names and faces of 14 famous and 14 unfamiliar British persons. For example, from a related study (Young, Ellis, Flude, McWeeny, & Hay, 1986; reprinted with permission) here are three pictures of Mick Jagger, one labeled properly and the other two labeled as the former Labor Party leader Neil Kinnock, and as the

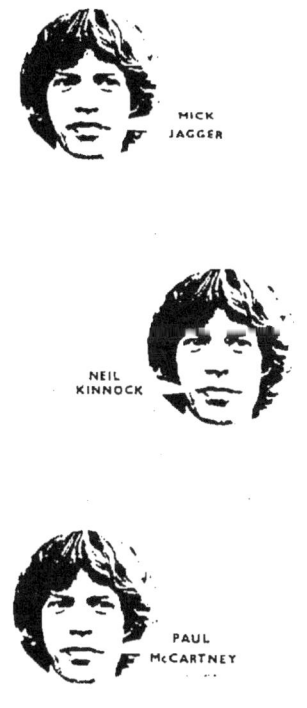

MICK
JAGGER

NEIL
KINNOCK

PAUL
McCARTNEY

famous Beatle, Paul McCartney. In the first study mentioned, pictures and names were presented separately. The A_1B_1 treatment combination required subjects to say "Yes" to pictures of familiar faces and "No" to unfamiliar ones. The A_1B_2 task was to say Yes" to names of familiar persons and "No" to names of unfamiliar ones. The A_2B_1 task was to give the correct name of each familar face or to say "Don't know" to unfamiliar faces. The A_2B_2 task was simply to read each name aloud. In all four tasks the subject was to respond as quickly and accurately as possible; mean latency of response to familiar stimuli was the basis of Young et al.'s major data analysis.

ANALYZING A 2×2 WITHIN-SUBJECTS EXAMPLE

Experimental Design and Statistical Model

From the aforementioned example, we follow Young et al. in thinking of one factor as a classification of tasks, categorization versus naming (A_1 and A_2). The other factor relates to type of stimulus, faces versus names (B_1 and B_2). Each of the four possible combinations of one A value and one B value was used with each subject. We also deal only with response latencies to pictures or names of familiar persons.

We simulate some aspects of this names and faces experiment by acting as if there were only 1 test for each subject under each treatment combination, not 14 tests because of the availability of 14 familiar faces in the actual experiment. This reduces the complexity of the data analysis, of course. Unfortunately, psychological research, including this experiment, is often reported without much information about the order in which different treatments were presented. For the moment, let us suppose that four different arrangements (stimulus sequences) are employed in our example. Also, we assume that four subjects in this experiment received each of the following treatment orders (sequences) below in an experimental session:

Sequence 1: A_1B_1 A_2B_2 A_1B_2 A_2B1

Sequence 2: A_1B_2 A_1B_1 $A_2 B_1$ A_2B_2

Sequence 3: A_2B_1 A_1B_2 A_2B_2 A_1B_1

Sequence 4: A_2B_2 A_2B_1 A_1B_1 A_1B_2

This design has two interesting properties: (a) every treatment combination (Task and Stimulus pair) such as A_1B_1, appears exactly once in each row (sequence) and once in each column (stage). This property makes it what is called a Latin square design. (b) Every treatment combination appears an equal number of times immediately before every other combination. For example, in Sequence 1 A_1B_1 precedes A_2B_2, in Sequence 2 it precedes A_2B_1, in Sequence 3 it is at the end of the session and does not precede anything, and in Sequence 4 it precedes A_1B_2. This pair of properties makes a design of this kind with one subject per sequence, a special kind of Latin square (i.e., a balanced Latin square or a so-called Williams square; Williams, 1949). With a constant number (more than one) of subjects for each of these sequences, we have a nicely replicated balanced Latin square. For squares with an odd number of treatments, two different squares are used to provide the sort of balance just defined.

Williams squares have a number of desirable properties, especially their usefulness in facilitating the assessment of carryover effects. See chapter 6 for programs and exercises using three other computer packages to assess data from balanced Latin squares (SYSTAT™, SPSS®, and BMDP™). Those methods are applicable here, but a bit of added complexity results because two treatment dimensions, task and stimulus, are used instead of only one with as many treatments as sequences.

In thinking about the current experimental design, we will let g and i refer to sequence and subject numbers, respectively, with g being only a notational device in case we wish to number subjects from 1 to 5 in each sequence rather than from 1 to 15 across groups as is done in the SAS® programs. Also j will refer to stage, k to Treatment Factor 1 — the task type (categorization vs. naming) — and m to Treatment Factor

2 — the stimulus type (faces vs. names). An apostrophe on k or m will mean that the treatment for the immediately prior stage is involved. A reasonable model equation for observations (Y_{gijkm}) from such a design might be:

$$Y_{gijkm} = \mu + s_{gi} + \pi_j + \gamma_k + \tau_m + (\gamma\tau)_{km} + \lambda_1 k' + \lambda_2 m' + (\lambda_1\lambda_2)_{k'm'}$$

$$+ e_{gijkm} \tag{5.1}$$

What do the many symbols in this model equation mean? To answer this question, let us illustrate how to apply the equation to performance of Subject 6 in Sequence 2 on Stage 2. We know that all subjects in Sequence 2 had A_1B_2 on Stage 1. We also know that these subjects have A_1B_1 on Stage 2. So Equation 5.1 implies that the score Y_{26211} for this case includes the following components:

an additive constant, μ;

a random subject effect, s_{26}, for Subject 6, Sequence 2;

a stage effect, π_2, for Stage 2;

an A_1 effect, γ_1, for Task 1;

a B_1 effect, τ_1, for Stimulus 1;

an interaction of A_1 and B_1 effects, $(\gamma\tau)_{11}$;

a carryover from A_1 on Stage 1, λ_{11} for the first type of carryover

when $k' = 1$;

a carryover from B_2 on Stage 1, λ_{22} for the second type of carryover

when $m' = 2$;

an interaction of λ_{11} and λ_{22} carryover effects, $(\lambda_1\lambda_2)_{12}$, and

an error component, e_{26211}.

Note that $(\gamma\tau)_{km}$ in Equation 5.1 is a mnemonic way to label the interaction between its two within-subject treatment factors, effects for the k-th level of A, and for the m-th level of B. The carryover terms are intended to reflect processes related to another kind of possible interaction, that between A values and stages ($\lambda_1 k'$) or between B values and stages ($\lambda_2 m'$). As in other carryover models, any carryover on Stage 1 is defined to have zero as its value. We have not found it possible to expand the present model to include subject by task, subject by stimulus, and subject by task by stimulus components without losing the capacity to assess stage effects and carryovers in (5.1).

As in earlier models, we assume that subject effects are i.i.d. $N(0, \sigma_s^2)$, error components have a Type H covariance structure, error scores from different subjects are independent, and subject and error components are independent. As a consequence, observed scores within any given treatment sequence group are normally distributed with an identical spherical (Type H) covariance structure for each subject across Stages m regardless of their other subscripts.

Method A: Crossover Model Analysis for a 2 × 2 Within-Subjects Design

Hypothetical Data and Program for Analyzing Them

Table 5.1 displays a hypothetical set of data for the specific design just mentioned.

TABLE 5.1

Hypothetical Data for a Balanced 2 × 2 Within-Subjects Experiment

(Responses are overall response quality in arbitrary units)

Sequence 1	Stage 1	Stage 2	Stage 3	Stage 4	
Subject	A_1B_1	A_2B_2	A_1B_2	A_2B_1	Subj Means
1	7.18	6.05	18.95	8.94	10.280
2	11.80	6.05	22.28	9.85	12.495
3	9.10	7.68	21.73	9.71	12.055
4	7.38	6.07	19.55	7.91	10.228
Seq 1 Stage Means	8.865	6.462	20.628	9.102	11.264
Sequence 2	A_1B_2	A_1B_1	A_2B_1	A_2B_2	Subj Means
5	7.36	10.75	11.70	20.85	12.665
6	8.10	11.49	11.31	21.87	13.192
7	7.62	9.98	12..23	19.90	12.432
8	6.40	9.89	11.15	19.83	11.818
Seq 2 Stage Means	7.370	10.528	11.598	20.612	12.527
Sequence 3	A_2B_1	A_1B_2	A_2B_2	A_1B_1	Subj Means
9	11.82	21.64	6.90	22.98	15.835
					(Continued)

TABLE 5.1
(Continued)

Sequence 3	A_2B_1	A_1B_2	A_2B_2	A_1B_1	Subj Means
10	8.63	18.65	9.28	23.26	14.955
11	12.52	21.32	10.01	24.42	17.068
12	10.76	20.40	6.93	23.46	15.388
Seq 3 Stage Means	10.932	20.502	8.280	23.530	15.811
Sequence 4	A_2B_2	A_2B_1	A_1B_1	$A1B_2$	Subj Means
13	5.96	21.95	24.63	6.73	14.010
14	4.81	22.07	25.43	6.11	14.605
15	4.93	21.87	24.17	4.24	13.802
16	10.43	26.12	26.80	7.08	17.608
Seq 4 Stage Means	6.532	23.002	25.258	6.040	15.208
Overall Stage Means	8.425	15.124	16.441	14.821	
Cell Means	(A_1B_1)	(A_1B_2)	(A_2B_1)	(A_2B_2)	(Overall Mean)
	17.045	13.635	13.659	10.472	13.702
Factor Means	(A_1) 15.340	(A_2) 12.065	(B_1) 15.352	(B_2) 12.053	

Now we turn to an analysis intended to measure any effects of each of the components included in the model of Equation 5.1. Table 5.2 is a SAS® GLM program developed for that purpose.

TABLE 5.2

A Program for Performing a Crossover Design Analysis
of the Hypothetical Within-Subjects Factorial Data of Table 5.1

```
*PROGRAM NAME IS 2WAYLAT.SAS; DATA WITHIN-S;
INPUT Y TASK STIM STAGE SUBJ CARRY1 CARRY2 @@; CARDS;
 7.18 1 1 1   1 0 0   6.05 2 2 2   1 1 1   18.95 1 2 3   1 2 2   8.94 2 1 4   1 1 2
11.80 1 1 1   2 0 0   6.05 2 2 2   2 1 1   22.28 1 2 3   2 2 2   9.85 2 1 4   2 1 2
 9.10 1 1 1   3 0 0   7.68 2 2 2   3 1 1   21.73 1 2 3   3 2 2   9.71 2 1 4   3 1 2
 7.38 1 1 1   4 0 0   6.07 2 2 2   4 1 1   19.55 1 2 3   4 2 2   7.91 2 1 4   4 1 2
 7.36 1 2 1   5 0 0  10.75 1 1 2   5 1 2   11.70 2 1 3   5 1 1  20.85 2 2 4   5 2 1
 8.10 1 2 1   6 0 0  11.49 1 1 2   6 1 2   11.31 2 1 3   6 1 1  21.87 2 2 4   6 2 1
```
(Continued)

TABLE 5.2

(Continued)

```
7.62 1 2 1    7 0 0   9.98 1 1 2   7 1 2   12.23 2 1 3    7 1 1  19.90 2 2 4   7 2 1
6.40 1 2 1    8 0 0   9.89 1 1 2   8 1 2   11.15 2 1 3    8 1 1  19.83 2 2 4   8 2 1
11.82 2 1 1   9 0 0  21.64 1 2 2   9 2 1    6.90 2 2 3    9 1 2  22.98 1 1 4   9 2 2
8.63 2 1 1   10 0 0  18.65 1 2 2  10 2 1    9.28 2 2 3   10 1 2  23.26 1 1 4  10 2 2
12.52 2 1 1  11 0 0  21.32 1 2 2  11 2 1   10.01 2 2 3   11 1 2  24.42 1 1 4  11 2 2
10.76 2 1 1  12 0 0  20.40 1 2 2  12 2 1    6.93 2 2 3   12 1 2  23.46 1 1 4  12 2 2
5.96 2 2 1   13 0 0  21.95 2 1 2  13 2 2   24.63 1 1 3   13 2 1   6.73 1 2 4  13 1 1
4.81 2 2 1   14 0 0  22.07 2 1 2  14 2 2   25.43 1 1 3   14 2 1   6.11 1 2 4  14 1 1
4.93 2 2 1   15 0 0  21.87 2 1 2  15 2 2   24.17 1 1 3   15 2 1   4.24 1 2 4  15 1 1
10.43 2 2 1  16 0 0  26.12 2 1 2  16 2 2   26.80 1 1 3   16 2 1   7.08 1 2 4  16 1 1
RUN; PROC GLM; CLASS SUBJ STAGE TASK STIM CARRY1 CARRY2;
MODEL Y = SUBJ STAGE TASK STIM TASK*STIM CARRY1 CARRY2
    CARRY1*CARRY2/SOLUTION E SS1 E2;
RANDOM SUBJ; MEANS SUBJ; MEANS STAGE; MEANS TASK;
    MEANS STIM; MEANS TASK*STIM;
ESTIMATE 'STAGE2-STAGE4' STAGE 0 1 0 -1;
ESTIMATE 'STAGE3-STAGE4' STAGE 0 0 1 -1;
ESTIMATE 'TASK EFFECT' TASK 1 -1/E;
ESTIMATE 'STIM EFFECT' STIM 1 -1/E;
ESTIMATE 'TASK STIM INTER' TASK*STIM .5 -.5 -.5 .5;
ESTIMATE 'CA1 1 - CA1 2' CARRY1 0 1 -1/E;
ESTIMATE 'CA2 1 - CA2 2' CARRY2 0 1 -1/E;
ESTIMATE 'CA INTER' CARRY1*CARRY2 0 .5 -.5 -.5 .5;
estimate 'task-solution' task 1 -1 task*stim 0 1 0 -1;
estimate 'stim-solution' stim 1 -1 task*stim 0 0 1 -1;
TITLE '2WAYLAT.SAS 4 STAGE, IN A BALANCED LS.'; RUN;
```

Interpreting What This SAS® Program Has to Say

We already understand most of this program because it is similar to those of previous chapters. An ESTIMATE command provides a new method of estimating those functions of parameters which can be estimated. For example, the first ESTIMATE command leads to an estimate of the STAGE 2 parameter minus STAGE 4 parameter ($\pi_2 - \pi_4$), coded as a 0 weight for Stage 1, a 1 for Stage 2, a 0 for Stage 3, and a −1 for Stage 4, and yields the same estimated value as our earlier method combining biased values.

This first "ESTIMATE" command begins with a label (surrounded by single quotes) for the parameter or function of parameters to be estimated. Then in a statement such as "ESTIMATE 'STAGE 2 – STAGE 4' STAGE 1 –1;" the name of a parameter family (STAGE) is displayed, followed by the weights for each level (1 for Stage 1 and –1 for Stage 2). Sometimes, as with "estimate 'task-solution'" in Table 5.2, there will be more than one parameter family name list, with each family name followed by weights for each of its levels. Use of "/E" at the end of an "ESTIMATE" command is asking for estimability information, like that of "E" and "E2" in the "MODEL" statement. Several "MEANS" statements were used here to generate summary data.

Interpretation of ANOVA Output From the SAS® Program

Significance tests for this 2-way within-subject design appear in Table 5.3, an analysis of variance table based on output from Table 5.2 presented earlier. Because we want to use mean squares whose expectations involve as few effects as possible (see the next section), a Type II analysis (= Type III = Type IV in this case) is most appropriate here.

TABLE 5.3

Crossover Design Type II Analysis of Variance Results for Table 5.1 Data, Based on the Program in Table 5.2

Source	Sum of Squares	df	Mean Square	F
Subjects	76.77	15	5.12	5.14****
Stages2_4	23.72	2	11.86	11.91****
Tasks	0.18	1	0.18	0.18
Stimuli	164.74	1	164.74	165.35****
Task × Stim	0.06	1	0.06	0.06
Carryover1	1,835.74	1	1,835.75	1,842.55****
Carryover2	0.72	1	0.72	0.40
Car1 × Car2	0.35	1	0.35	0.56
Error	38.86	39	1.00	—

Note.   **** $p < 0.0001$.

Table 5.3 tells us that all effects except those for tasks, task × stimuli interaction, carryover from stimuli (Carryover2), and Carryover1 × Carryover2 are highly significant ($p < 0.0001$). Nonsignificance for task effects is puzzling in view of the similarity of the mean difference between tasks to the mean difference between stimuli in Table 5.1.

Relation of E Option Output and Expected Mean Squares to Certain Estimates of Effects

The output giving "Estimate" values must be interpreted in the light of what we are told about estimability because of output from the E and E2 options (or E1, E3, or E4 when employed) and in the light of expected mean squares reported later for TASK and STIM and other quantities in the computer output. Because subjects are assumed random in our program, the best information about their effects comes from expected mean square values rather than the E2 information required with fixed effects. We know that this listing could also logically include "ERROR Var(Error):

Source	Type II Expected Mean Square
SUBJ	Var(Error) + 3.9273 Var(SUBJ)
STAGE	Var(Error) + Q(STAGE)
TASK	Var(Error) + Q(TASK,TASK*STIM)
STIM	Var(Error) + Q(STIM,TASK*STIM)
TASK*STIM	Var(Error) + Q(TASK*STIM)
CARRY1	Var(Error) + Q(CARRY1,CARRY1*CARRY2)
CARRY2	Var(Error) + Q(CARRY2,CARRY1*CARRY2)
CARRY1*CARRY2	Var(Error) + Q(CARRY1*CARRY2)

Comparing expected mean squares for subjects and for error later in this chapter suggests subtracting one from the other, yielding $E(MS_{subjects}) - E(MS_{error}) = 3.9273$ Var(Subjects). If we take our observed mean squares from Table 5.3 as approximations of expected mean square values, we can say $MS_{subjects} - MS_{error} = 5.12 - 1.00 = 4.12 \approx 3.9273$ Var(Subjects). In turn this suggests that Var(Subjects) is about 1.0491 or that the standard deviation of subjects is about 1.02.

Four other expected mean squares from this set also need special discussion here: those involving tasks, stimuli, carryover from tasks, and carryover from stimuli. Analysis of variance theory plus those expected mean squares imply, for example, that our reported test for task effects was in fact a test for task plus interaction effects. Analogous conclusions apply to our tests for stimulus, and the two kinds of carryover effects.

These conclusions are clarified by learning more precisely what fixed effect parameters or functions of fixed parameters can be estimated with this model, experimental design, and program. We omit discussion of the General Form of Estimable Functions (E) output from Table 5.2 (not shown here), except to mention four inferences we could make after thorough examination of it:

1. We cannot estimate the difference between Stage 1 and Stage 4 effects no matter which type of analysis we employ.

2. We cannot estimate any linear function composed only of CARRY1 0 and other CARRY1 values. The corresponding statement applies to CARRY2 estimates.

3. Output from the E option implies that we can estimate TASK 1 + TASK*STIM 1 2 – TASK 2 – TASK*STIM 22 = $\gamma_1 + (\gamma\tau)_{12} - \gamma_2 - (\gamma\tau)_{22}$ for tasks. This is actually what the SOLUTION option does for the biased estimate of tasks in the MODEL statement of the program in Table 5.2; the "estimate" commands at the end of this program are not needed in the data analysis itself, but they do lead to the same values (–0.177 and 3.301) as given in that option.

4. There is no way to estimate TASK 1 – TASK 2 = $\gamma_1 - \gamma_2$ alone within the effects model of Equation 5.1.

Type II Estimable Function Output

In order to clarify what we can estimate with a Type II analysis, let us now consider the Type II Estimable Functions (E2) output. This is like the General Form of Estimable Functions information available with the E option of the MODEL statement. However, it is specific to the type of analysis to be performed. What is estimable with Type II is often the same as for other types, but it is especially likely to be different from that for Type I when a crossover design is employed. In addition, a separate set of effects and coefficients is displayed for each family of parameters, such as stages. Here is part of the TYPE II output for stages, based on the program in Table 5.2:

Effect		Coefficients
INTERCEPT		0
SUBJ	1	0
	2	0
	3	0
	. . .	. . .
	16	0
STAGE	1	0
	2	L19
	3	L20
	4	-L19-L20

All other entries, such as for TASK, STIM, and TASK*STIM are zero and will not be shown here.   It can be shown that we can set any term or set of terms such as L19 or L19 and L20 to any desired numerical value or values and then develop an equation based on summing all effects multiplied by their coefficient values.

A term such as SUBJ 1 refers to the parameter value for the first subject. For example, if we set L19 = 1 and L20 = 0, the above tells us that 0 INT + 0 SUBJ 1 + 0 SUBJ 2 + 0 SUBJ 3 + . . . + 0 SUBJ 16 + 0 STAGE 1 + 1 STAGE 2 + 0 STAGE 3 – 1 STAGE 4 + 0 . . . + 0 is estimable. This simplifies to the statement that STAGE 2 – STAGE 4 = $\pi_2 - \pi_4$ is estimable in a Type II analysis.   Further, we can see from the E2 information that STAGE 3 – STAGE 4   (= $\pi_3 - \pi_4$) is estimable. Estimated values for STAGE 2 and STAGE 4 are 0.302B and 0.000 B, respectively, B meaning that each is biased. So the STAGE 2 – STAGE 4 estimate is 0.302 – 0.00 = 0.302 and, for similar reasons, the STAGE 3 – STAGE 4 estimate is 1.619 – 0.00 = 1.619. Notice that these conclusions from output of the SOLUTION option are also confirmed by output of specific "ESTIMATE" commands.   E2 information also tells us that, because the coefficient for STAGE 1 is 0 in the Effect table, no function of a STAGE 1 parameter is estimable.

Comparable reasoning about task, stimulus, and two kinds of carryover effects uses other little tables of the output, entitled "Type II Estimable Functions for: TASK" or for "STIM". The estimable function of task and interaction just noted under the discussion of the E option is not estimable under Type II. However, we can see from that information (mentioned earlier but not shown explicitly in this book) that TASK 1 – TASK 2 + .5 TASK*STIM 1 1   + .5 TASK*STIM 1 2 – .5 TASK*STIM 2 1 – .5 TASK*STIM 2 2 = $\gamma_1 - \gamma_2 + .5[(\gamma\tau)_{11} + (\gamma\tau)_{12} - (\gamma\tau)_{21} - (\gamma\tau)_{22}]$ is estimable. It forms the basis for the F-test for tasks reported in the Type II analysis of variance generated from Table 5.2.

Paradoxically, the "ESTIMATE 'TASK EFFECTS' 1 –1/E;" statement in our Table 5.2 program yielded an estimate of –0.113, which is the same value we would have obtained with the command: "ESTIMATE 'TASK 1 – TASK 2 + INT' TASK 1 – TASK*STIM .5 .5 –.5 –.5;" which follows from the Type II information just given. This result is partly explained by some new estimability information given by the "/E" option in our current statement. Despite apparently asking only for task effects, the "ESTIMATE 'TASK EFFECTS' 1 –1/E;" output tells us that the same function of task and interaction effects is being estimated as reported in the Type II estimability output just mentioned. Fulenwider (1989) discussed comparable properties of the SAS® GLM "CONTRAST" command. We view these properties as making SAS® GLM a hybrid system, with the E1, E2, and so on, estimability information focused on an effects model without special assumptions and commands like "ESTIMATE 'TASK EFFECTS' 1 –1/E;" yielding results requiring either sum-to-zero assumptions to be discussed next or development of appropriate cell means models in the tradition of Kirk (1995) and of Searle (1987), not considered further here.

Notice that crossover design programs sometimes must be run once before revision and then run again: We did not know which "ESTIMATE" commands to use until we had examined the output based on the "E" and "E2" commands or until we saw the results of "ESTIMATE" commands ending with "/E;". In the present example, the latter options would have sufficed, except that we would have needed an "E" option in the "MODEL" statement in order to learn what linear combinations of biased estimates from the "SOLUTION" option to use in order to do the didactically inspired comands written in lower case. Often, however, we may choose to use the "E"-type options with the "MODEL" statement in order to be sure of the estimability of each possible option.

Interpreting Hypothesis Tests in the Light of Estimability Informamation. Searle (1987) discusses a so-called Σ-restricted model for a between-subjects balanced 2-way factorial design in which row effects and column effects are recoded (reparameterized) to sum to zero, and interaction effects are similarly treated to sum to zero over rows and also over columns. Algebraically, nothing is changed; the model is restated in such a way that sum-to-zero constraints apply to the new parameters but that each observation can still be predicted to be the same combination of original parameters. We apply the same logic to the current within-subjects design: Since all combinations of row and columns in our design have the same sample size, we can rewrite the current task effects hypothesis as the Σ-restricted model hypothesis that

$$\gamma_1^* - \gamma_2^* = \left[\gamma_1 + .50\big((\gamma\tau)_{11} + (\gamma\tau)_{12}\big)\right] - \left[\gamma_2 + .50\big((\gamma\tau)_{21} + (\gamma\tau)_{22}\big)\right] = 0.$$

This makes sense because the recoded Task 1 effect is the original effect plus the average of interactions for that task; a comparable statement holds for Task 2. Notice that it really does not matter whether we state our hypothesis in terms of $\gamma_1^* - \gamma_2^*$ or of γ_1, γ_2, $(\gamma\tau)_{11}$, $(\gamma\tau)_{12}$, $(\gamma\tau)_{21}$, and $(\gamma\tau)_{22}$. Also, the same logic applies when interpreting the test of stimulus effects based on Table 5.2.

An alternate justification for conventional tests of main effects of treatments and effects of carryover occurs if the relevant interaction terms are equal to each other. Then $\gamma_1 - \gamma_2$, for example, becomes estimable and associated tests become legitimate tests of the original hypotheses, not the Σ-restricted hypotheses. Because we found no significance in our tests of interaction effects between tasks and stimuli or of interaction between carryovers from tasks and stimuli, it is probably safe to conclude that the original hypotheses about tasks, stimuli, and carryovers from those effects were tested here. One might even redo the analysis program of Table 5.2, excluding those interactions in order to permit including current contributions from interactions in a revised sum of squares for error, with the hope that power would be improved thereby.

Implications for Confidence Intervals or Post Hoc Tests. Ordinarily this book makes no comments on the computation of confidence intervals or performance of post hoc tests. In principle, there should be no change in the approach to this kind of task when one shifts from a traditional design to a crossover design. However, we believe that assessment of individual effects in factorial designs, whether crossover or not, have special problems related to the previous discussion. In brief, one must always ask if estimates, confidence intervals, or simultaneous confidence intervals for such effects stated in terms of reparameterized effects are really of interest given their meaning in the original model.

(1) 2 × 2 or Other Designs With Only One Degree of Freedom for an Effect. Ordinarily this sort of design uses family-wise rather than experiment-wise significance levels. Therefore, it can properly use confidence intervals rather than simultaneous confidence intervals and post hoc tests.

Difficulties noted for testing hypotheses in such designs also apply to the computation of confidence intervals. Since, for example, the Type II Expected Mean Square for Tasks given is $Var(Error) + Q(TASK,TASK*STIM)$, a $100(1 - \alpha)\%$ confidence interval for task effects will include interaction effects if present. From Table 5.2, we know that TASK 1 – TASK 2 + .5(TASK STIM$_{11}$ + TASK STIM$_{12}$ – TASK STIM$_{21}$ – TASK STIM$_{22}$) $= \gamma_1 - \gamma_2 + .5*[(\gamma\tau)_{11} + (\gamma\tau)_{12} - (\gamma\tau)_{21} - (\gamma\tau)_{22}]$ from Equation 5.1 is being estimated by an ESTIMATE command. We have already called this estimated quantity $\gamma_1{}^* - \gamma_2{}^*$, the difference in task parameters reparameterized by use of sum-to-zero constraints. Output from the program in that table yields an estimate of –0.113 with a standard error of 0.26. For $df_{error} = 39$, the 5% significance level for $|t|$ is 2.093. Accordingly, standard methods give the 95% confidence interval as –0.657 (= –0.113 – 2.093 × 0.26) to 0.431 (= –0.113 + 2.093 × 0.26), including 0 as it must when the effect in question is not statistically significant. The current example has a 95% confidence interval for $\gamma_1{}^* - \gamma_2{}^*$, the difference in reparameterized stimulus effects. Similarly, simpler sum-to-zero models for this design (e.g., that of Kirk, 1995, without stage and carryover effects) must be viewed as testing hypotheses and supporting post hoc tests or confidence intervals related to starred rather than unstarred parameters.

Similar calculations apply to confidence intervals for stimuli and for interaction, the latter having no special problems because it does not reflect more than one kind of effect. Of course, the interpretation of confidence intervals of this kind is simplified if interaction effects are not present.

(2) 2 × 3 or Other Designs With More Than One Degree of Freedom for an Effect. One needs to determine what is estimated by each 1-degree of freedom effect of interest for any factor with more than two levels. Then, simultaneous confidence intervals or associated post hoc tests can be computed by standard methods.

(3) Application to Between-S designs. The same issues also apply to between-subjects fixed effect factorial designs For example, Kirk

(1995) gives expected mean squares for a $p \times q$ design with n subjects per cell:

1. His expected mean squares for row and column effects can be used in confidence interval and post hoc testing concerning reparameterized effects.

2. For interpretive purposes it would be helpful to specify precisely what main effect and interaction components are estimated by a quantity such as the Row 1 mean minus Grand Mean, the traditional estimator for Row 1 effects in a reparameterized model with this design.

3. A final option, asserting that the traditional reparameterized model is the underlying model and that relevant parameters do sum to zero, does not seem viable to us. At least as long ago as in Scheffè's (1959) classic text, it has been known that the basic analysis of variance models begin without such reparameterization. However, Scheffè did not emphasize this point as strongly with complex designs as with the model for one-way analysis of variance. The issue may have seemed less important in earlier days when hand calculations were simplified by this kind of reparameterization. But, when expected mean squares obtained with SAS® GLM are based on the underlying model, it is incumbent on us to come to grips with the implications of sum-to-zero reparameterization.

Method B: Determining Efficiencies of Estimates of Different Effects From This Design

Relevant Theory for Determining Variability of Estimates of Effects (in $\frac{\sigma^2}{n}$ Units)

Introductory Remarks. In chapter 3, we displayed the approximate variances and efficiencies of estimates of effects in $\frac{\sigma^2}{n}$ units for a specific randomized block design with carryover effects in its model. However, no method was shown for their calculation or for efficiency calculations associated with them. Now it is time to present each of these kinds of information.

If we can relax our sphericity assumption to compound symmetry, a variety of formulas and computer programs become appropriate for our calculations. Let us define a set of observed means $Y_{g.j..}$ related to

Equation 5.1 and representing combinations of sequence groups and stages. Now consider a minor adaptation of Kershner and Federer's (1981) estimation and variance formulas, applicable under set-to-zero modeling:

$$\hat{\theta} = \sum \sum a_{gj} \overline{Y}_{g.j..} \text{ and} \tag{5.2}$$

$$var(\hat{\theta}) = [s\sum \sum a_{gj}^2]\frac{\sigma^2}{sn} = [\sum \sum a_{gj}^2]\frac{\sigma^2}{n} \tag{5.3}$$

for a parameter θ estimated as a function of the observed means for each combination of Sequence Group g and Stage j, given a design with s sequence groups of n subjects each. To develop the previous variance equation from Kershner and Federer's (4.3) or (4.4), we set their correlation between error components for the same subject, ρ, to equal zero. Direct calculation of the a_{gj} weights for a given design is possible; such weights for treatment and carryover effects of 16 crossover designs appear in Kershner and Federer's Table 3. For an even larger set of designs, their Table 4 presents $s\sum \sum a_{gj}^2$ values. For many crossover designs, Jones and Kenward (1989) presented variance of parameter estimates in units that are multiples of $\frac{\sigma^2}{n}$, these values also being equal to $\sum \sum a_{gj}^2$; occasionally they reported multiples of $\frac{\sigma^2}{N}$, with $N = ns$ being the total number of subjects involved. So long as the divisor for this multiplier is constant, Equation 5.3 tells us that we can compare reported (dimensionless) variances of parameter estimates knowing that all are proportional to the actual variances. Another option would be to report multiples of $\frac{\sigma^2}{\left(\frac{Np}{T}\right)}$ where T = number of treatments and p = number of stages, so that the variability per average number of observations per treatment is reported. Later we will use a further symbol, N_{tot}, $= nps = Np$, for the total number of observations in the experiment.

Effects of Sum-to-Zero and Set-to-Zero on Estimation Equations. With sum-to-zero reparameterization of a model equation such as (5.1), a 2-level effect such as carryover from treatments is represented in a form like $\hat{\lambda}^*_{11} = \hat{\lambda}_{11} - \hat{\lambda}_1$ and $\hat{\lambda}^*_{12} = \hat{\lambda}_{12} - \hat{\lambda}_1$, making $\hat{\lambda}^*_{11} = -\hat{\lambda}^*_{12}$ and

$\hat{\lambda}^*_{11} + \hat{\lambda}^*_{12} = 0$, showing the sum-to-zero property. Note also that $\hat{\lambda}^*_{11} = 0.5\hat{\lambda}_{11} - 0.5\hat{\lambda}_{12}$, implying $Var(\hat{\lambda}^*_{11}) = 0.25Var(\hat{\lambda}_{11} - \hat{\lambda}_{12})$. It is easy to see also that the a_{gj} weights for this sum-to-zero example using $\hat{\lambda}^*_{11}$ are exactly one-half those for the corresponding set-to-zero example using $\hat{\lambda}_{11} - \hat{\lambda}_{12}$, making $\sum \sum a^2_{gj}$ one-fourth as large for sum-to-zero as for set-to-zero cases. Corresponding relations can be found between sum-to-zero (Jones & Kenward, 1989) and set-to-zero estimates (Kershner & Federer, 1981) and weights in cases with factors having more than two levels, possiby affecting some examples later in this book. Rather than introducing a new set of symbols, we use a_{gj} both in sum-to-zero and set-to-zero examples, pointing out which is involved when necessary.

Further Introductory Remarks. The strategy for our computations is to use information from analysis of a dataset but correct it to omit values of sample variances, just as Equation 5.4 using $\sum \sum a^2_{gj}$ will justify. Although it is mathematically equivalent to a traditional method and the same efficiency values are obtained as with such a method, this approach lacks the elegance of a method like that of Kershner and Federer or of Jones and Kenward using design features but no empirical data. However, because it is computationally more convenient, we use it in this book.

We know from chapter 3 that we are using the quantity $\sum \sum a^2_{gj}$ as an index of variability of any estimate of a parameter value such as the quantity $\hat{\theta}$ just shown. Out of many algebraically equivalent methods for estimating this quantity, one seems specially convenient if we are working with SAS® GLM:

$$\text{Variance of } \hat{\theta} \text{ in } \frac{\sigma^2}{n} \text{ units } = \frac{n\,(s.e.e.[\hat{\theta}])^2}{MS_{error}} = \sum \sum a^2_{gj} \text{ for } \hat{\theta} \qquad (5.4)$$

For the case of a difference $\hat{\pi}_2 - \hat{\pi}_4$ from Equation 5.1, this means:

$$\text{Variance of } \hat{\pi}_2 - \hat{\pi}_4 \text{ in } \frac{\sigma^2}{n} \text{ units} = \sum \sum a^2_{gj} = \frac{n\,(s.e.e.[\hat{\pi}_2 - \hat{\pi}_4])^2}{MS_{error}} \qquad (5.5)$$

where the standard error of estimate, $s.e.e.[\hat{\pi}_2 - \hat{\pi}_4]$, and the mean square for error, MS_{error}, are computed from output of a program such as the one in Table 5.2. Sometimes a published source tells us the value of $\Sigma \Sigma a_{gj}^2$ for a certain parameter estimate. In other cases we can employ some other kind of computer program to yield that quantity.   Or we can calculate it from its theoretical definition.

Example of Computing Variances of Estimated Effects With SAS® GLM

Now it is time to illustrate our SAS®-based way to compute the variance of estimators of parameter differences of interest, using information generated with Table 5.2 as our basic source.   Our computational procedure begins by noting that each ESTIMATE command in Table 5.2 generates both an estimate of something like the Stage 2 – Stage 4 effect, $\pi_2 - \pi_4$, and a standard deviation called the *standard error of estimate* (s.e.e.; see A, Table 5.4). (For the reason that parenthesized values appear in the Task or Stim row of this table, see a later paragraph.) The s.e.e. values are squared in Table 5.4 to yield variances of estimate, called B values. Also, the Mean Square for Error, called D, appears at the bottom of the table. Column C uses a ratio of variances to cancel out estimates of σ^2 and thus permit generation of $\Sigma \Sigma a_{gj}^2$ values for a given effect.

TABLE 5.4

Determining Variability of Estimates (in $\dfrac{\sigma^2}{n}$ Units) of Effects From a 2×2

Within-Subjects Factorial Design, Using Output of the Program in Table 5.2

Type of Effect	A = Standard Error of Estimate (s.e.e.)	B = A^2 = Variance of Estimate	C = 4B/ MSerror = nB/D = $\Sigma\Sigma\alpha^2_{gj}$ = Estimator Variance in multiples of $\dfrac{\sigma^2}{n}$
Stage 2 – Stage 4 or Stage 3 – Stage 4	0.35290114	0.124539215	0.50000

(Continued)

TABLE 5.4

(Continued)

Task + Task × Stim or Stim + Task × Stim or Task × Stim	0.26171849 (with ESTIMATE) (0.37012584 for main effects with SOLUTION)	0.068496568 (0.136993137)	0.2750 (0.5500)
Carry1 + CA1 × CA2 or Carry2 + CA1 × CA2 or CA1 × CA2	0.31564438	0.099631375	0.4000
MSerror			D = 0.996314

Note. $n = 4$ for each of four sequence groups in this design.

Table 5.4 shows that our measure of variability of estimates is small-est for the complicated task (or stimulus) main effect combined with interaction or for interaction alone, each using "ESTIMATE", and larger for stage or carryover effects, showing that the factors of primary inter-est are measured with relatively high sensitivity.

Theory and Computation of Efficiency Values From SAS® GLM Output

We know from chapter 3 that efficiency calculations for a crossover design depend on the relative variances of estimators for a reference design and model compared to a current crossover design and model:

$$Efficiency = E = 100 \frac{Var(Estimator_{Reference\ Model})}{Var(Estimator_{Current\ Model})} \tag{5.6}$$

Let us ask exactly what designs and models are to be invoked in these calculations. The current model is simply the one applying to our cur-rent within-subjects design; we know the dimensionless variances of its estimators from Table 5.4. The definition of the numerator will become more clear if we first present in our own terminology Jones and Kenward's (1989) equation for the efficiency of estimating the differ-ence between two treatment effects, k and k^*:

$$E_t = 100 \, \frac{2 \left(\dfrac{\sigma^2}{r} \right)}{V[\hat{\tau}_k - \hat{\tau}_{k*}]} \qquad (5.7)$$

Here the variance σ^2 is the population value for the crossover design and model of current interest. But the numerator as a whole is the squared variance of differences between two independent groups' sample means in a t-test procedure. It can be thought of as coming either from a 2-group experiment or representing two groups from a multi-group design (such as a Latin square) with equal numbers of observations per treatment. Also

$$r = \frac{N_{tot}}{no. \, levels} = \frac{nps}{no. \, levels} \qquad (5.8)$$

per group, where N_{tot} is the total number of observations in the experiment and the number of levels is the number of treatments or of some other factor whose effects are to be estimated. In either case the variance of such a design is minimal among all possible designs with that σ^2 and that number of observations. Accordingly, the only way to attain maximal efficiency ($E_t = 100$) in a crossover design is for $V[\hat{\tau}_k - \hat{\tau}_{k*}]$ to be so small as to equal $\dfrac{\sigma^2}{r}$.

If the numbers of stages and treatments are different, comparable measurement of efficiencies for stages will require use of a different r value, in effect involving a different reference experiment for the two kinds of effects. There is no special problem about the number of carryovers, which is also the number of treatments of a given kind. Even though, for most models, there is no carryover on Stage 1, it is conventional to let the number of replications, r, for carryovers be the same as its number for the corresponding type of treatments.

For treatments or carryovers, the number of replications becomes

$$r = \frac{N_{tot}}{T} = \frac{nps}{T} \qquad (5.9)$$

and for stages, the number of replications becomes

$$r = \frac{N_{tot}}{p} = ns \tag{5.10}$$

Because our computational procedure for estimating variances is dimensionless, we want the numerator of any efficiency formula like (5.7) to be dimensionless as well. This means that we must define a new variable $r* = \frac{r}{n}$ where n = number of subjects per treatment sequence. Accordingly, we have

$$r* = \frac{ps}{no.\ levels} \tag{5.11}$$

in general, so that

$$r* = \frac{ps}{T} \tag{5.12}$$

applies for treatments and usually also for carryover and

$$r* = s \tag{5.13}$$

for stages. Equations 5.7 through 5.13 apply even for within-subject factorial designs, so long as the value of T is the same for each factor, such as tasks and stimuli in the present example.

With Equation 5.4 and a close cousin of (5.7) applicable to any estimated parameter or parameter difference $\hat{\theta}$, this leads to a convenient formula for application here:

$$E\hat{\theta} = \frac{\left(\frac{200}{r*}\right)}{\frac{n(s.e.e.[\hat{\theta}])^2}{MS_{error}}} = \frac{\left(\frac{200}{r*}\right)}{\Sigma\Sigma\alpha^2_{gj}} \tag{5.14}$$

To compute efficiencies from earlier results, we repeat the last column of Table 5.4, which is equal to denominator values of (5.14) for different effects. Next we add a column for replications: Our value of $r*$ for treatments (tasks or stimuli) and also for their respective carryovers is $\frac{ps}{T} = \frac{4(4)}{2} = \frac{16}{2} = 8$, and our $r*$ value for stages is $s = 4$. The last column of Table 5.5 shows the resulting efficiencies.

TABLE 5.5

Calculation of Efficiency Values from Equation 5.14 and Table 5.4

Type of Effect	$C = 4B/$ MSerror $= nB/D =$ $\Sigma\Sigma\alpha^2_{gj} =$ Estimator Variance in multiples of $\frac{\sigma^2}{n}$	$r*$	Efficiency = E $\dfrac{200}{r*\Sigma\Sigma\alpha^2_{gj}}$
Stage 2 – Stage 4 or Stage 3 – Stage 4	0.50000	4	100.00
Task + Task × Stim or Stim + Task × Stim or Task × Stim	0.27500 (with ESTIMATE) (0.55000 for main effects with Solution)	8	90.91 (45.45)
Carry1 + CA1 × CA2 or Carry2 + CA1 × CA2 or CA1 × CA2	0.40000	8	62.50

Table 5.5 shows that a maximum possible efficiency of 100 applies to each estimable stage effect difference. A near-maximum efficiency appears for complicated estimated task or stimulus effects or their interactions only if an appropriate ESTIMATE command is used; a moderately sized efficiency appears for each estimable carryover effect difference. However, ESTIMATE and SOLUTION usually yield the same results.

There are various equivalent methods of computing efficiency values, such as data-free methods using a matrix manipulation package such as GAUSS (Aptech Systems, 1993). The present method has the advantage of computational simplicity. Note also that there may be no previous publications giving efficiency measures for stage effects, which may be of greatest interest in behavioral science.

ANALYZING A 2 × 2 WITHIN-SUBJECTS EXAMPLE WITHOUT COMPLETE BALANCE

Revised Design and Hypothetical Data

We saw earlier that our first data set for this chapter has the advantages coming from replicated orthogonal Latin squares. Now suppose that much of this balance were destroyed and that a different response measure, latency in making a response, were employed. Let us keep only the first three of the four sequences shown earlier, and let there be five subjects assigned to each sequence:

Sequence 1: A_1B_1 A_2B_2 A_1B_2 A_2B_1
Sequence 2: A_1B_2 A_1B_1 A_2B_1 A_2B_2
Sequence 3: A_2B_1 A_1B_2 A_2B_2 A_1B_1

Now each sequence has each treatment combination exactly five times, but the other properties of orthogonal Latin squares or even of a single balanced Latin square (Williams square) do not hold. The same model as used with Table 5.1 data, Equation 5.1, will be applied here as well. Table 5.6 shows a set of hypothetical data for the current design.

TABLE 5.6
Hypothetical Data for a 3-Sequence 2 × 2 Within-Subjects Experiment

Sequence 1	Stage 1	Stage 2	Stage 3	Stage 4	
Subject	A_1B_1	A_2B_2	A_1B_2	A_2B_1	Subj Means
1	341.7	570.4	997.7	393.4	575.80
2	583.9	645.5	1,111.5	644.4	746.32
3	440.7	597.6	1,048.4	608.2	673.72
4	1,049.6	1,124.8	1,664.2	1,096.1	1,233.68
5	1,298.0	712.5	762.0	637.8	852.58
					(Continued)

TABLE 5.6
(Continued)

Seq 1 Stage Means	742.78	730.16	1,116.76	675.98	816.42

Sequence 2	A_1B_2	A_1B_1	A_2B_1	A_2B_2	Subj Means
6	613.2	773.1	675.9	1,172.7	808.72
7	573.9	701.2	664.5	1,176.8	779.10
8	1,042.7	1,138.8	1,122.3	1,569.0	1,218.20
9	1,007.4	941.0	977.6	1,498.3	1,106.08
10	837.7	697.3	841.4	1,267.9	911.08
Seq 2 Stage Means	814.98	850.28	856.34	1,336.94	964.64

Sequence 3	A_2B_1	A_1B_2	$A2B2$	A_1B_1	Subj Means
11	840.8	1,292.1	688.3	723.3	886.12
12	993.6	1,446.9	936.5	988.2	1,091.30
13	358.4	585.7	464.0	1,059.9	617.00
14	684.5	804.1	790.9	1,260.6	885.02
15	982.2	920.0	1,043.6	1,424.6	1,092.60
Seq 3 Stage Means	771.90	1,009.76	784.66	1,091.32	914.41

Overall Stage Means	776.55	863.40	919.25	1,034.75	
Cell Means	A_1B_1: 894.79	A_1B_2: 980.50	A_2B_1: 768.07	A_2B_2: 950.59	Overall Mean
Factor Means	A_1: 937.65	A_2: 859.33	B_1: 831.43	B_2: 965.54	898.49

Note. Responses are latencies in ms.

Method C: A Type III ANOVA

Program for Analyzing Data From a 3-Sequence Design

Table 5.7 presents a program for performing an analysis of these data for the 3-sequence design, using a similar basic approach to that before.

TABLE 5.7

for Performing a Crossover Design Analysis of Hypothetical 3-Sequence Within-Subjects Fa

AME IS 3SEFAC2A.SAS; DATA WITHIN_S;

: STIM STAGE SUBJ CARRY1 CARRY2 @@; CARDS;

```
1 0 0   570.4 2 2 2   1 1 1   997.7 1 2 3   1 2 2   393.4 2 1 4   1 1 2
2 0 0   645.5 2 2 2   2 1 1  1111.5 1 2 3   2 2 2   644.4 2 1 4   2 1 2
3 0 0   597.6 2 2 2   3 1 1  1048.4 1 2 3   3 2 2   608.2 2 1 4   3 1 2
4 0 0  1124.8 2 2 2   4 1 1  1664.2 1 2 3   4 2 2  1096.1 2 1 4   4 1 2
5 0 0   712.5 2 2 2   5 1 1   762.0 1 2 3   5 2 2   637.8 2 1 4   5 1 2
6 0 0   773.1 1 1 2   6 1 2   675.9 2 1 3   6 1 1  1172.7 2 2 4   6 2 1
7 0 0   701.2 1 1 2   7 1 2   664.5 2 1 3   7 1 1  1176.8 2 2 4   7 2 1
8 0 0  1138.8 1 1 2   8 1 2  1122.3 2 1 3   8 1 1  1569.0 2 2 4   8 2 1
9 0 0   941.0 1 1 2   9 1 2   977.6 2 1 3   9 1 1  1498.3 2 2 4   9 2 1
0 0 0   697.3 1 1 2  10 1 2   841.4 2 1 3  10 1 1  1267.9 2 2 4  10 2 1
1 0 0  1292.1 1 2 2  11 2 1   688.3 2 2 3  11 1 2   723.3 1 1 4  11 2 2
2 0 0  1446.9 1 2 2  12 2 1   936.5 2 2 3  12 1 2   988.2 1 1 4  12 2 2
3 0 0   585.7 1 2 2  13 2 1   464.0 2 2 3  13 1 2  1059.9 1 1 4  13 2 2
```

(Continued)

TABLE 5.7
(Continued)

14 0 0 804.1 1 2 2 14 2 1 790.9 2 2 3 14 1 2 1260.6 1 1 4 14 2 2
15 0 0 920.0 1 2 2 15 2 1 1043.6 2 2 3 15 1 2 1424.6 1 1 4 15 2 2
LM: CLASS SUBJ STAGE TASK STIM CARRY1 CARRY2;
UBJ STAGE TASK STIM TASK*STIM CARRY1 CARRY2 CARRY1*CARRY2/SOLUTIC

IJ; MEANS SUBJ; MEANS STAGE; MEANS TASK; MEANS STIM; MEANS TASK*STIM
rAGE2-STAGE4' STAGE 0 1 0 –1; ESTIMATE 'STAGE3-STAGE4' STAGE 0 0 1 –1;
\SK TYPE III' TASK 1 –1 TASK*STIM .5 .5 –.5 –.5; ESTIMATE 'STIM TYPE III' STIM
 –.5 .5 –.5; ESTIMATE 'TREAT INTER' TASK*STIM .5 –.5 –.5 .5; ESTIMATE 'CA1 TYF
1*CARRY2 0 .5 .5 –.5 –.5;
\2 TYPE III' CARRY2 0 1 –1 CARRY1*CARRY2 0 .5 –.5 .5 –.5; ESTIMATE 'CA1 X CA
.RY2 0 .5 –.5 –.5 .5;
\SK TYPE II' TASK 1 –1 TASK*STIM .5625 .4375 –.5625 .4375;
rIM TYPE II' STIM 1 –1 TASK*STIM .4063 -.4063 .5938 –.5937;
\1 TYPE II' CARRY1 0 1 –1 CARRY1*CARRY2 0 .4286 .5714 –.4286 –.5714;
\2 TYPE II' CARRY2 0 1 –1 CARRY1*CARRY2 0 .7143 –.7143 .2857 –.2857;
C2A 4 STAGE, TASK = CATEGORIZATION OR NAMING TASK';
= FACE OR NAMES STIMULUS. DESIGN HAS 3 SEQUENCES'; RUN;

Results of New Hypothesis Tests

Table 5.8 summarizes two analyses of variance based on output from the program above. Since they are different and important, both the Type II and Type III analyses are presented.

TABLE 5.8
Type II and III ANOVA Results for Hypothetical Data
from a 3-Sequence 2 × 2 Factorial Design

Source	Type II SS	df	Mean Square	F
Subjects	2,496,536.14	14	178,324.01	5.12****
Stages 2:4	27,013.52	2	13,506.76	0.39
Tasks	47,205.34	1	47,205.34	1.36
Stimuli	257.89	1	257.89	0.01
Task×Stim	64,958.50	1	64,958.50	1.87
Carry1	566,765.14	1	566,765.14	16.27***
Carry2	16,286.96	1	16,286.96	0.47
CA1*CA2	127.08	1	127.08	0.00
Error	1,253,709.40	36	34,825.26	—

Source	Type III SS	df	Mean Square	F
Tasks	54,183.03	1	54,183.03	1.56
Stimuli	2,927.66	1	2,927.66	0.08
Carry1	564,579.19	1	564,579.19	16.21***
Carry2	14,096.34	1	14,096.34	0.40

Note. *** $p < 0.001$. **** $p < 0.0001$.

Only four lines of results appear in the Type III section of Table 5.8; for all other effects, the same entries as for Type II apply. Regardless of the type of analysis, this table shows no statistically significant effects other than those for subjects and for carryovers from previous tasks (each $p < 0.001$ or better). More important differences between Type II and Type III results will appear in our discussion of estimation of parameters in this data set.

As usual, extensive examination of the data and SAS® GLM program output is required. First, we turn again to expected mean squares and related questions about what parameters we can estimate here:

Source	Type II Expected Mean Square = Type III = Type IV
SUBJ	Var(Error) + 3.8206 Var(SUBJ)
STAGE	Var(Error) + Q(STAGE)
TASK	Var(Error) + Q(TASK,TASK*STIM)
STIM	Var(Error) + Q(STIM,TASK*STIM)
TASK*STIM	Var(Error) + Q(TASK*STIM)
CARRY1	Var(Error) + Q(CARRY1,CARRY1*CARRY2)
CARRY2	Var(Error) + Q(CARRY2,CARRY1*CARRY2)
CARRY1*CARRY2	Var(Error) + Q(CARRY1*CARRY2)

Again we give special attention to two expected mean squares: E(MS Categorization vs. Naming) = E(MS TASK) = Var(Error) + Q (TASK,TASK*STIM) and E(MS Faces vs. Names) = E(MS STIM) = Var(Error) + Q(TASK,TASK*STIM). As before, these equations are consistent with the output (not shown here) for the E2 option in the MODEL statement of this program, saying that neither the task effect difference $\gamma_1 - \gamma_2$ nor the stimulus effect difference $\tau_1 - \tau_2$ is estimable.

Estimation of Effects and Interpretation of Related Hypothesis Tests

Stage Effects. The output giving "Estimate" values must be interpreted in the light of what we know about estimability because of output from E2 and E3 output (not shown fully here), and of the expected mean squares (shown previously) for various quantities in the computer output. For each type of output, we find that no function of the STAGE 1 parameter with other STAGE parameters is estimable. Both with analysis types II and III, STAGE 2 – STAGE 4 ($= \pi_2 - \pi_4$) is estimable, yielding an estimated but nonsignificant value of 70.470. For similar reasons, the STAGE 3 – STAGE 4 effect ($= \pi_3 - \pi_4$) is estimated as a nonsignificant 86.190.

Treatment Effects. In view of other estimability information from this SAS® GLM run, our Type II analysis test of task effects in Table

5.9 is testing and accepting the hypothesis that $\gamma_1^* - \gamma_2^* = \gamma_1 - \gamma_2 +$ $[.5625((\gamma\tau)_{11} - (\gamma\tau)_{21}) + .4375 ((\gamma\tau)_{12} - (\gamma\tau)_{22})] = 0$. Using the corresponding "ESTIMATE 'TASK TYPE II'. . ." command in Table 5.7 yields -122.665 as the estimated quantity; but, despite the large size of this estimate, we cannot reject the null hypothesis. Because of the variations in numbers such as .5625 and .4375, this Type II hypothesis is not of much interest to us. Fortunately, Type III estimability information, if displayed here, would show that we can estimate task effects $= \gamma_1^* - \gamma_2^* = \gamma_1 - \gamma_2 + .50 [(\gamma\tau)_{11} + (\gamma\tau)_{12} - (\gamma\tau)_{21} - (\gamma\tau)_{22}]$. This was performed with the "ESTIMATE 'TASK TYPE III'. . ." command in Table 5.9, obtaining a nonsignificant -131.676. Similar logic yields 5.621 for our estimate of composite stimulus effects,

$$\tau_1^* - \tau_2^* = \tau_1 - \tau_2 + [.4063((\gamma\tau)_{11} - (\gamma\tau)_{12}) + .5938(\gamma\tau)_{21} - .5937 (\gamma\tau)_{22}],$$

based on a Type II analysis. However, the non-significance of the stimulus effect in the Type II section of Table 5.8 or, equivalently in the t-test reported with the estimated value, would suggest that this quantity is equal to 0. Similar logic yielded a nonsignificant 19.130 for stimulus effects in a Type III analysis estimating the quantity $\tau_1^* - \tau_2^* = \tau_1 - \tau_2 + .50 [(\gamma\tau)_{11} + (\gamma\tau)_{21} - (\gamma\tau)_{12} - (\gamma\tau)_{22}]$. The interaction of tasks and stimuli, $.50 [(\gamma\tau)_{11} - (\gamma\tau)_{12} - (\gamma\tau)_{21} + (\gamma\tau)_{22}]$, is estimated as a nonsignificant 72.088 regardless of whether a Type II or a Type III analysis is performed.

Carryover Effects. Examination of E2 information for carryover from tasks and carryover from stimuli yields complicated hypotheses like those just encountered with task and stimulus effects. We find the Type II estimate of carryover from tasks, $\lambda_{11}^* - \lambda_{12}^* = \lambda_{11} - \lambda_{12} + .4286$ $((\lambda_1\lambda_2)_{11} - (\lambda_1\lambda_2)_{21}) + .5714((\lambda_1\lambda_2)_{12} - (\lambda_1\lambda_2)_{22})$, with value -509.012, which is highly significant ($p < 0.0003$). We also can show with a Type III procedure that the carryover from tasks, $\lambda_{11}^* - \lambda_{12}^* = \lambda_{11} - \lambda_{12} + .50$ $[(\lambda_1\lambda_2)_{11} + (\lambda_1\lambda_2)_{12} - (\lambda_1\lambda_2)_{21} - (\lambda_1\lambda_2)_{22}]$ is -509.614. We reject the hypothesis that this more interesting version of $\lambda_{11}^* - \lambda_{12}^*$ is zero ($p < 0.001$).

Similarly, E2 information tells us that we can estimate $\lambda_{21}^* - \lambda_{22}^* = \lambda_{21} - \lambda_{22} + .7143(\lambda_1\lambda_2)_{11} - (\lambda_1\lambda_2)_{12}) + .2857((\lambda_1\lambda_2)_{21} - (\lambda_1\lambda_2)_{22})$, the second carryover effect, obtaining a nonsignificant -66.838 value. Also we find that $\lambda_{21}^* - \lambda_{22}^* = \lambda_{21} - \lambda_{22} + .50[(\lambda_1\lambda_2)_{11} - (\lambda_1\lambda_2)_{12} + (\lambda_1\lambda_2)_{21} -$

$(\lambda_1\lambda_2)_{22}$] is estimated with a Type III procedure as a nonsignificant −65.030, showing no effect of the immediately previous stimulus on current performance.

Other Comments. Notice that, for any effect with only one degree of freedom (everything but subjects and stages in the present example), the analysis of variance table reports an equivalent significance test to that performed with the "ESTIMATE" command for that effect. Careful examination of computer outputs like this one leads us to draw the conclusion that in cases where Type II and III results differ, it is the Type III analysis that constitutes use of a Σ-restricted model. For this reason, a Type III analysis is said to test a sum-to-zero or Σ-restricted model. We still have the problem that estimates of task effects include interaction effects as well. But at least there is balance in our comparison: What we call the task effect in a Type III analysis is the sum of the task effect plus the unweighted average interaction of task and stimulus effects. Both for treatment and carryover effects, a Type III analysis is equivalent to ignoring interactions and stating "ESTIMATE 'TASK1 − TASK2' TASK 1 −1;", for example, with or without "/E" preceding the semi-colon.

Method D: A Multisample Sphericity Test Using a Saturated Multigroup Split-Plot Design Model

Could It Be That Nonsphericity With These Data Would Be a Problem Only for Testing Stage Effects?

If instead of using Equation 5.1, we had a more traditional model for this design, there would be two crossed treatment factors but no stage effects. This also means that we might replace an overall test of sphericity (a *global sphericity* test) by a test that a certain segment of the data exhibits sphericity (*local sphericity*). For example, Crowder and Hand (1990) analyzed data from a 7-subject, 2 eyes × 4 lenses factorial within-subjects design but ignored stage effects. They performed a test of local sphericity for visual acuity scores on the four levels of lenses rather than performing a test of global sphericity for the eight (stage) scores generated for each subject of the experiment. Because there is no required assumption of equal variances or of local sphericity for a *t*-test of the hypothesis that the mean difference between two scores for the same people is zero, Crowder and Hand were able to compare mean on right and left eyes without further assumptions.

Unfortunately, Equation 5.1 for our within-subjects factorial crossover design in which stage and/or carryover effects are also potentially involved precludes the simple local sphericity test technique invoked by Crowder and Hand. The present design has four stages for which sphericity is desired. One might hope by analogy to Crowder and Hand's work that sphericity would not be required for the two-level variables such as task and stimuli being compared within those four stages. However, testing task effects, for example, would use difference scores for subjects in different sequence groups. The hypothesis tested would be that the average population mean difference score across different sequence groups is zero. But, if different sequence groups have different variances for their difference scores, this would need to be taken into account. Accordingly, a test of global sphericity is required in order to be certain that stage, carryover, and the two kinds of treatment effects can be assessed. Because subject effects are assumed random and because multivariate statistics (including the Mauchly test) use subjects as its experimental unit, we need not question the suitability of our previous F-test of subject effects.

A Saturated Split-Plot Design Model

We now illustrate a pair of tests for multisample sphericity in a multigroup split-plot design. For observations from s sequence groups in this design, the model for such a design is as follows:

$$Y_{gij} = \mu + \alpha_g + s_{gi} + \pi_j + (\alpha\pi)_{gj} + e_{gij} \qquad (5.15)$$

where α_g is a Group g effect, $(\alpha\pi)_{gj}$ is interaction of group and stages, and all other terms have obvious definitions. (For pragmatic reasons, we are contravening our earlier decision not to model sequence effects.) This model predicts exact means for the 12 main cells of the three sequences by four-stage design, as well as for the 15 subjects in the design. We report tests of equality of error variance in different groups and of sphericity of the pooled covariance matrix across groups (also called more precisely, the pooled variance-covariance matrix across groups). Each is relevant to traditional split-plot designs, but the latter is of more interest in the assessment of data from our within-subject factorial crossover design. Even here, we must consider the issue of equating evidence from a split-plot design model to a saturated model for a crossover design, as discussed in chapter 3.

Testing the Equality of Covariance Matrices for Different Groups

Kirk (1995) recommended a more modern test rather than routine use of the Mauchly test of sphericity. Nonetheless, we want to illustrate the earlier test again, primarily because all stages of a multisample test of sphericity are feasible here, making it possible to show slightly different techniques than before.

Again, but now using Equation 5.15, we employ a saturated multigroup split-plot design model that could be paralleled with a saturated crossover design model analogous to that in chapter 3. If there is a suggestion of non-sphericity in the current data set and if significance tests of added terms in the latter model suggest that a saturated model is unnecessary, we should pursue the question of conservative testing as in chapter 3.

Because every sequence has more than one subject in it, a sample covariance matrix for each sequence can be obtained with SAS® GLM and its REPEATED command. As Kirk (1982) pointed out, such matrices from a conventional multigroup split-plot design can be examined separately for sphericity and then tested for equality with each other. Later these matrices are combined into a pooled covariance matrix prior to performing an overall sphericity test using a test statistic whose distribution under the null hypothesis is approximately chi-square with an appropriate degrees of freedom value.

Table 5.9 is a SAS® GLM program needed to test the hypothesis of equal covariance matrices for the data of Table 5.6. After presenting a bit of theory related to its use, we show relevant results from running this program and report further calculations required to test this hypothesis. If the hypothesis of equal population covariance matrices proves tenable, then one can proceed to test the hypothesis of sphericity of the pooled covariance matrix. Only if both tests prove nonsignificant does one conclude that the Type H covariance structure is present in the population generating the data being studied. However, failure of robustness may lead to a false rejection of this hypothesis, as noted by Kirk (1982) and others. Accordingly, we are at risk in both directions, fearing the possibility of both Type I and Type II errors in assessing whether the Type H assumption holds.

TABLE 5.9

A Program Computing Separate Weighted SSCP Matrices for Sequence Groups of Table 5.6 and Performing a Pooled Groups Sphericity Test

```
* PROGRAM IS 3SESPHER.SAS;
DATA SEQ1;  INPUT Y1 Y2 Y3 Y4 SEQ SUBJ @@;  CARDS;
341.7  570.4  997.7  393.4 1 1  583.9  645.5 1111.5  644.4 1 2
440.7  597.6 1048.4  608.2 1 3 1049.6 1124.8 1664.2 1096.1 1 4
1298.0  712.5  762.0  637.8 1 5
RUN;  PROC GLM; MODEL Y1–Y4=/NOUNI;
REPEATED STAGE 4 POLYNOMIAL/SUMMARY PRINTE;
TITLE 'ANALYSIS OF SEQUENCE 1 ALONE.'; RUN;
DATA SEQ2;  INPUT Y1 Y2 Y3 Y4 SEQ SUBJ @@;  CARDS;
613.2  773.1  675.9 1172.7 2 6  573.9  701.2  664.5 1176.8 2 7
1042.7 1138.8 1122.3 1569.0 2 8 1007.4  941.0  977.6 1498.3 2 9
837.7  697.3  841.4 1267.9 2 10
RUN;  PROC GLM; MODEL Y1–Y4=/NOUNI;
REPEATED STAGE 4 POLYNOMIAL/SUMMARY PRINTE;
TITLE 'ANALYSIS OF SEQUENCE 2 ALONE.';  RUN;
DATA SEQ3;  INPUT Y1 Y2 Y3 Y4 SEQ SUBJ @@;  CARDS;
840.8 1292.1  688.3  723.3 3 11  993.6 1446.9  936.5  988.2 3 12
358.4  585.7  464.0 1059.9 3 13  684.5  804.1  790.9 1260.6 3 14
982.2  920.0 1043.6 1424.6 3 15
RUN;  PROC GLM; MODEL Y1–Y4=/NOUNI;
REPEATED  STAGE 4 POLYNOMIAL/SUMMARY  PRINTE;
TITLE 'ANALYSIS OF SEQUENCE 3 ALONE.'; RUN;
* SUBPROGRAM FOR POOLING DATA ACROSS SEQUENCE GROUPS;
PROC  APPEND BASE = SEQ1 DATA = SEQ2;
PROC  APPEND BASE = SEQ1 DATA = SEQ3;
PROC  PRINT  DATA = SEQ1;
TITLE 'SEQ1 DATA SET WITH ALL OTHER SEQUENCES APPENDED.';
RUN; PROC  GLM DATA = SEQ1; CLASS SEQ; MODEL
Y1–Y4=SEQ/NOUNI;
REPEATED  STAGE  4 POLYNOMIAL/SUMMARY PRINTE;
TITLE  'ANALYSIS OF 3 SEQUENCES AT ONCE'; RUN;
```

Interpreting What This SAS® GLM Program Says and Yields.
For each data set with a constant size n for each group, this table can generate what SAS® output refers to as the Error SS&CP matrix for three contrasts of stage scores ($Y_1 - Y_4$, $Y_2 - Y_4$, and $Y_3 - Y_4$) for the sequence group involved or, more generally, for any transformation C forming a $p \times (p - 1)$ matrix with each column summing to zero.

Without the "POLYNOMIAL" constraints in the "REPEATED" commands of Table 5.9, SAS® would readily perform Mauchly tests for each group in the experiment under analysis. However, use of an orthonormal C such as that invoked with "POLYNOMIAL" also facilitates our going on to test the hypothesis of equal covariance structures for all sequence groups. SAS® yields what it calls Error SS&CP matrices (sums of squares and sums of cross-products) which are equal to $(n-1)C'\hat{\Sigma}_g C$, where $\hat{\Sigma}_g$ is the estimated covariance matrix of the p stage scores of each subject receiving Sequence g.

Interpreting What the Final Subprogram Has to Say. The major new feature of this sub-program is the merging of three datasets from earlier in the program. Because there are three sequence groups whose data is to be combined for an overall analysis, two successive "PROC APPEND" commands are employed to add one SAS® data set at a time to the first one, SEQ1. Once the total data set is available, a "PROC PRINT" command is employed to show that the proper combination of data is available. In the "PROC GLM" command it is essential that the revised operative data set is identified by adding "DATA = SEQ1;". Also notice the "POLYNOMIAL" constraint in "REPEATED STAGE 4 POLYNOMIAL/PRINTE;" just as was true for separate analyses of individual sequences. Notice that "MODEL Y1–Y4 = SEQ;" has "SEQ" on its right hand side. This permits testing for sequence and sequence × stage effects from Equation 5.15. Because linear, quadratic, and cubic trends of stage effects do not appear in our original model, Equation 5.1, for this design and would be contaminated by task, stimulus, and two kinds of carryover effects if taken seriously here, the results of these sequence and sequence × stage effect tests are not reported here.

Theory. Kirk (1982) discusses the Box test of the hypothesis that $C'\Sigma_1 C, = C'\Sigma_2 C, = C'\Sigma_3 C$ or, more generally, that $C'\Sigma_1 C, = C'\Sigma_2 C, = \ldots = C'\Sigma_s C$ for s groups. We illustrate the first and simpler of two test procedures provided by Kirk even though the last of its three assumptions fails: (a and b) that the number of parameters for groups $(s - 1)$ and number of stages (p) each is less than 5 or 6 and that (c) each group's sample size is 20 or more. (Note differences in symbols and definitions just used from those of Kirk.) Let

$$\chi^2 = (1 - E_1)M \text{ with } M = \sum_{g=1}^{s}(n_g - 1)\,[\ln(|C'\hat{\Sigma}_{pooled}\,C\,|/|C'\hat{\Sigma}_g\,C|)]$$

$$\text{and } E_1 = \frac{2p^2 + 3p - 1}{6(p+1)(s-1)} \left(\sum_{g=1}^{s} \frac{1}{n_g - 1} - \frac{1}{\sum_{g=1}^{s}(n_g - 1)} \right)$$

where $|A|$ is the determinant of *any matrix called A* and $ln(B)$ is the natural logarithm of any scalar called B. The degrees of freedom for this chi-square statistic are set at $df = \frac{p(p+1)(s-1)}{2} = \frac{(4)(5)(2)}{2} = 20.$

Here are the Error SS&CP matrices reported by the program in Table 5.9:

Error SS&CP Matrix for Sequence Group $1 = (n_1 - 1)\, C' \hat{\Sigma}_1 C$

$$= \begin{pmatrix} 284,196.3560 & -260,012.6364 & -53,772.3430 \\ -260,012.6364 & 259,992.1880 & 50,480.6500 \\ -53,772.3430 & 50,480.6500 & 15,389.2540 \end{pmatrix},$$

Error SS&CP Matrix for Sequence Group $2 = (n_2 - 1)\, C' \hat{\Sigma}_2 C$

$$= \begin{pmatrix} 3,148.0606 & -4,220.0797 & 6,076.6022 \\ -4,220.0797 & 14,812.1350 & -15,204.9022 \\ 6,076.6022 & -15,204.9022 & 22,027.8014 \end{pmatrix},$$

and Error SS&CP Matrix for Sequence Group $3 = (n_3 - 1)\, C' \hat{\Sigma}_3 C$

$$= \begin{pmatrix} 374,104.1906 & 260,691.3546 & -139,754.4298 \\ 260,691.3546 & 191,445.8150 & -114,003.3633 \\ -139,754.4298 & -114,003.3633 & 88,593.6034 \end{pmatrix},$$

Pooled Error SS&CP Matrix for All Sequence Groups

$$= \left(\sum_{g=1}^{s}(n_g - 1) \right) C' \hat{\Sigma}_{pooled} C$$

$$= \begin{pmatrix} 661,448.6072 & -3,541.3615 & -187,450.1706 \\ -3,541.3615 & 466,250.1380 & -78,727.6155 \\ -187,450.1706 & -78,727.6155 & 126,010.6588 \end{pmatrix}.$$

With these formulas and Error SS&CP values, matrix program or hand calculation of the test statistics is possible, yielding $M = 98.13$, $E_1 = 0.4778$, $df = 20$, and $\chi^2 = 51.25$, which exceeds $\chi^2_{0.001}(20) = 45.32$. Accordingly, the assumption of equal covariance matrices is rejected.

Testing Sphericity of Data From a Multisequence Group Design

A pooled groups sphericity test combining covariance information from the different sequence groups was performed with the subprogram of Table 5.9 already discussed. With the POLYNOMIAL setting for the REPEATED command, a significant χ^2 of 14.85 with 5 degrees of freedom ($p = 0.0110$) is obtained, yielding the same result as if that transformation were omitted and the consequently recommended one of two resulting Mauchly tests, a test for orthogonal components, was used (SAS Institute Inc., 1989d).

Overall Conclusions About Suitability of ANOVA For the Present Data

The test of equal covariance matrices suggests that the assumption of multigroup sphericity does not hold, as does the multigroup Mauchly test. Nonetheless, one reason to be hopeful about use of ANOVA here is that output from another part of the program of Table 5.9, parallelling the Mauchly test, suggests little or no correction for sphericity: the G-G correction is 0.6953, and the generally more satisfactory H-F correction is 0.9848, very close to the unity for no correction.

Method E: Checking for a Further Possible Difficulty: Presence of Outliers

Because there are five replications of data in each treatment-sequence group of Table 5.6, we are able to invoke a more robust method of identifying outliers than was presented in chapter 3. The earlier method had a bit of contamination: With only one observation per combination of treatment-sequence and stage, possible outliers had to be used in estimating parameters for computing standardized residuals, conceivably reflecting discrepancies from normality and distorting those estimates. For example, in the current search for outliers, one abnormally large score in a sample of five could badly shift both the sample mean and the sample standard deviation, making all five standardized residuals greatly inaccurate. In contrast, Rousseeuw (1991) provided methods employing medians and thus prevented changes in estimators due to outliers unless at least half of the observations are questionable. This half may be called a breakdown point of 50% for the median. Unless there are only two observations, the sample mean and standard deviation each have smaller breakdown points equal to the reciprocal of the sample size.

The Rousseeuw method for a single replicated univariate sample is to compute an analogue of standardized residuals based on raw scores together with the median and the weighted median of absolute distances (*MAD*) from the median:

$$z = \frac{Y - mdn(Y)}{MAD} = \frac{Y - mdn(Y)}{1.483(mdn \, |Y - mdn(Y)|)} \tag{5.16}$$

where MAD is implicitly defined. For the Sequence 1 data of Table 5.6, we use Table 5.10 to show calculation of the largest z-values for different stages.

By Rousseeuw's (1991) arbitrary cutoff of 2.5 in absolute value for the largest z in a cell of the design, there is one significant outlier for Stage 2 and two each for Stages 3 and 4 in this sequence group. The arbitrarily constructed data of Table 5.6 for Sequence 1 at least would seem questionable because of this result. If these were real data, we might well consider the possibility of excluding the raw scores yielding z values above 2.5 and seeking a new analysis of the remaining data. For further sophistication, we might want to try to extend Rousseeuw's (1991) and Rouseeuw and Leroy's (1987) regression and multivariate approaches for outlier detection to the kinds of designs considered in this book.

JUDGING IF A GIVEN WITHIN-SUBJECTS FACTORIAL DESIGN WILL LEAD TO INTERPRETABLE RESULTS

The two experimental designs just discussed were both 2×2 within-subjects factorial designs. However, the four-sequence design forming a Williams square functioned quite differently than the less balanced three-sequence design. One thing that can always be done when considering using a certain design (with a given number of specific sequences

TABLE 5.10
Identifying Outliers in the Hypothetical Data for Sequence 1
of the 3-Sequence 2 ×2 Within-Subjects Experiment

Stage 1 A₁B₁		Stage 2 A₂B₂		Stage 3 A₁B₂		S
Y	$Y - Mdn(Y)$	Y	$Y - Mdn(Y)$	Y	$Y - Mdn(Y)$	Y
341.7	−242.2	570.4	−75.1	997.7	−50.7	393.4
583.9	0	645.5	0	1,111.5	63.1	644.4
440.7	−143.2	597.6	−47.9	1,048.4	0	608.2
)49.6	465.7	1,124.8	479.3	1,664.2	615.8	1,096.1
298.0	714.1	712.5	67.0	762.0	−286.4	637.8
	583.9		645.5		1,048.4	

TABLE 5.10
(Continued)

242.2	67.0	63.1	
359.1826	99.361	93.5773	
$\dfrac{714.1}{359.1826} = 1.99$	$\dfrac{479.3}{99.361} = 4.82$	$\dfrac{615.8}{93.5773} = 6.58$	$\dfrac{45}{43.8}$
—	—	$\dfrac{-286.4}{93.5773} = -3.06$	$\dfrac{-24}{43.8}$

of treatments and a specific distribution of numbers of subjects per sequence) is to make up some data that could have been obtained with it and perform a data analysis like one of those here. If the expected mean squares and the other estimability information produced by an E2 option (for example) in the MODEL statement make the results of the hypothetical experiment statistically interpretable, then it would be reasonable to keep that precise design for the actual experiment to be performed. Otherwise, a new candidate design should be developed and tested in this way.

A quicker method is to restrict oneself to designs that are balanced Latin squares, replications of balanced Latin square designs, an orthogonal set of Latin squares, or combinations of such squares. See Cotton (1993) and Jones and Kenward (1989) for recent discussions of ways to find such squares. If there are many subjects available, it might be possible to include every possible treatment sequence. Thus, with four treatments in the current experiment, there are 4! = 24 available treatment sequences. At least one subject should receive each sequence, and all sequences should have the same number of subjects. See also chapter 13, this volume, for information on efficient but complicated designs not often used by psychologists.

THINGS TO REMEMBER

Major Analysis Options

1. Analyzing data from 2-way factorial within-subject designs in a fashion that looks for the following kinds of effects: Factor 1, factor 2, interaction of factor 1 and factor 2, stage of practice, subject, carryover from factor 1, carryover from factor 2, and interactions of those carryovers.

2. Supplementing the above analysis by a multisample sphericity test for a multigroup split-plot repeated measurements design.

3. Using output from the ESTIMATE commands of our basic data analysis program in computing the dimensionless variance of each such estimate of parameter differences.

4. Using output from the ESTIMATE commands of our basic and supplementary data analysis programs in computing the efficiency of each such estimate of parameter differences.

5. Using medians of raw scores and of absolute distances of scores from their medians to perform a robust search for outliers in observed data.

Interpreting Results of Computational Methods Not Previously Discussed

1. Understanding the notation $(\gamma\tau)_{11}$ for an interaction of A1 and B1 effects.

2. Knowing the potential problem indicated by an expected mean square result such as E(MS STIM) = Var(Error) + Q(STIM, TASK* STIM) where the quadratic term Q is a function of one variable plus an interaction of the variable with another.

3. Knowing how to read and apply other estimability information from a SAS® GLM analysis, for example. As a consequence, being able to state implications of the estimability information from the E2 option in the MODEL statement for the four-sequence 2×2 within-subjects factorial design discussed in this chapter. Being able to move from the printed output for E2 or E3 above to an inference, for example that 0 INT + ... + 0 TASK 2 + STIM 1 − STIM 2 + 0.5 TASK* STIM 11 − 0.5 TASK*STIM 12 + 0.5 TASK*STIM 2 1 − TASK* STIM 2 2 + 0 + ... + 0 = $\tau_1^* - \tau_2^* = \tau_1 - \tau_2 + 0.5\big((\gamma\tau)_{11} - (\gamma\tau)_{12} + (\gamma\tau)_{21} - (\gamma\tau)_{22}\big)$ is estimable and knowing how to interpret a significant F for stimuli when this information is available.

4. Knowing that E2 estimability information for our three-sequence 2×2 within-subjects factorial design implies we can estimate a stimulus effect difference of $\tau_1^* - \tau_2^* = \tau_1 - \tau_2 + [0.4063\big((\gamma\tau)_{11} - (\gamma\tau)_{12}\big) + 0.5938\,(\gamma\tau)_{21} - 0.5937(\gamma\tau)_{22}]$, but that the Type III estimability information for this design tells us that we can estimate a more interesting quantity: $\tau_1^* - \tau_2^* = \tau_1 - \tau_2 + 0.5000[(\gamma\tau)_{11} - (\gamma\tau)_{12} + (\gamma\tau)_{21} - (\gamma\tau)_{22}]$. Comparing the information here and in Point 3 shows that interpreting the result of a significance test for stimulus effects or other main effects and carryover effects requires less caution for the balanced Latin square form of a 2-way factorial crossover design than for this less balanced 3-sequence, 2-way factorial crossover design.

5. Remembering that these analysis methods are built around a specific set of treatment combination sequences for the different subjects of the experiment. The variances of estimators of functions of

parameters and the interpretability of the analyses are affected by the specific sequences employed and the relative number of subjects used with each.

EXERCISES

1. Run the SAS® GLM programs in this chapter. Do you obtain the same results reported here?

2. Modify the SAS® GLM program of Table 5.2 to include estimation of power for all effects tested in it.

3. How would you re-program Table 5.2 to compare performance under A_1B_1, A_1B_2, A_2B_1, and A_2B_2 as four treatments in a replicated Latin square design having 3 df for treatments and 3 df for carryover effects without reference to TASK and STIM variables?

4. How would the task in Exercise 2 be affected if you were working with Table 5.7?

6

Pretest–Posttest Control Group Designs: Comparing Different Treatment Groups After Pretesting

INTRODUCTION

Sometimes psychologists want to perform an experiment in which two groups of randomly assigned subjects are first checked for equivalent performance on one treatment (Treatment A). Then one group is measured again under Treatment A and the other group is measured under a second treatment (Treatment B). For example, Treatment A might be instruction to focus on the exact words in a psychology lecture when trying to learn its content. Treatment B might be instruction on how to recognize the most important ideas in the lecture in order to learn its content. This may be called a pretest–posttest control group design (Campbell & Stanley, 1966) and schematized as:

Group 1	R O_1	O_2
Group 2	R O_3 X	O_4

with each line representing a time sequence of events for differently treated group in the experiment. The R means that members of the two groups were randomly assigned, and a subscripted O represents a response measurement at a given stage of the experiment. X represents Treatment B, the feature that is different for the different groups in the experiment. Group 1 members are measured on O_1 and on O_2, both times under Treatment A, whereas Group 2 members are measured on O_3 under Treatment A and on O_4 under Treatment B.

Under Method A (next) we discuss one of three statistical analysis methods advocated by Campbell and Stanley for the simplest form of the pretest–posttest control group design. Later in the chapter we consider an expansion of this design that switches treatments in blocks (anticipating chapter 7 material):

Group 1   R O_1^3 O_2^3

Group 2   R O_3^3 $(XO_4)^3$

Here we have three observations at each stage and three applications of the differentiating treatment X. Clearly there are many variants of the pretest–posttest control group design; related statistical analyses for many of them can be inferred from the following illustrations.

METHOD A: ANALYZING DATA FROM A SIMPLE
DESIGN — AA VERSUS AB SEQUENCES

Example of an AA Versus AB Design

For $n = 3$ subjects in each group, we can represent a pretest–posttest control group design as in Table 6.1 below:

TABLE 6.1

A Design for Comparing Performance Under an AA Sequence
and an AB Sequence

	Phase 1 (Stage 1)	Phase 2 (Stage 2)
Group 1		
Subject 1	A	A
Subject 2	A	A
Subject 3	A	A
Group 2		
Subject 4	A	B
Subject 5	A	B
Subject 6	A	B

As planned, Group 1 members are tested under Treatment A twice, but Group 2 members receive one test under Treatment A and then a test under Treatment B. (Phases 1 and 2 mean the same as Stages 1 and 2 here; in the next design they have different meanings.)

Model: What Should We Try to Learn From Data Obtained With This Design?

We would like to assess treatment effects, the performance difference due to receiving Treatment A rather than B. Because of the Phase 1 test under Treatment A, we can take into account any correlation between performance under A and B to generate a more sensitive estimate of treatment effects than if the experiment had begun with Phase 2 for members of each group.

Let us call X_i the score for Subject i on Phase 1 with Treatment A and Y_{ik} the score for a Subject i on Phase 2 with Treatment k. That treatment can be either A or B, of course. Here is a model involving this kind of effect:

$$Y_{ik} = \mu + \tau_k + \beta_1 X_i + e_{ik} \qquad (6.1)$$

The parameters in Equation 6.1 have the following interpretations: μ is an arbitrary constant, and τ_k is the effect of Treatment k. Also, β_1 is the slope of a straight line for predicting Y_{iB} from X_i for a subject receiving B on Phase 2 and also for a different straight line with the same slope for predicting Y_{iA} from X_i for a subject receiving A on Phase 2, and e_{ik} is the random error for Y_{ik}. This error is $N(0, \sigma^2)$; no special assumption about $Cov(e_{ik}, e_{ik'})$ for different treatments k and k' is required. However, the errors for different subjects, e_{ik} and $e_{i'k'}$, are assumed independent of each other regardless of which treatments are involved. The slope constant is crucial to the analysis of covariance because it allows us to take out the effects of initial differences in Phase 1 behavior before assessing treatment effects on Phase 2.

Hypothetical Data

Here is a possible data set for the design just presented (see Table 6.2). Scores and treatments are shown for each subject in each group on each phase (stage) of the experiment.

TABLE 6.2
Hypothetical Data for Three Subjects Each
From an AA Versus AB Experiment

	Group 1			Group 2	
	Phase 1	Phase 2		Phase 1	Phase 2
Treatment	A	k = A		A	k = B
Subject i	X_i	Y_{ik}	i	X_i	Y_{ik}
1	110.0	60.0	4	90.0	40.0
2	103.0	59.0	5	112.0	35.0
3	96.0	57.0	6	102.0	37.0
Mean	103.00	58.67		101.33	37.33

Note. The symbol equated to *k* specifies the Phase 2 treatment.

Analysis Program and Results

The Phase 1 data show a slightly higher mean for Group 1 than for Group 2. On Phase 2 all means are lower than on Phase 1, possibly because of practice effects. Also, the Phase 2 mean for Group 1 with Treatment A is much higher than the Phase 2 mean for Group 2 with Treatment B. We will now perform an analysis of covariance to test the Phase 2 mean difference ($\bar{Y}_A - \bar{Y}_B$) for significance. For this data set and experimental design, it is easy to do this analysis with a hand calculator or to employ the analysis of covariance program in almost any statistical package. However, we may as well employ SAS® GLM here as usual. Here is a program that yields desired results (see Table 6.3):

TABLE 6.3
Program for Analyzing Data from Table 6.2

```
*PROGRAM NAME IS AB_COV.SAS FOR AN AA VERSUS AB
 COVANOVA DESIGN;
 DATA AB_COV; INPUT TREAT $ X Y @@;  CARDS;
```

(Continued)

TABLE 6.3

(Continued)

A 110 60 A 103 59   A 96 57 B 90 40   B 112 35 B 102 37
RUN; PROC GLM; CLASS TREAT;
MODEL Y = TREAT X/SS1 E2 SS3 SS4 SOLUTION;
MEANS TREAT; ESTIMATE 'TREAT A – TREAT B' 1 –1;
TITLE 'COVANOVA FOR AN AA VS AB CROSSOVER DESIGN
  EXPERIMENT'; RUN;

Because all subjects received Treatment A on Phase 1, the TREAT variable in this SAS® program refers only to the treatment on Phase 2. This program yields identical analysis of variance tables for Types II, III, and IV analyses (see Table 6.4):

TABLE 6.4
ANOVA Table (Type II = III = IV Results) Obtained
With Program of Table 6.3

Source	Sum of Squares	df	Mean Square	F
Treatments	685.08	1	685.08	148.15**
X (Phase 1 Performance)	3.46	1	3.46	0.75
Error	13.87	3	4.62	—

Note. ** $p < 0.01$.

This table shows that the only significant effects are treatment effects.

Estimation of Effects

From E2 output on the Type II Estimable Functions (not shown) and what we know already, we see that we can estimate the size of the treatment effect difference, $\tau_A - \tau_B$. Both with the SOLUTION option and with the ESTIMATE command, we find TREAT A – TREAT B = 21.50, an unbiased estimate of $\tau_A - \tau_B$. We mention now that efficiency of this design need not be computed. When analysis of covariance is used with the present design, it is a between-S design and therefore has $E = 100$ (compared with a comparable between-S design!). On the one hand, power may be increased because a positive correlation between Phase 1 and Phase 2 performance reduces the standard error of $\hat{\tau}_A - \hat{\tau}_B$ on Phase 2. On the other hand, we know that the experimental design is as efficient as possible because there is no within-subjects manipulation of treatments that could inflate that standard error when compared to the reference design with between-subjects variation only.

METHOD B: COMPARING A^3A^3 AND A^3B^3 SEQUENCES

Design

Instead of using the simplest pretest–posttest control group structure, the AA versus AB design just shown, the experimenter could add a certain constant number of stages to each subject on each phase, using the last treatment that subject received in that phase. For example, having three stages on Phase 1 and three stages on Phase 2 of the previous experiment yields the following design for three subjects in each sequence group (see Table 6.5):

TABLE 6.5
An A^3A^3 Versus A^3B^3 Design With Six Subjects

	Phase 1			Phase 2		
	Stage 1	Stage 2	Stage 3	Stage 4	Stage 5	Stage 6
Subject 1	A	A	A	A	A	A
Subject 2	A	A	A	A	A	A
Subject 3	A	A	A	A	A	A
Subject 4	A	A	A	B	B	B
Subject 5	A	A	A	B	B	B
Subject 6	A	A	A	B	B	B

Hypothetical Data

A possible set of data for this design appears in Table 6.6. Each score is the number of minutes required to learn the material of a lecture. Different lectures occurred on successive stages. If the lectures have been pretested and shown to be equally difficult to master, we can consider differences in performance on Treatment A from stage to stage to be primarily due to stage effects, not lecture effects. Similarly for Treat-

TABLE 6.6
Hypothetical Data for an A^3A^3 Versus A^3B^3 Design With Six Subjects

| | Phase 1 | | | | Phase 2 | | |
Stage 1	Stage 2	Stage 3	Phase Mean	Stage 4	Stage 5	Stage 6	Phase Mea
110 (A)	60 (A)	51(A)	73.67	48 (A)	47 (A)	45 (A)	46.6
103 (A)	59 (A)	48 (A)	70.00	49 (A)	47 (A)	46 (A)	47.3
96 (A)	57 (A)	50 (A)	67.67	51 (A)	48 (A)	48 (A)	49.0
103.00	58.67	49.67	70.45	49.33	47.33	46.33	47.6
90 (A)	56 (A)	49 (A)	65.00	40 (B)	45 (B)	46 (B)	43.6
112 (A)	61 (A)	55 (A)	76.00	35 (B)	39 (B)	37 (B)	37.0
102 (A)	60 (A)	44(A)	68.67	37 (B)	42 (B)	41 (B)	40.0
101.33	59.00	49.33	69.89	37.33	42.00	41.33	40.2
102.17	58.83	49.50	70.17	43.33	44.67	43.83	43.9

ment B. (Alternatively, we might want to balance lectures across stages and include both lectures and stages as tested effects in a more complex design.) There is also the possibility of performing a between-subjects comparison of Subjects 1 through 3 with one sequence of treatments and Subjects 4 through 6 with the other. However, this would require assuming that the two groups would perform differently on Stages 1 through 3 even though they were treated identically then.

The means in this table show a trend toward better scores (lower means) for later stages of the experiment. They also suggest that overall performance on Phase 2 is slightly better on Treatment B than Treatment A (43.94 minutes to learn rather than 47.67).

Model: What Should We Try to Learn From Data Obtained With This Design?

1. Are there any significant differences in performance for different subjects of this experiment?

2. We want to look for effects of the stage variable: Is there a change in performance as subjects gain more practice with this task?

3. Are there different effects of different treatments?

4. Is there a change in performance as a function of what treatment occurred on the previous stage (i.e., a carryover effect of previous treatments)?

These data need to be analyzed statistically. A plausible model for data from this design is:

$$Y_{ijk} = \mu + s_i + \pi_j + \tau_k + \lambda_{k'} + e_{ijk} \tag{6.2}$$

where s_i is the random subject effect for Subject i, π_j is the effect for Stage j, τ_k is the effect of Treatment k, $\lambda_{k'}$ is the carryover from Treatment k' on the previous stage, and e_{ijk} is random error for Subject i on Stage j with Treatment k. We assume that the s_i are i.i.d. $N(0, \sigma_s^2)$ and that the e_{ijk} for different subjects are i.i.d normally distributed with mean zero. However, their covariances across treatments are assumed to have a Type H structure that is the same for each treatment-sequence group, A^3A^3 or A^3B^3. Also, the s_i and $e_{i'jk}$ are assumed independent whether or not $i = i'$. Thus multisample sphericity of the observations is implied.

TABLE 6.7
A Program for Analyzing Hypothetical Results From an A^3A^3 Versus A^3B^3 Design

```
B3; INPUT GROUP SUBJ STAGE TREAT $ CARRY $ Y @@; CARDS;
 1 1 2 A A 60    1 1 3 A A 51    1 1 4 A A 48    1 1 5 A A 47   1 1 6 A A 45
 1 2 2 A A 59    1 2 3 A A 48    1 2 4 A A 49    1 2 5 A A 47   1 2 6 A A 46
 1 3 2 A A 57    1 3 3 A A 50    1 3 4 A A 51    1 3 5 A A 48   1 3 6 A A 48
 2 4 2 A A 56    2 4 3 A A 49    2 4 4 B A 40    2 4 5 B B 45   2 4 6 B B 46
 2 5 2 A A 61    2 5 3 A A 55    2 5 4 B A 35    2 5 5 B B 39   2 5 6 B B 37
 2 6 2 A A 60    2 6 3 A A 44    2 6 4 B A 37    2 6 5 B B 42   2 6 6 B B 41
LM; CLASS SUBJ STAGE TREAT CARRY;
UBJ STAGE TREAT CARRY/E SS1 E2 SS3 SS4 SOLUTION;
3J; MEANS SUBJ; MEANS STAGE; MEANS TREAT;
TAGE2 – STAGE6' STAGE 0 1 0 0 0 –1;
TAGE3 – STAGE6' STAGE 0 0 1 0 0 –1;
TAGE4 – STAGE6' STAGE 0 0 0 1 0 –1;
TAGE5 – STAGE 6' STAGE 0 0 0 0 1 –1;
REAT A – TREAT B' TREAT 1 –1; ESTIMATE 'CARRY A – CARRY B' CARRY 0 1 –1;
SAS FOR COMPARING A3A3 TO A3B3 CONDITION.'; RUN;
```

Analysis Program and Results

Here is a SAS® program for analyzing the data for this experiment (see Table 6.7):

Note that GROUP and group values need not really be included in the INPUT line or in the data set. The only advantage of such inclusion would come if we added "PROC MEANS; VAR Y; BY GROUP;" and perhaps other similar series of commands in order to compute means relating to groups for Table 6.6.

As in earlier chapters, we are not actually sure which ESTIMATE commands to employ in this program until we have seen the estimability output based on the E2 option associated with the MODEL statement. So, in setting up this kind of analysis, you would probably run it first with E2 but no ESTIMATE commands and second without E2 but with ESTIMATE commands that make sense in view of output from the first run. Table 6.8 summarizes the Type II analysis of variance performed with the previous program; in this example, Types III and IV give the same results as Type II.

TABLE 6.8

Analysis of Variance Table Resulting From the Table 6.7 Program

Source	Sum of Squares	df	Mean Square	F
Subjects	31.61	5	6.32	0.30
Stages 2:6	459.67	4	114.92	5.52**
Treatments	147.35	1	147.35	7.08*
Carryovers	46.69	1	46.69	2.24
Error	478.97	23	20.82	—

Note. $* p < .05.$ $** p < 0.01.$

This table indicates that, working at the 0.05 level, stage and treatment effects are significant but that subject and carryover effects are not.

Estimation of Effects

Estimation of subject effects has problems because they are not significant and the F for them is less than one. Our usual method of estimating random subjects effects using expected mean squares from our program's output would lead us to the following negative value: $Var(Subj) \approx \dfrac{MS_{subj} - MS_{error}}{5.4} = \dfrac{6.32 - 20.82}{5.4} = -2.69$. The most natural solution may be to say that the variance of subject effects may well be zero, implying that the s_i term could be omitted from Equation 6.2 in this case.

Because we used a SOLUTION option in the MODEL statement of our SAS® program, and we have appropriate estimability information from the E2 command, we can estimate the size of specific significant effects of our statistical model (or, of course, from the ESTIMATE command outputs once they are included in the program). Either method yields TREAT A – TREAT B = 11.44 as an unbiased estimate of $\tau_A - \tau_B$, the difference between the effects of the two treatments.

Similarly, Type II Estimable Functions information (not shown) tells us that the Stage 1 effect (π_1) effect and all any differences between Stage 1 and other stage effects cannot be estimated with Type II. This is why there are only four degrees of freedom for Stages in Table 6.8 instead of the five degrees of freedom we would expect for six stages. We can estimate four stage effect differences, however: $\pi_2 - \pi_6$ is estimated either with the SOLUTION option or the ESTIMATE command as STAGE 2 – STAGE 6 = 12.69, $\pi_3 - \pi_6$ is estimated as STAGE 3 – STAGE 6 = 3.36, $\pi_4 - \pi_6$ is estimated as STAGE 4 - STAGE 6 = 2.92, and $\pi_5 - \pi_6$ is estimated as STAGE 5 – STAGE 6 = 0.83. Because subject and carryover effects are not statistically significant, we need not examine estimates for them.

Measuring Efficiencies and Variances of Estimated Effects in This Example

We use the estimated variance formula (5.4) of chapter 5 here as well:

$$\Sigma \Sigma a_{gj}^2 = \text{Estimator Variance in multiples of } \frac{\sigma^2}{n} = \frac{n \, (s.e.e.[\hat{\theta}])^2}{MSerror} \qquad (6.3)$$

with $n = 3$ being the number of subjects for each of two sequence groups, a_{gj} being the weight in the estimate of the effect in question, based on the observed mean for sequence group g on stage j, and s.e.e.[$\hat{\theta}$] being the standard error of the estimated quantity. Other constants are $s = 2$ sequences, $p = 6$ stages, $N = ns = 6$ subjects and $N_{tot} = nps = 36$ observations.

Efficiency calculations are performed with the aid of (5.14) from chapter 5:

$$E\hat{\theta} = \frac{\left(\dfrac{200}{r*}\right)}{\dfrac{n(s.e.e.[\hat{\theta}])^2}{MS_{error}}} \tag{6.4}$$

where $r* = \dfrac{ps}{T}$ for treatments or carryover and $r* = s$ for stages from (5.12) and (5.13) in that chapter.

Table 6.9 shows the greatest efficiency and lowest variance for estimates of Stage 5 – Stage 6 effects; the opposite holds for estimates of treatment and carryover differences.

GENERALIZING THIS DESIGN

Obviously, the use of three stages per phase of this experiment is just one possibility; an experimenter can add any desired number n for every phase for each subject, producing an A^mA^m versus A^mB^m design. Our first design used $m = 1$ and our second design used $m = 3$. No new principles are invoked when using any other m.

A possible alternative to the AA versus AB design is the 2-stage crossover design with some subjects receiving an AB sequence and others receiving its reverse, a BA sequence. Because this design (also called a 2 × 2 Latin square design) balances treatment orders, it would seem useful as a vehicle for separating treatment effects, stage effects, and carryover effects. However, various authors have pointed out that such a complete separation is not possible with a 2-stage design if carryover is present. See Cotton (1989) for one review of this problem.

One definition of a repeated measurements Latin square is that it is a design with n rows for different subjects, with n columns for stages, and

TABLE 6.9

Calculating Efficiencies and Variances of Estimators in σ^2/n Units
for a A^3A^3 Versus A^3B^3 Design From Output of the Program in Table 6.7

	Model with Carryovers				
	Standard Error of estimate (s.e.e)	Variance of Estimate (s.e.e. squared) = A	$3A/MS_{error} = nA/C = \Sigma\Sigma\alpha^2_{gj}$ = Estimator Variance in multiples of $\dfrac{\sigma^2}{n}$	$r^* = $ dimensionless number of replications of effect in an ideal experiment	I
6 or Stage 3 –	3.13591625	9.83397073	1.4167	2	
6	3.48537605	12.14784621	1.7500	2	
6	2.63469664	6.94162638	1.0000	2	
B	4.30244160	18.51100372	2.6667	6	
' B	4.56342845	20.82487922	3.0000	6	
			C = 20.82488		

r each of 2 sequences.

with every row and every column involving each of n treatments exactly once. Fortunately, when n is greater than 3 for such a repeated measurements Latin square, it is commonplace to test its data for treatment, stage, and subject effects; this book emphasizes that carryover effects can also be assessed for such a design.

EXERCISES

1. Run each of the programs in this chapter to be sure you are comfortable with your computer's SAS® facilities for these problems and that the programs yield the values reported above.

2. Modify the design in Table 6.5 to have some other number of m for the $A'''A'''$ versus $A'''B'''$ design. Possibly use a different m in the first stage of each subject's treatment than in the second. Or change the number of subjects per group or even make different numbers of subjects per group. Then make up possible data for this new design, modify the related program and run it.

3. The SAS® GLM manual's (SAS Institute Inc., 1989d) example of an analysis of covariance does not include a test for equality of slopes for different treatment groups. Can you devise a SAS® GLM modification of the program in Table 6.3 that would include such a test? Can you find a way to test the assumption of equal variances of the Y's in each group or to correct for unequal variances if necessary?

OPTIONAL THEORY, EXAMPLES, AND EXERCISES
INVOLVING BMDP™, SPSS®, and SYSTAT™

Introduction

This book avowedly focuses on SAS® as the most informative available statistical package that can be used with crossover designs. However, many investigators prefer to use other statistical packages. Now that you know how SAS® GLM can be used for the analysis of a few crossover designs, you are ready to learn related methods employing other statistical packages if you wish to do so. The current set of exercises gives a very brief point of entry to analysis methods using BMDP™ (Dixon, Brown, Engelman, Hill, & Jennrich, 1990), SPSS® (Norusis,

1990b), and SYSTAT™ (Wilkinson, 1989). Our theoretical discussion of programming with those packages is limited, as is our set of procedural instructions. We assume that, if you plan to do the next exercises for a certain package, you are already somewhat comfortable with the BMDP™, SPSS®, or SYSTAT™ implementation available to you. Anyone wishing to employ packages other than SAS® probably should run the current example programs and perform related exercises while reading the references provided with them. Note that, although some information about estimation is provided, not all packages can provide all estimates available with SAS® GLM. Also, we do not explore methods of estimating efficiency with other packages. Cotton (1993) and Edwards and Bland (1993) have demonstrated the use of various computer packages for the analysis of the hypothetical Latin square data in Table 6.10 (with the term *Period* used instead of *Stage* in order to keep two factors from starting with S and complicating certain computer programs):

TABLE 6.10
Hypothetical Data From a Balanced Latin Square

	Period 1	Period 2	Period 3	Period 4
Subject 1	68 (A)	74 (B)	93 (D)	94 (C)
Subject 2	60 (B)	66 (C)	59 (A)	79 (D)
Subject 3	69 (C)	85 (D)	78 (B)	69 (A)
Subject 4	90 (D)	80 (A)	80 (C)	86 (B)

Source: Adapted from Cotton, J. W. (1993). Latin square designs. In L. K. Edwards (Ed.), *Applied analysis of variance in behavioral science*. New York: Marcel Dekker, p. 177, with the permission of the author and editor.

Recoding (= Reparameterizing) Analysis of Variance Models

Here is an abbreviated model statement for the previous data set:

$$Y_{ijk'k} = \mu + s_i + \pi_j + \tau_k + \lambda_{k'} + e_{ijk'k} \tag{6.5}$$

We can understand certain differences between SAS® and other statistical packages such as SYSTAT™ if we look at two ways of recoding

Equation 6.5 in an attempt to eliminate unknowable parameters.

Set-to-Zero Recoding (Set-to-Zero Reparameterization)

Consider just the first two observations for Subject 1, based on Equation 6.5:

$$Y_{110A} = \mu + s_1 + \pi_1 + \tau_A + \lambda_0 + e_{110A} \quad \text{and}$$

$$Y_{12AB} = \mu + s_1 + \pi_2 + \tau_B + \lambda_A + e_{12AB}$$

where μ is an additive constant or intercept, s_1, and $e_{1jk'k}$ are random effects for Subject 1 and for error on a given observation; and π_j, τ_k, and $\lambda_{k'}$ are the fixed effects for Period j, Treatment k, and carryover from Prior Treatment k', with λ_0 applying on Period 1 where there is no prior treatment. Let us first recode the first two observations for Subject 1:

$$Y_{110A} = (\mu + s_4 + \pi_4 + \tau_D + \lambda_D) + (s_1 - s_4) + (\pi_1 + \lambda_0 - \pi_4 - \lambda_D)$$

$$+ (\tau_A - \tau_D) + 0 + e_{110A}$$

$$= \mu^+ + s_1^+ + \pi_1^+ + \tau_A^+ + \lambda_0^+ + e_{110A}$$

$$= \mu^+ + s_1^+ + \pi_1^+ + \tau_A^+ + e_{110A} \tag{6.6}$$

with $\mu^+ = \mu + s_4 + \pi_4 + \tau_D + \lambda_D$, $s_1^+ = s_1 - s_4$, $\pi_1^+ = \pi_1 + \lambda_0 - \pi_4 - \lambda_D$, $\tau_A^+ = \tau_A - \tau_D$, and λ_0^+ identically zero as we would like it to be because no treatment preceded Period 1. Also

$$Y_{12AB} = (\mu + s_4 + \pi_4 + \tau_D + \lambda_D) + (s_1 - s_4) + (\pi_2 - \pi_4) + (\tau_B - \tau_D)$$

$$+ (\lambda_A - \lambda_D) + e_{12AB}$$

$$= \mu^+ + s_1^+ + \pi_2^+ + \tau_B^+ + \lambda_A^+ + e_{12AB} \tag{6.7}$$

with implicit definitions of its new elements. Notice that the initial and final forms of Equations 6.6 and 6.7 are algebraically equivalent. Equation 6.7 has an obvious counterpart for Period 3. However, if we were to write an equation for the observation on Period 4 with Subject 1, we would obtain the interesting result that $\pi_4^+ = \pi_4 - \pi_4 = 0$. Similarly, we could show that the last recoded subject, treatment, and carryover parameters are all zero: $s_4^+ = \tau_D^+ = \lambda_D^+ = 0$.

Originally we had 18 parameters in our model. Our recoding procedure has set five parameters to zero (π_4^+, s_4^+, τ_D^+, λ_D^+, and λ_0^+), leaving only 13 to estimate. But μ^+, and π_1^+ are of little interest. This leaves us with 11 parameters (non-error degrees of freedom) of interest, just as would be reported in a SAS® GLM Type II analysis of data from a balanced Williams 4×4 Latin square conforming to Equation 6.5 above. That SAS® analysis appears in Cotton (1993) and is not repeated here.

Using a recoding procedure like that above may be called a *set-last-to-zero* procedure. Some people and programs set the first parameter in each group to zero, making a *set-first-to-zero* procedure. But SAS® GLM uses a set-last-to-zero procedure, and it is commonly labeled simply a set-to-zero procedure, a set-to-zero recoding, or a set-to-zero reparameterization. Its purpose, of course, is to simplify an over-parameterized model, so that interesting functions of the original parameters can be estimated.

Sum-to-Zero Recoding (Sum-to-Zero Reparameterization)

The reason to discuss an alternate recoding is twofold: (a) Alternate solutions should be algebraically equivalent, and (b) our SYSTAT™ program employs an alternate recoding called sum-to-zero reparameterization. Again, we begin with Equation 6.5 for a 4×4 Latin square design:

$$Y_{ijk'k} = \mu + s_i + \pi_j + \tau_k + \lambda_{k'} + e_{ijk'k}$$

Consider just the first two observations for Subject 1, based on this equation:

$$Y_{110A} = \mu + s_1 + \pi_1 + \tau_A + \lambda_D + e_{110A} \text{ and}$$

$$Y_{12AB} = \mu + s_1 + \pi_2 + \tau_B + \lambda_A + e_{12AB},$$

where parameter definitions are as before except that, because of special features of SYSTAT 5.02, we let $\lambda_0 = \lambda_D$ on Period 1 where there is no prior treatment. Let us first recode the first two observations for Subject 1:

$$Y_{110A} = (\mu + \bar{s} + \bar{\pi} + \bar{\tau} + \bar{\lambda}) + (s_1 - \bar{s}) + (\pi_1 + \lambda_D - \bar{\pi} - \bar{\lambda}) + (\tau_A - \bar{\tau}) +$$

$$0 + e_{110A}$$

$$= \tilde{\mu} + \tilde{s}_1 + \tilde{\pi}_1 + \tilde{\tau}_A + \tilde{\lambda}_0 + e_{110A}$$

$$= \tilde{\mu} + \tilde{s}_1 + \tilde{\pi}_1 + \tilde{\tau}_A + e_{110A} \tag{6.8}$$

because $\tilde{\lambda}_0$ is identically zero as we would like it to be because no treatment preceded Period 1 and $\bar{\lambda}$ is $0.25(\lambda_A + \lambda_B + \lambda_C + \lambda_D)$, not 0.2 $(\lambda_0 + \lambda_A + \lambda_B + \lambda_C + \lambda_D)$. Also,

$$Y_{12AB} = (\mu + \bar{s} + \bar{\pi} + \bar{\tau} + \bar{\lambda}) + (s_1 - \bar{s}) + (\pi_2 - \bar{\pi}) + (\tau_B - \bar{\tau}) +$$

$$(\lambda_A - \bar{\lambda}) + e_{12AB}$$

$$= \tilde{\mu} + \tilde{s}_1 + \tilde{\pi}_2 + \tilde{\tau}_B + \tilde{\lambda}_A + e_{12AB} \tag{6.9}$$

Notice that new terms with tilde signs are implicitly defined in (6.8) and (6.9). For example, $\tilde{\pi}_1 = \pi_1 + \lambda_D - \bar{\pi} - \bar{\lambda}$ is shown in (6.8) and $\tilde{\pi}_2 = \pi_2 - \bar{\pi}$ in (6.9). Comparable equations to (6.9) apply for Periods 3 and 4. Note that $\Sigma \tilde{s}_i = \Sigma \tilde{\tau}_k = \Sigma \tilde{\lambda}_{k'} = 0$. Also, perhaps surprisingly, $\Sigma \tilde{\pi}_j = \lambda_D - \bar{\lambda}$.

As before, we started with 18 parameters in our model. Our recoding procedure has set four parameters ($\tilde{s}_4$, $\tilde{\pi}_4$, $\tilde{\tau}_D$, and $\tilde{\lambda}_D$) to linear functions of other parameters, and one ($\tilde{\lambda}_0$) explicitly to zero. This leaves only 13 to estimate. But $\tilde{\mu}$, and $\tilde{\pi}_1 = \pi_1 + \lambda_D - \bar{\pi} - \bar{\lambda}$ are of little interest even though the initial run of SYSTAT™ for this data set will include $\tilde{\pi}_1$ in its significance test for period effects. Omitting $\tilde{\mu}$ from the ANOVA table leaves us with 12 parameters (non-error degrees of freedom) until we modify the analysis by comparing only Periods 2 through 4, yielding 11 parameters to assess. Alternatively, we could assume that $\lambda_D = \lambda$, making $\Sigma\tilde{\pi}_j = 0$ and having a completely justified sum-to-zero recoding with 12 parameters plus μ. Note that assumptions like this one were not needed in our set-to-zero example.

A BMDP™ P4V Program for Latin Square Data

Here is a slight modification of a BMDP™ P4V program presented by Edwards and Bland (1993) for the analysis of these data (Table 6.11). You may want to run it yourself.

TABLE 6.11

A BMDP™ 4V Program for Analyzing the Data From Table 6.10

```
/INPUT  VARIABLES = 5.
    CASES = 16.
    FORMAT = 'X1,2(I1,X2),2(A1,X2),F2.0'.
/VARIABLE   NAMES = SUBJ, PERIOD, TREAT, CARRY, Y.
/TRANSFORM  IF(CARRY EQ CHAR(A)) THEN CARRY = 1.
        IF(CARRY EQ CHAR(B)) THEN CARRY = 2.
        IF(CARRY EQ CHAR(C)) THEN CARRY = 3.
        IF(CARRY EQ CHAR(D)) THEN CARRY = 4.
        IF(CARRY EQ CHAR(0)) THEN CARRY = 5.
        IF(TREAT EQ CHAR(A)) THEN TREAT = 1.
        IF(TREAT EQ CHAR(B)) THEN TREAT = 2.
        IF(TREAT EQ CHAR(C)) THEN TREAT = 3.
        IF(TREAT EQ CHAR(D)) THEN TREAT = 4.
/BETWEEN    FACTORS = SUBJ, PERIOD, TREAT, CARRY.
        CODES(SUBJ) = 1, 2, 3, 4.
        CODES(PERIOD) = 1, 2, 3, 4.
        CODES(TREAT) = 1, 2, 3, 4.
        CODES(CARRY) = 1, 2, 3, 4, 5.
/WEIGHTS    BETWEEN=EQUAL.
/END
  1  1  A  0  68
  1  2  B  A  74
  1  3  D  B  93
  1  4  C  D  94
  2  1  B  0  60
  2  2  C  B  66
```

(Continued)

TABLE 6.11

(Continued)

```
2  3  A  C  59
2  4  D  A  79
3  1  C  0  69
3  2  D  C  85
3  3  B  D  78
3  4  A  B  69
4  1  D  0  90
4  2  A  D  80
4  3  C  A  80
4  4  B  C  86
DESIGN   FACTOR = SUBJ, PERIOD, TREAT, CARRY.
      TYPE = BETWEEN.
      REGRESSION.
      PRINT./
ANALYSIS PROCEDURE = STRUCTURE.
      BFORM = 'SUBJ + PERIOD + TREAT + CARRY'.
      ESTIMATES./
END/
```

Source: Adapted from Edwards, L. K., & Bland, P. C. (1993). Some computer programs for selected ANOVA programs. In L. K. Edwards (Ed.), *Applied analysis of variance in behavioral science*. New York: Marcel Dekker, pp. 586-587, with the permission of the authors and editor.

The most important thing to know about typing this program is that, if the FORMAT line is exactly as shown, the beginning points and spacing of data lines beginning: 1 1 A 0 68 must be exactly as shown, with one space before the first entry and two spaces between each pair of entries. Suppose that you entitled this program **lat.bmd**. Then one way to run it would be to type: **bmdp** at the prompt for a computer having access to BMDP™ at the level where your program is located. Later, when asked for a BMDP™ program name, you would type **4v** at the prompt. Next, when asked for an instruction language file name, you would type **lat.bmd**. Finally, when asked for an output file name, you would type something like: **lat.out**. To retain all relevant information, you may want to print out both **lat.bmd** and **lat.out**.

This program yields correct values for a Latin square analysis of variance with carryover effects. Its last five sums of squares and associated tests on the last page of output are the most useful, with (for example) "S | P,T,C" signaling an analysis of subjects conditional (indicated by the vertical bar "|") on periods, treatments, and carryover, just as provided in a Type II analysis for SAS® GLM. However, BMDP™ is not very flexible for this kind of design and reports that it cannot estimate period and carryover effects. Estimated values for fixed subject and treatment effects seem to be based on sum-to-zero logic and thus are equal to those obtained with SYSTAT™. See Edwards and Bland (1993) for further discussion of this example and for further discussion of the logic justifying writing of the BMDP™ program just shown. The current BMDP™ manual (Dixon et al., 1990) will be useful for formatting rules and methods of using the program P4V. However, this manual will not help much to understand the use of BMDP™ for analyzing crossover design data.

Exercise 5 (A BMDP™ P4V Program for an A^3A^3 Versus A^3B^3 Design)

Try to write a BMDP™ P4V program program for the analysis of data from Table 6.7 based on the A^3A^3 versus A^3B^3 design of Table 6.6. Can you obtain the same analysis of variance table as shown in Table 6.8?

An SPSS® Program for Latin Square Data

We are finding that most programs can perform data analyses for crossover design experiments provided that appropriate care is taken in that programming. However, lack of full information about estimatibility in non-SAS® programs makes us believe that a model program in SAS® should be developed before other statistical packages are employed.

Here is a slight modification of an SPSS® MANOVA program presented by Edwards and Bland (1993) for the analysis of these data (see Table 6.12). You may want to run it yourself. If you have a menu-driven SPSS® system such as resides on a Power Macintosh computer or an IBM Windows machine, the procedure shown here will require expansion to keep it as a programming approach or adaptation to permit interactive control of the computational task. However, the same results for this data analysis should be obtained with any current SPSS® system.

TABLE 6.12

An SPSS® MANOVA Program for Analyzing the Data From Table 6.10

```
DATA LIST
/SUBJ 1–2 PERIOD 5 TREAT 8 (A) CARRYO 11 (A) Y 14–15.
BEGIN DATA.
 1 1 A 0 68
 1 2 B A 74
 1 3 D B 93
 1 4 C D 94
 2 1 B 0 60
 2 2 C B 66
 2 3 A C 59
 2 4 D A 79
 3 1 C 0 69
 3 2 D C 85
 3 3 B D 78
 3 4 A B 69
 4 1 D 0 90
 4 2 A D 80
 4 3 C A 80
 4 4 B C 86
END DATA.
RECODE  CARRYO('A'=1) ('B'=2) ('C'=3) ('D'=4) ('0'=5)
 INTO
 CARRY.
RECODE  TREAT('A'=1) ('B'=2) ('C'=3) ('D'=4)
 INTO
TREATMNT.
MANOVA  Y BY SUBJ,PERIOD,TREATMNT(1,4),CARRY(1,5)/
PRINT = CELLINFO(MEANS) PARAM(EST)/
 METHOD = SSTYPE(UNIQUE)/
 CONTRAST(PERIOD) = SPECIAL
 (1 1 1 1
  1 0 0 –1
  0 1 0 –1
```

(Continued)

TABLE 6.12
(Continued)

```
  0 0 1 –1)/
PARTITION(PERIOD) = (1,2)/
 CONTRAST(TREATMNT) = SPECIAL
 (1 1 1  1
  1 0 0 –1
  0 1 0 –1
  0 0 1 –1)/
 CONTRAST(CARRY) = SPECIAL
 (1 1 1 1  1
  1 0 0 0 –1
  0 1 0 0 –1
  0 0 1 0 –1
  0 0 0 1 –1)/
DESIGN = SUBJ VS RESIDUAL,
 PERIOD(1)  VS WITHIN,
 PERIOD(2)  VS RESIDUAL,
 CARRY VS RESIDUAL,
 TREATMNT VS RESIDUAL.
FINISH.
```

Source: Adapted from Edwards, L. K., & Bland, P. C. (1993). Some computer programs for selected ANOVA programs. In L. K. Edwards (Ed.), *Applied analysis of variance in behavioral science*. New York: Marcel Dekker, pp. 584-585, with the permission of the authors and editor.

Suppose that you entitled this program **lat.cmd**. Then, if your computer has access to SPSS® at the level where your program is stored, one way to run it would be to type: **spss lat.cmd** at the prompt. Next the SPSS® double window will appear, with the end of your program appearing in the bottom window. You can use the up arrow on your keyboard to move the cursor to the top line of the program and, if necessary, the left arrow to move it to the beginning of that line. Now you can press the esc key, release it, and press 0. Hit ENTER in response to a highlighted message: "run from Cursor". If properly typed in, the program should run and output should appear in the top window, where your activity is now moved. You can examine the output or error reports in lieu of output by using the up and down arrows on your keyboard as needed. To save the output, press esc again and then 9. The screen will give an option to write the file, so press ENTER. When asked for an output file name, type something like lat.out and press ENTER again. Leave SPSS® with esc and 0, choosing the option to exit.

Important considerations in typing this program are to type **CARRYO** (not **CARRY0**) and **TREATMNT** (not **TREATMENT**). Also be sure to use periods and slashes exactly where shown.

Notice that matrices in the CONTRAST sections of Table 6.12 reflect the set-to-zero nature of the SPSS® analysis procedure. For example, the contrast matrix for the four treatments has four rows standing for four "contrasts" and four columns standing for four treatment effects or τ_k values. We already know that in vector multiplication, one can cross-multiply the entries in a row of the matrix by the entries in a row vector of treatment parameters: $\tau_1 \ \tau_2 \ \tau_3 \ \tau_4$. For the vector multiplication involving the first row $(1 \ 1 \ 1 \ 1)$, we have $(1 \times \tau_1) + (1 \times \tau_2) + (1 \times \tau_3) + (1 \times \tau_4) = \tau_1 + \tau_2 + \tau_3 + \tau_4$, which is of little interest because the other three rows reflect all three degrees of freedom for treatments. More importantly, the vector multiplication for the second row uses $(1 \times \tau_1) + (0 \times \tau_2) + (0 \times \tau_3) + (-1 \times \tau_4) = \tau_1 - \tau_4$. Similarly, the third and fourth row processes yield $\tau_2 - \tau_4$ and $\tau_3 - \tau_4$, respectively, yielding three estimable parameter differences for treatments in the form implied by set-to-zero recoding. Similar reasoning applies to carryover and period estimation, with the provision that aliasing of Period 1 effects makes estimation of functions of it more complicated, leading to its PARTITION command as a way to separate Period 1 from other periods in the analysis.

This program yields correct values for a Latin square analysis of variance with carryover effects. Estimates of period, treatment, and carryover effects are the same as with SAS®, but fixed effect estimates of subject effects match SAS® only after taking into account sum-to-zero recoding comparable to that of SYSTAT™. Accordingly, SPSS® seems to employ both set-to-zero and sum-to-zero logic, depending on whether between subject effects are or are not involved! See Edwards and Bland (1993) for further discussion of this SPSS® program. Recent SPSS® manuals (Norusis, 1990a, 1990b) will be useful for formatting rules and methods of using this program as run in the all-purpose version as opposed to a pure PC version.

Exercise 6 (SPSS® Program for A^3A^3 Versus A^3B^3 Design)

Try to write an SPSS® program for the analysis of data from Table 6.6 based on the $A^3 A^3$ versus A^3B^3 design of Table 6.5. Can you obtain the same analysis of variance table as shown in Table 6.8? (Hints: Be sure that you understand when to put parentheses and what to include between them in various parts of a "MANOVA Y SUBJ ..." command. Also be sure that you know the meaning of the parenthesized numbers in a "PARTITION" command and how to select them.)

SYSTAT™ Programming for a Latin Square Design

A SYSTAT™ 4.0 Method

You may want to analyze the data of Table 6.10 as described here. Cotton (1993) has presented a SYSTAT™ 4.0 MGLH program for the analysis of these data. It is still useable with that variety of SYSTAT™, but a typographical error does exist in it: The MODEL statement requires the addition of a missing expression + SUBJ.

A SYSTAT™ 5.02 or 5.03 Data File and Method

If you have a newer IBM version (SYSTAT™ 5.02) or an IBM WINDOWS version (SYSTAT™ 5.03), you may want to make the SYSTAT™ data file or .SYS file (not an ASCII file!) represented in Table 6.13 and place it on a diskette on your A drive before running a slightly revised program necessitated by the upgrading of SYSTAT™. The following instructions apply directly to SYSTAT 5.02 but are easy to adapt by WINDOWS users: With SYSTAT 5.02 or 5.03, CARRY cannot be coded as 0 for Period 1; rather, it must be coded as the last carryover, 4 (or D), in the present example. This equating of Period 1 and Treatment D carryover is preferred by Ratkowsky, Evans, and Alldredge (1993) in order to facilitate contrast tests using an LSMEANS command not presented by us. Note that with SYSTAT™, as well as some other packages, it is convenient to use numerals 1 through 4 in place of letters A through D.

See Cotton (1993) for a discussion of the method of relating Latin square design parameter estimates using sum-to-zero recoding to estimates made with SAS® using set-to-zero recoding. Algebraic formulas permit calculating SAS® estimates from SYSTAT™ estimates and vice versa. Either is satisfactory so long as one is clear which recoding is employed. However, hypothesis testing sometimes yields different conclusions with the two methods.

TABLE 6.13

Entries in a SYSTAT™ 5.02 Data File (Named LAT5.02.SYS, for example) for the Latin Square Design and Data From Table 6.10

SUBJ	PERIOD	TREAT	CARRY	RESP
1	1	1	4	68
1	2	2	1	74
1	3	4	2	93
1	4	3	4	94
2	1	2	4	60
2	2	3	2	66
2	3	1	3	59
2	4	4	1	79
3	1	3	4	69
3	2	4	3	85
3	3	2	4	78
3	4	1	2	69
4	1	4	4	90
4	2	1	4	80
4	3	3	1	80
4	4	2	3	86

Source: Written using Table 6.10 information. Data from Cotton, J. W. (1993). Latin square designs. In L. K. Edwards (Ed.), *Applied analysis of variance in behavioral science*. New York: Marcel Dekker, p. 177, with the permission of the author and editor.

Commands for a SYSTAT™ 5.02 Analysis

To perform a SYSTAT™ 5.02 Latin square analysis of these data, follow the instructions in the table below, reflecting minor changes from the procedures employed with SYSTAT™ 4.0. They do not make a permanent program file but rather are used when they are typed and then disappear. Output files and printing procedures may be unique to your computer installation.

TABLE 6.14

Commands to Be Typed Into a Computer to Perform a SYSTAT™ 5.02
Analysis of the Latin Square Data of Table 6.10

Type in: **SYSTAT**
You will enter a menu-driven version of SYSTAT™. Feel free to use the menu if desired; the following instructions presume that you will disable the menu by accessing COMMANDS via UTILITIES and pressing ENTER when Menu On is displayed.

Type in: USE 'A:\ LAT502.SYS' followed by pressing ENTER.
Type in: MGLH followed by pressing ENTER.
Now you will see a ">" prompt from SYSTAT MGLH. Now give the commands, separated by **ENTER** commands:
CATEGORY SUBJ, PERIOD, TREAT, CARRY
MODEL RESP = CONSTANT + SUBJ + PERIOD + TREAT
    + CARRY
OUTPUT LAT.DAT
PRINT = LONG
ESTIMATE

This concludes one section of the analysis, but to get a proper test of period effects and leave SYSTAT™ you need to type in seven more lines of commands:

HYPOTHESIS
EFFECT = PERIOD
CONTRAST
0 1 –.5 –.5
0 0   .5 –.5
TEST

QUIT

Source: Program in Table 6.11 and seven additional lines adapted from Cotton, J. W. (1993). Latin square designs. In L. K. Edwards (Ed.), *Applied analysis of variance in behavioral science*. New York: Marcel Dekker, pp. 183-184, with the permission of the author and editor.

Note that the two lines of numbers following the CONTRAST command have a vector product of zero based on the vector multiplication operation defined in chapter 1 and illustrated in the previous SPSS®

example.   Therefore, two orthogonal 1-degree-of-freedom sums of squares are combined into the 2 df sum of squares desired for periods. This program yields correct values for a Latin square analysis of variance with carryover effects. See Cotton (1993) for further discussion of the SYSTAT™ analysis of these data. A SYSTAT™ manual (Wilkinson, 1989, or newer, such as for the SYSTAT 6.1 for Windows released in December, 1996) will be useful for formatting rules and methods of using this program. Note a related discussion and sample program (Wilkinson, 1989) in connection with the Williams data file provided by Wilkinson of an alternate analysis method (Cochran & Cox, 1957) for data from two Latin square designs with carryover effects in the model. It should run with SYSTAT™ 4.0 but not with SYSTAT™ 5.02 or 5.03.

Exercise 7 (Writing a SYSTAT™ Program for a Pretest–Posttest Control Group Design)

Try to write a SYSTAT™ MGLH program for the analysis of data from Table 6.6 based on the A^3A^3 versus A^3B^3 design of Table 6.5.   Can you obtain the same analysis of variance table as shown in Table 6.8? (Hint: How many lines of numbers do you need for the CONTRAST process?   How can you make all their vector products equal to zero?)

THINGS TO REMEMBER

Major Analysis Options

1. Using a SAS® GLM program to perform an analysis of covariance with data from a replicated 2-group, 2-phase design (pretest–posttest control group design) with members of one group receiving Treatment A in each phase and one group receiving Treatment A in Phase 1 and Treatment B in Phase 2 (A^1A^1 versus A^1B^1 design.) Testing effects of treatments on Phase 2 and also assessing predictability of performance on Phase 2 from performance on Phase 1.

2 Using a SAS® GLM program to perform an ANOVA of data from a replicated 2-group, 6-stage A^3A^3 versus A^3B^3 design testing differences among subjects and effects of stages, treatments, and carryovers.

3. Using SAS®, BMDP™, SPSS®, or SYSTAT™ to analyze data from an unreplicated 4 × 4 Latin square design with methods previously

discussed by Cotton (1993) and Edwards and Bland (1993). The analysis of variance breakdowns and estimated parameter values from these programs are or can be made comparable, except that BMDP™ gives no estimates for period and carryover effects. Estimability information in general seems more clear with SAS® than with other packages. Computation of variances of estimators in $\frac{\sigma^2}{n}$ terms or of corresponding efficiencies with BMDP™, SPSS®, and SYSTAT™ is not described.

Interpreting Results of Computational Methods Not Previously Discussed

A significant F for treatment effects in an analysis of covariance is interpreted as suggesting that mean performance differences between the treatment groups are not attributable to random sampling nor to pre-existing group differences in the predictor variable.

7

Switching Treatments in Blocks: $A^m A^m$, $A^m B^m$, $B^m A^m$, or $B^m B^m$ Patterns With m Stages

INTRODUCTION

The famous "Hawthorne effect" experiments, named for the Chicago area Hawthorne works of Western Electric Company where they were conducted, suggested beneficial effects on employee's work efficiency when there was an experimental change in the work environment. The authors of the report on this research (Roethlisberger & Dickson, 1939) found indications that almost any change led to increased work output, regardless of whether it could be interpreted as inherently helpful or pleasant. For example, in the so-called Illumination Studies of that series, decreasing room lighting from 10-foot candles in a control group to as low as 1-foot candle in an experimental group (or to .06-foot candles —like moonlight in an informal experiment) proved favorable! In another part of this series, the Relay Assembly Test Room Study, taking over a year to conduct, several variables were manipulated: the basis for determining a worker's wages, the length of the work day or work week, the length and timing of rest periods, and whether or not the employer provided lunch or something to drink. Productivity increased with most changes and did not drop when there was a change back to the original full work schedules without breaks or free lunches.

Later authors (Adair, 1984; Cook & Campbell, 1983) have suggested that the Hawthorne effect or effects are not as strong in the original article nor as reproducible as in textbook descriptions of them. If present they could also be attributed to one or more of a variety of variables such as (a) workers' interpretations of the changes supervisors were making, (b) special attention to experimental group members, and (c) a human need for varied experience (see psychological studies of sensory deprivation and of curiosity drive). Let us assume that there are some verifiable Hawthorne effects. We will focus on explanation (c). We might hypothesize that a need for varied experience could be satiated with extended fluctuation in conditions. Then the advantage of stimulus change in a factory environment would decline with extended experience of such changing patterns. So, there might be more beneficial effects of experimental changes in the work environment early in a study than later on. We could explore this hypothesis by looking for an interaction between stages and treatments but choose the related approach of looking for carryover effects from previous treatments.

A reasonable way to test this hypothesis is to make the following comparison at least twice, once early in an experiment and once later on: Compare Treatment A (4 weeks in a widget factory with stable work conditions throughout) to Treatment B (4 weeks in a widget factory with a different pattern of lighting, rest periods, and so on, from week to week). Let us call a 4-week period a month for convenience in discussion; this eliminates problems of comparing performance during months having different numbers of work days. Our experimental plan might be to use an $A^m A^m$ versus $A^m B^m$ versus $B^m A^m$ versus $B^m B^m$ design, with m being the number of "months" in a block of the experiment and a performance measure being taken at the end of every month. In its $m = 1$ form the statistical aspects of this kind of design have been studied by Balaam (1968) for whom it is now named, by Jones and Kenward (1989), and by Ratkowsky, Evans, and Alldredge (1993), among others.

METHOD A: ANALYZING DATA FROM AN AA VERSUS AB VERSUS BA VERSUS BB EXPERIMENT

Orientation

To make different measurements in any one month independent, we might like to perform an experiment in which we modify the Relay Assembly Test Room study design to use several identically treated work areas (rooms or even separate buildings or widget factories) and make the mean performance for a month by all workers in a work area be our basic measure. Instead of having subjects as our experimental unit, we have work areas or shops. It will be simple to say *Shop* or *Unit* rather than *Subject* throughout the rest of this chapter. Here is a more precise statement of the experimental design for such an experiment.

A Specific Experimental Design

For $n = 2$ work areas (shops or experimental units) in each treatment sequence group, we obtain the design in Table 7.1.

TABLE 7.1

A Design for Comparing Effects of AA, AB, BA, and BB Treatment Sequences

Sequence Group 1 (Shops 1 and 2)		
Stage 1	Stage 2	
A	A	
Sequence Group 2 (Shops 3 and 4)		
Stage 1	Stage 2	
A	B	
Sequence Group 3 (Shops 5 and 6)		
Stage 1	Stage 2	
B	A	
Sequence Group 4 (Shops 7 and 8)		
Stage 1	Stage 2	
B	B	

Notice that Group 1 members are tested under Treatment A twice and Group 4 members under Treatment B twice, but Group 2 members receive one test under Treatment A and then a test under Treatment B with Group 3 members being tested under both treatments once but in opposite order.

What Should We Try to Learn From Data Obtained With This Design?

1. Are there any significant differences in performance for different work areas or shops of this experiment?

2. Is there a change in performance as shops gain more practice with this task? So, we want to look for effects of the stage variable. (It turns out that this cannot be done unless carryover effects and their interactions with treatment effects are absent).

3. Are there different effects of different treatments?

TABLE 7.2
Number of Widgets Constructed for Two Shops Per Sequence Group
From a Hypothetical AA Versus AB Versus BA Versus BB Experiment

AA Sequence		AB Sequence			BA Sequence			BB Sequ		
Shop 2	Mean	Shop 3	Shop 4	Mean	Shop 5	Shop 6	Mean	Shop 7	Shop 8	N
45.7	43.750	41.8	45.5	43.650	55.0	56.9	55.950	55.0	57.3	5
52.6	49.650	56.6	58.6	57.600	46.0	43.7	44.850	52.4	52.9	5
49.150	46.700	49.200	52.050	50.625	50.500	50.300	50.400	53.700	55.100	5

an 45.475   Treatment B Mean 55.588

4. Is there a change in performance as a function of what treatment occurred on the previous stage (i.e., a carryover effect of previous treatments or even an interaction of treatment and carryover effects?) These effects are similar to an interaction of treatments and shops, so they could reflect changes in the effectiveness of treatments as the experiment progresses.

Hypothetical Data From an AA Versus AB Versus BA Versus BB Experiment

Here is a possible data set for the design just presented. Information is shown for each subject on each stage (see Table 7.2). Preliminary answers to the previous questions come from means displayed in or computable from this table: (1) Except in Treatment Sequence BA there is a substantial difference between performance of different units in the same treatment sequence group; (2) the Stage 2 data show a slightly higher mean than for Stage 1, suggesting improvement with practice; (3) the Treatment B data show a substantially higher mean than for Treatment A, suggesting improvement due to varying the working conditions during application of Treatment B; and (4) the mean Stage 2 performance for the AA and AB groups is 53.625 compared to the corresponding mean for the BA and BB groups of 48.750. This suggests that there is a larger carryover effect from Treatment A than from Treatment B. However, the corresponding Stage 2 mean difference between AB and AA is $57.6 - 49.65 = 7.95$, almost exactly the same as the $52.65 - 44.85 = 7.8$ difference between BB and BA. This suggests that there is no treatment by carryover interaction.

An Initial Model for Data From This Experiment

A more refined set of answers to the previous questions can be obtained by further analysis of the data in Table 7.2. One model for data from this design is closely allied to one of Kershner and Federer's (1981) general equations for two-treatment crossover designs:

$$Y_{ijk} = \mu + s_i + \pi_j + \tau_k + \lambda_{k'} + (\tau\lambda)_{kk'} + e_{ijk} \qquad (7.1)$$

where μ is an arbitrary constant, s_i is the random effect for Shop (experimental unit) i, π_j is the effect for Stage j, τ_k is the effect of Treatment k, $\lambda_{k'}$ is the carryover from Treatment k' on the previous stage,

$(\tau\lambda)_{kk'}$ is an interaction of Treatment k and carryover from k' effects, and e_{ijk} is random error for Shop i on Stage j with Treatment k.

A Possibly Relevant Computer Program

The SAS® GLM program of Table 7.3 is based on the model of Equation 7.1.

TABLE 7.3
A Possible Program for Analyzing Hypothetical Data
From Table 7.2

```
* PROGRAM BALAAM.SAS;
DATA WIDGET;
INPUT Y UNIT STAGE TREAT CARRY @@; CARDS
41.8 1 1 1 0        46.7 1 2 1 1        45.7 2 1 1 0        52.6 2 2 1 1
41.8 3 1 1 0        56.6 3 2 2 1        45.5 4 1 1 0        58.6 4 2 2 1
55.0 5 1 2 0        46.0 5 2 1 2        56.9 6 1 2 0        43.7 6 2 1 2
55.0 7 1 2 0        52.4 7 2 2 2        57.3 8 1 2 0        52.9 8 2 2 2
RUN ; PROC GLM;  CLASS UNIT STAGE TREAT CARRY;
MODEL Y = UNIT STAGE TREAT CARRY TREAT*CARRY/SOLUTION
E E2;
RANDOM UNIT;
ESTIMATE 'TREAT A – TREAT B' TREAT 1 –1 TREAT*CARRY 0 .5 .5 0
–.5 –.5;
ESTIMATE 'CARRY1 – CARRY2' CARRY 0 1 –1 TREAT*CARRY –1 1 0
1 0 –1;
ESTIMATE 'TREAT*CARRY' TREAT*CARRY 0 1 –1 0 –1 1;
TITLE 'BALAAM.SAS WITH CARRYOVERS AND DIRECT BY CARRY
INTERACTION.';
RUN;
```

This SAS® program is intended to use the same model employed by Jones and Kenward (1989) for a different data set. Units, our analogue of subjects, are the only random factors other than error. So, stages, treatments, carryovers, and any interactions among them have fixed effects. Inclusion of a treatment × carryover interaction is an attempt to expand the kinds of carryover that can be explored statistically. Use of "ESTIMATE" commands provides a supplement to the hypothesis testing with the "MODEL" statement. To obtain more satisfactory expected mean squares and estimation results (thus facilitating interpretation of hypothesis tests and parameter estimates), we perform Type II analyses instead of what appears to be a Type I analysis by Jones and Kenward. (Note that extra spacing between columns just before each Y is for ease of reading but does not affect the operation of this program.)

Difficulties Observed With Significance Tests Based on the Previous Program

Most output from the previous program is not shown here because so many difficulties arise when it is run. As expected from previous examples in which the first stage effect is contaminated by carryover effects, the two stage effects and even their difference are not estimable. Furthermore, Type II expected mean squares in the output include:

$$E(MS_{TREAT}) = Var(ERROR) + Q(TREAT, TREAT*CARRY) \text{ and}$$

$$E(MS_{CARRY}) = Var(ERROR) + Q(CARRY, TREAT*CARRY).$$

The Q terms of these equations tell us that we cannot estimate differences of TREAT or CARRY parameters separately from parameters of their interaction. Nonetheless, as in chapter 5 for factorial within-subject designs, it seems reasonable to see exactly what is estimable about these factors. (Obviously, the ESTIMATE commands in our program were based on estimability information from prior runs of the program.)

The nonzero part of the TYPE II Estimable Function output for treatments is as follows:

TREAT	1		L12
	2		–L12
TREAT*CARRY	1	0	0
	1	1	0.5*L12
	1	2	0.5*L12
	2	0	0
	2	1	–0.5*L12
	2	2	–0.5*L12

A similar examination of the TYPE II Estimable Function outputs for carryover and for treatment times carryover (not shown) tell us that the Table 7.3 ESTIMATE commands for "CARRY1 – CARRY2" and for "TREAT*CARRY" yield unbiased estimates of $\lambda_A - \lambda_B - (\tau\lambda)_{A0} + (\tau\lambda)_{A1} + (\tau\lambda)_{B0} - (\tau\lambda)_{B2}$ and $(\tau\lambda)_{A1} - (\tau\lambda)_{A2} - (\tau\lambda)_{B1} + (\tau\lambda)_{B2}$, respectively, with values 9.400 for the carryover term and –0.450 for the interaction term. The estimate of treatment effects could be taken as the basis for assessing an interpretable combined effect of treatment and interaction of treatment and carryover effects, just as main effects and interaction effects were combined in the main effects estimates and tests of the within-subjects factorial design of chapter 5. However, it is harder to justify estimating a combined effect of carryover and interaction of treatment and carryover that includes terms such as $(\tau\lambda)_{A0}$ and $(\tau\lambda)_{B0}$ because of our desire to exclude nonzero carryovers from Period 1 (λ_0).

Using a Revised Program to Test a Model Without Interaction

Because output from the data analysis based on the program of Table 7.3 would show no significance for interaction of treatment × carryover effects, we need a new model in which that factor is deleted:

$$Y_{ijk} = \mu + s_i + \pi_j + \tau_k + \lambda_{k'} + e_{ijk} \tag{7.2}$$

with all elements defined as before. This equation is the basis for the program of Table 7.4. As a consequence, we expect estimability to hold for subject, treatment, and carryover effects, but not for stage effects.

TABLE 7.4

Final Program for Analyzing Hypothetical Data From Table 7.2

```
PROGRAM BALAAM2.SAS;
DATA WIDGET; INPUT Y UNIT STAGE TREAT CARRY @@;  CARDS;
41.8 1 1 1 0      46.7 1 2 1 1      45.7 2 1 1 0      52.6 2 2 1 1
41.8 3 1 1 0      56.6 3 2 2 1      45.5 4 1 1 0      58.6 4 2 2 1
55.0 5 1 2 0      46.0 5 2 1 2      56.9 6 1 2 0      43.7 6 2 1 2
55.0 7 1 2 0      52.4 7 2 2 2      57.3 8 1 2 0      52.9 8 2 2 2
RUN ; PROC GLM;  CLASS UNIT STAGE TREAT CARRY;
MODEL Y = UNIT STAGE TREAT CARRY/SOLUTION E E2;
RANDOM UNIT; MEANS UNIT; MEANS STAGE; MEANS TREAT;
ESTIMATE 'TREAT A – TREAT B' TREAT 1 –1;
ESTIMATE 'CARRY1 – CARRY2' CARRY 0 1 –1;
TITLE 'BALAAM2.SAS WITHOUT DIRECT BY CARRY INTERACTION';
RUN;
```

Table 7.5 shows the results of the significance tests performed with the program of Table 7.4. There is no testable stage effect. However, shops, treatments, and carryover effects all show significant differences. Most of the relevant means associated with those differences were reported previously in Table 7.2. We report that $\hat{\tau_A} - \hat{\tau_B} = -7.825$ and $\hat{\lambda_1} - \hat{\lambda_2} = 9.400$.

TABLE 7.5
Type II ANOVA Table Obtained with Program of Table 7.4

Source	Sum of Squares	df	Mean Square	F
Shops (Units)	54.17	7	7.74	5.53*
Stages	—	0	—	—
Treatments	61.23	1	61.23	43.78**
Carryovers	44.18	1	44.18	31.59**
Error	6.99	5	1.40	—

Note. * $p < 0.05$.   ** $p < 0.01$.

Computing Efficiencies and Variances of Estimators for Parameter Differences in This Example

We remind ourselves that we are looking for the following quantity for each estimable parameter difference of interest in the present chapter:

$$Variance\ of\ Estimator\ in\ \frac{\sigma^2}{n}\ units = \Sigma\Sigma\ \alpha_{gj}^2 = \frac{n(s.e.[\hat{\theta}])^2}{MS_{error}} \qquad (7.3)$$

We also want to compute efficiencies of estimating those parameter differences using our earlier formula:

$$E\hat{\theta} = \frac{\left(\dfrac{200}{r*}\right)}{\dfrac{n(s.e.[\hat{\theta}])^2}{MS_{Error}}} \qquad (7.4)$$

with $r* = \frac{ps}{T}$ for treatments or carryover. No efficiency calculations are possible for stages, which are not estimable. This Balaam design has $n = 2$ shops per sequence, $s = 4$ sequences, $T = 2$ treatments, and $p = 2$ stages. The standard errors of estimate for parameter differences computed with the Table 7.4 program are shown in Table 7.6, together with computation of the dimensionless variances and efficiencies of the current design for estimating various differences among parameter values.

TABLE 7.6

Calculation of Efficiencies and Variances of Estimators
for Parameter Differences for an AA Versus AB Versus BA Versus BB Design,
Using Table 7.4 Program Output

	A = Standard Error of Estimate = s.e.e.	B = A² = Variance of Estimate	C = 2B/MSerror = nB/MSerrror = nB/D = $\sum \sum a_{gj}^2$ = Estimator Variance in multiples of $\dfrac{\sigma^2}{n}$	D = 200/r* = 200/(ps/T) = 200/4	Effi E =
	not estimable	—	—	—	—
3	1.18263477	1.398624999	2.0000	50.00	25.0
B	1.67249813	2.797249995	4.0000	50.00	12.5
				F = 1.398625	

Table 7.6 shows that this Balaam design using Equation 7.2 is not very efficient at all. It is most sensitive for estimating treatment effects and least sensitive for carryover effects. As mentioned earlier, stage effects cannot even be estimated with this design. Ratkowsky, Evans, and Alldredge (1993) have pointed out that, though the two-treatment Balaam design is by some criteria as efficient a crossover design as can be obtained for two treatments with only two stages, it is not a very useful design. In fact, two-stage crossover designs generally have a so-called Variance Inflation Factor (VIF) much larger than the 100% which would have indicated that the variance of an estimate of a treatment parameter was not increased by adding a carryover parameter to the model (Ratkowsky et al., 1993). Kershner and Federer (1981) warn that efficient crossover designs need to have more than two stages or periods, for example ABB for one sequence and BAA for another.

METHOD B: ANALYZING DATA
FROM THREE-STAGE BLOCKS:
A^3A^3, A^3B^3, B^3A^3, AND B^3B^3 SEQUENCES

Specific Experimental Design

Table 7.7 shows an expanded design with addition of two stages of identical treatments at each point in the original plan.

TABLE 7.7
An A^3A^3 Versus A^3B^3 Versus B^3A^3 Versus B^3B^3 Design With Two
Experimental Units (Shops) Per Treatment Sequence Group

	Phase 1			Phase 2		
	Stage 1	Stage 2	Stage 3	Stage 4	Stage 5	Stage 6
Sequence 1 Shops 1&2	A	A	A	A	A	A
Sequence 2 Shops 3&4	A	A	A	B	B	B
Sequence 3 Shops 5&6	B	B	B	A	A	A
Sequence 4 Shops 7&8	B	B	B	B	B	B

Now there are three stages like the original Stage 1 and three stages like the original Stage 2 of the previous experiment. Again, each of the four sequence groups includes two shops as experimental units.

Hypothetical Data for This Design

A possible set of data for this design appears in Table 7.8. Each score is the number of do-hickeys built in an experimental unit (a shop, do-hickey factory, or other work area) in a month.

Assessing the Findings of This Hypothetical Experiment

What Should We Try to Learn From Data Obtained With This Design?

1. Are there any significant differences in performance for different work areas (units) of this experiment?

2. Is there a change in performance as units gain more practice with this task? So, we want to look for effects of the stage variable.

3. Are there different effects of different treatments?

4. Is there a change in performance as a function of the current pair of treatments (immediately prior and current treatments)? These effects are similar to an interaction of treatments and stages, but they are more specific in their operation. The sum of squares for such an effect will be larger than the sum of squares for classical carryover like that in Equation 7.1, now including additional effects of prior and current treatments and having a larger number of degrees of freedom than before.

Preliminary answers to these questions come from means displayed or computable from Table 7.8: (a) There are noticeable differences in mean number of do-hickeys produced by different shops within each treatment sequence; (b) the mean number of do-hickeys produced declines from stage to stage, except for an increase on Stage 5; (c) there is an approximately 2.6 increase in number of do-hickey produced under Treatment B (changing conditions) than under Treatment A (constant conditions); and (d) the mean of nine stage means on an A stage following an A stage (an AA pair) is 48.533, the one stage mean for a B following an A (AB pair) is 52.150, the one stage mean under BA is 43.300, and the mean of nine stage means under BB is 47.844. Interactions among differences among these means as a function of prior and current treatments is suggestive of carryover differences but do not represent refined estimates of them.

TABLE 7.8
Hypothetical Data for an A^3A^3 Versus A^3B^3 Versus B^3A^3 Versus B^3B^3 Design With Two Shops Per Group

equence		A^3B^3 Sequence			B^3A^3 Sequence			B^3B^3 Sequence		
Shop 2	Mean	Shop 3	Shop 4	Mean	Shop 5	Shop 6	Mean	Shop 7	Shop 8	N
44.0	42.050	42.2	44.6	43.400	57.5	57.5	57.500	56.0	56.9	5
46.8	45.300	44.9	47.7	46.300	52.1	50.0	51.050	49.6	53.0	5
48.9	46.950	47.2	49.7	48.450	47.5	47.8	47.650	48.2	52.4	5
46.567	44.767	44.767	47.333	46.050	52.367	51.767	52.067	51.267	54.100	5
51.0	49.200	49.0	55.3	52.150	45.3	41.3	43.300	47.4	49.1	4
53.7	49.700	45.1	47.9	46.500	52.4	49.6	51.000	46.9	49.9	4

TABLE 7.8
(Continued)

51.2	48.800	**40.3**	**44.0**	42.150	**52.1**	**50.1**	51.100	**43.3**	**46.7**	4
51.967	49.233	44.800	49.067	46.933	49.933	47.000	48.467	45.867	48.567	4
49.267	47.000	44.783	48.200	46.492	51.150	49.383	50.267	48.567	51.333	4

an   47.129   Treatment B Mean 49.725

A Model Appropriate to the Present Experimental Design

The present design is complex enough to permit introducing a model in which there are more carryover parameters than before and in which treatment effects are not aliased with carryover as with Equation 7.1. A reasonable model for data from this design is given by Equation 7.5:

$$Y_{ijk} = \mu + s_i + \pi_j + \tau_k + \lambda_{k'k} + e_{ijk} \qquad (7.5)$$

with parameters defined as in Equation 7.1 except that, in place of separate terms for carryover and interaction of treatment and carryover, we now have a carryover expression $\lambda_{k'k}$ indexed on both the preceding and current treatments. Thus, there are four carryovers for the second stages of different two-stage patterns: λ_{AA} for an AA pattern, λ_{AB} for AB, λ_{BA} for BA, and λ_{BB} for BB (coded as 1, 2, 3, and 4 for λ_1, λ_2, λ_3, and λ_4, respectively, in the following computer program).

A SAS® GLM Program for Assessing Current Data

In our program for this study, the first stage of experimentation for any experimental unit (shop here) has a carryover coding of λ_0 as usual. Here is the program proposed for analyzing the data for this experiment (see Table 7.9):

Table 7.9

A Program for Analyzing Table 7.8 Data

From an A^3A^3 Versus A^3B^3 Versus B^3A^3 Versus B^3B^3 Design

---

```
* PROGRAM DOHICKEY.SAS; DATA DOHICKEY;
INPUT Y SHOP STAGE TREAT CARRY SEQ PHASE @ @; CARDS;
40.1 1 1 1 0 1 1        43.8 1 2 1 1 1 1        45.0 1 3 1 1 1 1
47.4 1 4 1 1 1 2        45.7 1 5 1 1 1 2        46.4 1 6 1 1 1 2
44.0 2 1 1 0 1 1        46.8 2 2 1 1 1 1        48.9 2 3 1 1 1 1
51.0 2 4 1 1 1 2        53.7 2 5 1 1 1 2        51.2 2 6 1 1 1 2
42.2 3 1 1 0 2 1        44.9 3 2 1 1 2 1        47.2 3 3 1 1 2 1
49.0 3 4 2 2 2 2        45.1 3 5 2 4 2 2        40.3 3 6 2 4 2 2
44.6 4 1 1 0 2 1        47.7 4 2 1 1 2 1        49.7 4 3 1 1 2 1
55.3 4 4 2 2 2 2        47.9 4 5 2 4 2 2        44.0 4 6 2 4 2 2
57.5 5 1 2 0 3 1        52.1 5 2 2 4 3 1        47.5 5 3 2 4 3 1
45.3 5 4 1 3 3 2        52.4 5 5 1 1 3 2        52.1 5 6 1 1 3 2
57.5 6 1 2 0 3 1        50.0 6 2 2 4 3 1        47.8 6 3 2 4 3 1
41.3 6 4 1 3 3 2        49.6 6 5 1 1 3 2        50.1 6 6 1 1 3 2
```
(Continued)

TABLE 7.9
(Continued)

```
56.0 7 1 2 0 4 1        49.6 7 2 2 4 4 1        48.2 7 3 2 4 4 1
47.4 7 4 2 4 4 2        46.9 7 5 2 4 4 2        43.3 7 6 2 4 4 2
56.9 8 1 2 0 4 1        53.0 8 2 2 4 4 1        52.4 8 3 2 4 4 1
49.1 8 4 2 4 4 2        49.9 8 5 2 4 4 2        46.7 8 6 2 4 4 2
RUN ; PROC GLM; CLASS SHOP STAGE TREAT CARRY;
MODEL Y = SHOP STAGE TREAT CARRY/SOLUTION E SS1 E2 SS3;
MEANS SHOP; MEANS STAGE; MEANS TREAT; RANDOM SHOP;
ESTIMATE 'STAGE2 – STAGE6' STAGE 0 1 0 0 0 –1;
ESTIMATE 'STAGE3 – STAGE6' STAGE 0 0 1 0 0 –1;
ESTIMATE 'STAGE4 – STAGE6' STAGE 0 0 0 1 0 –1;
ESTIMATE 'STAGE5 – STAGE6' STAGE 0 0 0 0 1 –1;
ESTIMATE 'TREAT A – TREAT B' TREAT 1 –1;
ESTIMATE 'CARRY AA – CARRY BB' CARRY 0 1 0 0 –1;
ESTIMATE 'CARRY AB – CARRY BB' CARRY 0 0 1 0 –1;
ESTIMATE 'CARRY BA – CARRY BB' CARRY 0 0 0 1 –1'
PROC MEANS; VAR Y; BY SEQ; PROC SORT; BY SEQ STAGE;
PROC MEANS; VAR Y; BY SEQ STAGE; PROC SORT; BY STAGE
TREAT;
PROC MEANS; VAR Y; BY STAGE TREAT; PROC SORT; BY PHASE
SEQ;
PROC MEANS; VAR Y; BY PHASE SEQ; PROC SORT; BY PHASE;
PROC MEANS; VAR Y; BY PHASE; PROC SORT; BY PHASE SHOP;
PROC MEANS; VAR Y; BY PHASE SHOP;
TITLE 'DOHICKEY.SAS FOR 6 TRIAL SEQUENCES A3A3,A3B3, B3A3,
B3B3'; RUN;
```

As usual, tests of hypotheses about families of parameters and specification of expected means squares and other estimability information
are evoked by the "MODEL" statement. Specific effects in the data are
pinpointed by the "ESTIMATE" commands just shown. The
"MEANS", "PROC MEANS", and "PROC SORT" commands in this
program are not essential to the estimation and significance testing procedure in it. However, they were helpful in providing means for Table
7.8, which in turn were useful in providing initial answers to questions
asked with this experiment.

ANOVA for the Current Dataset

Table 7.10 summarizes the Type II analysis of variance just performed; the Type I analysis appears in the output but can be ignored
here; the Type III significance tests also appear there and are identical to

those obtained with Type II.

TABLE 7.10

Type II ANOVA Table for the Do-Hickey Experiment

Source	Sum of Squares	df	Mean Square	F
Shops	224.31	7	32.04	8.52****
Stages 2:6	22.43	4	5.61	1.49
Treatments	164.16	1	164.16	43.66****
Carryover	418.05	3	139.35	37.06****
Error	116.57	31	3.76	—

Note. **** $p < 0.0001$.

This table indicates that all effects tested except for stages two through six are significant and that all significant effects reached the 0.0001 level.

Estimation of Effects

Estimability information and expected mean squares (not shown here) for our Type II analysis tell us that most parameter differences of interest are estimable. This means that our use of a SOLUTION option in the MODEL statement of the previous SAS® GLM program can be used to obtain those estimates. The same answers are given with our ESTIMATE commands, needed in the efficiency computations described next.

Significance values for individual parameter differences are reported both in SOLUTION and ESTIMATE output. Even though they yield identical results here, except when Stage 1 effects are involved, we know, and Searle (1987) warned readers, to be careful with the former. The estimates of Stage 2 – Stage 6 $(\pi_2 - \pi_6)$, Stage 3 – Stage 6 $(\pi_3 - \pi_6)$, Stage 4 – Stage 6 $(\pi_4 - \pi_6)$, and Stage 5 – Stage 6 effects $(\pi_5 - \pi_6)$ are 1.725, 1.575, 2.005, and 2.1375, respectively, with Stage 5 – Stage 6 having the only significance for stages, $t(31) = 2.20$, $p = 0.0350$.

The treatment effect is already known to be significant, with the estimate of Treatment A – Treatment B effect $(\tau_A - \tau_B)$ being –10.498. There are two separate significant carryover differences: Carry AA – Carry BB $(\lambda_{AA} - \lambda_{BB})$ estimated as 13.022 with $t(31) = 8.22$, $p =$

0.0001, and Carry AB – Carry BB ($\lambda_{AB} - \lambda_{BB}$) estimated as 6.702 with $t(31) = 3.50$, $p = 0.0014$. A nonsignificant estimate of Carry BA – Carry BB ($\lambda_{BA} - \lambda_{BB}$) is 4.150. Because the last two estimates are smaller than their predecessor, it seems that standing pat with AA has a greater effect relative to standing pat with BB than does any switching from one treatment to another.

Computing Efficiencies and Variances of Estimators for Specific Parameter Differences in This Example

The variance and efficiency definitions of (7.2) and (7.3) are used again, now with $n = 2$ shops per sequence, $p = 6$ stages, $s = 4$ sequences and $T = 2$ treatments. Associated formulas for replications yield $r* = s = 4$ for stages and $r* = \dfrac{ps}{T} = 12$ for treatments. For carryover, a more general formula from chapter 5 must be applied: $r* = \dfrac{ps}{no.\ levels} = 6$ because there are four levels of carryover, λ_{AA}, λ_{AB}, λ_{BA}, and λ_{BB}, rather than two levels as would be true with a classical carryover model. Table 7.11 presents the desired variances in $\dfrac{\sigma^2}{n}$ terms and uses them to yield corresponding efficiency values.

This table shows that the variances in $\dfrac{\sigma^2}{n}$ terms of parameter differences and efficiencies for the present design range from 0.5000 ($E = 100.00$) for several stage effect differences to 3.2833 ($E = 10.15$) for one of the carryover effect differences, with the efficiency of estimation of the treatment effect difference also being extremely small. By comparison to the AA versus AB versus BA versus BB Balaam design, this design has the advantages of permitting estimates of differences between stage effect and of lower variances (greater sensitivity) for treatment and carryover effect differences. But, much of the improvement must be due to use of more observations in the current design. Efficiency of estimating treatment effects has declined after changing to an A^3A^3 versus A^3B^3 versus B^3A^3 versus B^3B^3 design. However, the typical efficiency and richness of estimating carryover effects has improved with an increase in the number of them that can be estimated with the new design. Thus, $E = 12.50$ for Carry A – Carry B in Table 7.6, but the different carryover Es for the current design are 25.00, 17.09, and 10.15.

TABLE 7.11

ncies and Variances of Estimators of Parameter Differences for an A^3A^3 Versus A^3B^3 Versus B^3B^3 Design, Using Table 7.9 Output

	A = Standard Error of Estimate = s.e.e.	B = A^2 = Variance of Estimate	C = 2B/MSerror = n B/D= $\sum \sum a_{gj}^2$ = Estimator Variance in multiples of $\dfrac{\sigma^2}{n}$	r*	Effi $\dfrac{2}{r*\sum}$
ï,	0.96958245	0.940090127	0.5000	4	100.
ï	1.22643557	1.504144207	0.8000	4	62.5
}	1.58880964	2.524316072	1.3426	12	12.4
y	1.58332151	2.506907004	1.3333	6	25.0
y	1.91477192	3.666351506	1.9500	6	17.0
y	2.48460430	6.173258528	3.2833	6	10.1
		D = 3.7603605			

FINAL THOUGHTS

Obviously, an experimenter can employ any desired number m for every phase for each subject, producing an $A^m A^m$ versus $A^m B^m$ versus $B^m A^m$ versus $B^m B^m$ design. Our first example used $m = 1$, and our second example used $m = 3$. No new principles are invoked when using any other positive value of m.

THINGS TO REMEMBER

Major Analysis Options

1. Using a SAS® GLM program to perform an ANOVA of data from a Balaam design (replicated AA versus AB versus BA versus BB design) appropriate in looking for a "Hawthorne effect".

2. Using a SAS® GLM program to perform an ANOVA of data from an $A^3 A^3$ versus $A^3 B^3$ versus $B^3 A^3$ versus $B^3 B^3$ design.

3. Using SAS® GLM programs to compute the efficiency of the designs in #1 and #2.

Interpreting Results of Computational Methods Not Previously Discussed

1. With a model for the AA versus AB versus BA versus BB design including interaction of treatment and carryover effects as well as a carryover from an immediately prior treatment, there is the possibility of more complex carryover effects than discussed with previous experimental designs.

2. With a model for the $A^3 A^3$ versus $A^3 B^3$ versus $B^3 A^3$ versus $B^3 B^3$ design including four carryover parameters, one each as a function of all possible combinations of immediately prior and present treatments, there is the possibility of a refined analysis of carryover effects in complex designs. Carryover from A to B or from B to A may be thought of as a switching effect such as psychologists identify with transfer of training or changes in food reward in studies of animal motivation.

EXERCISES

1. Run each of the programs in this chapter to be sure you are comfortable with your computer's SAS® GLM facilities for these examples and that the programs yield the values previously reported. Delete E and E2 options and re-run the programs; you know what can be estimated properly.

2. Modify one of the examples in this chapter to have a different number of subjects per sequence group and change the relevant program as necessary to analyze the new set of hypothetical data.

3. Modify the second example in this chapter to have an A^2A^4 versus A^2B^4 versus B^2A^4 versus B^2B^4 design with two subjects per sequence group. Change the program slightly and run it again with the new example.

4. Suppose that you had included four sequence group parameters in Equation 7.2 for the second example in this chapter. Forgetting about all other parameters, what would this model predict for Stages 1, 2, and 3 for the A^3A^3 and A^3B^3 sequence groups? What does this tell you about the usefulness of sequence effects in a crossover design model?

8

Analyzing Data From Variants
of Alternating
Treatment Designs

INTRODUCTION

Sometimes a design with alternating treatments may be attractive for psychological reasons. For example, in their Experiment 1 with eight subjects, Ingham and Andrews (1973) studied two methods of therapy for stutterers. In Treatment A (token reward method), subjects were given tokens that had value like money for having a low or reduced percentage of stuttered syllables in a 45-minute therapy session. In Treatment B (token reward and penalty method), they were given tokens for appropriate speech behavior but lost tokens after an increased rate of stuttering. Ingham and Andrews alternated blocks of sessions with these two treatments in order to learn whether one reward structure led to superior performance compared to the other. Inspection of a graph of average performance in this experiment suggests that Treatment B was more effective than Treatment A in reducing stuttering.

A special reason for using an $A^8B^6A^4B^3$ pattern as Ingham and Andrews did (or, in general, an $A^{m1}B^{m2}A^{m3}B^{m4}$ alternation pattern) rather than a pattern such as $A^{10} B^{10}$ is that one can study effects of switching from one treatment to another more than once. Barlow and Hersen (1984) discussed a variety of other ABAB or $A^{m1}B^{m2}A^{m3}B^{m4}$ experiments, focusing on the interpretation of data from single subjects in them. Gentile, Roden, and Klein (1972) proposed a replicated two-way ANOVA procedure for analysis of group data from an $A^{m1}B^{m2}A^{m3}B^{m4}$ design. Here, subjects and treatments (A and B) were the main effects, with replications being observations for a given subject in a stated phase (e.g., A^{m1} of the experiment). In one of several follow-up articles in the originating journal, Hartmann (1974) warned of the possibility of failure of assumptions such as normality of error components, homogeneity of variance of error components, and independence of error components.

ANALYZING DATA FROM AN ABAB VERSUS BABA REVERSAL DESIGN

Orientation

Henceforth we always consider mirror-image pairs of treatment patterns, such as ABAB versus BABA. In this section of the chapter we require all m values to be 1 in the $A^{m1}B^{m2}A^{m3}B^{m4}$ and $B^{m1}A^{m2}B^{m3}A^{m4}$ designs under consideration; alternation or reversal of treatments then occurs after each stage of experimentation. We pay attention to the question of sphericity related to Hartman's second and third issues, leaving the question of normality for the reader to ponder. More importantly, before one can legitimately test for failures of the three assumptions just mentioned, we believe it vital to develop statistical models including more realistic components of the processes that may be taking place in ABAB versus BABA experiments and their variants.

A Model for Data From This Design

For example, with an ABAB versus BABA design for n subjects in each treatment sequence group, one might assume that the score for Subject i on Stage j with Treatment k and with Treatment k' on Stage $j - 1$, called Y_{ijk}, is

$$Y_{ijk} = \mu + s_i + \pi_j + \tau_k + \lambda_{k'} + e_{ijk} \tag{8.1}$$

where μ is an additive constant, s_i is a random effect for Subject i, π_j is the effect of Stage j, τ_k is the effect of Treatment k, $\lambda_{k'}$ is the carryover effect from previous treatment k', and e_{ijk} is the random error component for Subject i, Stage j, and Treatment k. From Cochran and Cox (1957) we learn that this design may first have been called a "reversal" or "switchback" design. Distributional assumptions for this model will additionally be made comparable to those in earlier chapters, yielding multisample sphericity. However, note a relaxation of those assumptions when Method B is invoked.

Hypothetical Data for a Dual Balanced ABAB Versus BABA Design

Using models in the spirit of Equation 8.1, Jones and Kenward (1989) consider such treatment sequences as ABA and BAB which are mirror images of each other. If an equal number of subjects, n, receives each of these treatment sequences, we know that the overall mirror-image design is a dual balanced design, with excellent properties under certain models of behavior. Let us consider a pair of sequences for a 4-stage balanced design, ABAB and BABA. The data presented in Table 8.1 are intended to be similar to what Ingham and Andrews (1973) might have obtained with only this specific design.

TABLE 8.1

Hypothetical Data for a Dual Balanced Design Using ABAB and BABA Sequences With Four Subjects per Sequence

ABAB Sequence	Stage and Treatment				Mean for One or More
Subject	1 (A)	2 (B)	3 (A)	4 (B)	Subjects
1	14.0	11.5	12.8	9.9	12.05
2	12.9	11.1	10.9	8.9	10.95
3	15.6	12.9	12.1	11.2	12.95
4	13.8	11.4	11.5	9.8	11.62
Stage Mean for ABAB Seq.	14.08	11.72	11.82	9.95	11.89

BABA Sequence	Stage and Treatment				
Subject	1 (B)	2 (A)	3 (B)	4 (A)	Mean
5	12.5	11.3	10.6	10.8	11.30
6	14.1	13.4	12.7	11.2	12.85
7	12.3	12.6	10.5	9.1	11.12
8	13.6	11.3	11.9	10.7	11.88
Stage Mean for BABA Seq.	13.12	12.15	11.42	10.45	11.79
Stage Mean	13.60	11.94	11.62	10.20	11.84
Treatment Mean		12.125 (A) 11.556 (B)			

Method A: ANOVA for Data From an ABAB Versus BABA Design

A Relevant Computer Program

Here is a SAS® PROC GLM program for analyzing the data presented on the previous page. Notice the inclusion in Table 8.2 of the "proc sort" and "proc means" commands to facilitate computation of means related to sequences in the experiment. Overall means for subjects, stages, and treatments can be computed with the "means" command inside "proc glm" because subjects and treatments are included in the model. However, because sequences are not included in the model, separate procedures were needed to sort and find means for them.

TABLE 8.2

A Program For Analyzing Hypothetical Data From an ABAB
Versus BABA Reversal Design Taking Into Account
Possible Time-Related Effects

```
* PROGRAM ABAB.SAS;
data speak; input seq subj stage treat  $ carry $ y @@; cards;
1 1 1 A 0 14.0    1 1 2 B A 11.5    1 1 3 A B 12.8    1 1 4 B A   9.9
1 2 1 A 0 12.9    1 2 2 B A 11.1    1 2 3 A B 10.9    1 2 4 B A   8.9
1 3 1 A 0 15.6    1 3 2 B A 12.9    1 3 3 A B 12.1    1 3 4 B A 11.2
1 4 1 A 0 13.8    1 4 2 B A 11.4    1 4 3 A B 11.5    1 4 4 B A   9.8
2 5 1 B 0 12.5    2 5 2 A B 11.3    2 5 3 B A 10.6    2 5 4 A B 10.8
2 6 1 B 0 14.1    2 6 2 A B 13.4    2 6 3 B A 12.7    2 6 4 A B 11.2
2 7 1 B 0 12.3    2 7 2 A B 12.6    2 7 3 B A 10.5    2 7 4 A B   9.1
2 8 1 B 0 13.6    2 8 2 A B 11.3    2 8 3 B A 11.9    2 8 4 A B 10.7
run; proc glm; class subj stage carry treat;
model y = subj treat stage carry/c1 c2 ss3 ss4 solution; random subj;
estimate 'stage2 – stage3' stage 0 1  0 –1;
estimate 'stage3 – stage4' stage 0 0 1 –1;
estimate 'treat A – treat B' treat 1 –1;
estimate 'carry A – carry B' carry 0 1 –1;
means subj; means stage; means treat;
proc sort; by seq stage;
proc means; var y; by seq; proc means; by seq stage;
title 'ABAB vs. BABA design data. ABAB.SAS with carryovers.';run;
```

Significance Test Results Based on the Aforementioned Program

Running this program yields the makings of Table 8.3 next, which makes it clear that subjects and stages exhibit significant differences in performance and that carryover effects are not significant. Treatment effects are significant ($p < 0.05$) with Type I analysis and approach significance with the Type II analysis.

TABLE 8.3

ANOVA Results Based on Hypothetical Data for an ABAB Versus
BABA Design With Four Subjects Per Sequence of Treatments

Type I

Source	Sum of Squares	df	Mean Square	F
Subjects	15.75	7	2.25	6.95***
Treatments	2.59	1	2.59	8.00*
Stages 1:4	46.74	3	15.58	48.15****
Carryovers	0.30	1	0.30	0.93
Error	6.15	19	0.32	—

Type II
(Numbers given are also equal to Type III and IV resuls in this case)

Source	Sum of Squares	df	Mean Square	F
Subjects	15.67	7	2.24	6.92***
Treatments	1.40	1	1.40	4.33†
Stages 2:4	13.73	2	6.86	21.21****
Carryovers	0.30	1	0.30	0.93
Error	6.15	19	0.32	—

Note. † $p = 0.0513$. * $p < 0.05$. ** $p < 0.01$. *** $p < 0.001$.

**** $p < 0.0001$.

Because the Type I expected mean square for treatments is $\sigma^2 +$ Q(TREAT,CARRY), rather the the $\sigma^2 +$ Q(TREAT) associated with a Type II analysis, there is possible contamination of treatments and carryovers in the Type I analysis of treatment effects. However, because carryover effects were not significant in either analysis, it seems reasonable to trust the Type I conclusion that treatment effects are significant (higher mean for A than for B) even though the Type II analysis does not quite reach statistical significance. This conclusion is confirmed if one reruns the program of Table 8.2 with carryover effects omitted from the model being tested.

Estimation of Effects

The output giving "Estimate" values, usually labeled "B" for Bias, may be interpreted once we know the output from our E2 option in the MODEL statement. Except for random subject effects, estimates are the same with any type number of analysis. However, what is estimated with a certain reported estimation depends on what parameters are present in the model. For the current analysis, E2 estimability information and related output shows that $\tau_A - \tau_B$ or TREAT A – TREAT B is estimable as the difference between 0.98125 for TREAT A and 0.00000 for Treat B, yielding a rounded 0.981 as the amount Y should be greater under Treatment A than under Treatment B, all other factors being held constant. Similarly, $\pi_j - \pi_4$ = STAGE j – STAGE 4 is estimable as the difference between biased estimates of STAGE j and STAGE 4 provided that $j > 1$. This causes us to estimate $\pi_2 - \pi_4$ as 1.738 and $\pi_3 - \pi_4$ as 1.425.

What we do about estimation for nonsignificant effects depends on our purpose. We say fairly casually that we believe CARRY A – CARRY B is zero because of this nonsignificance. But, if we want to make a predicted value for each observation based on the original model (Equation 8.1), we can use a "P" option in our "MODEL" statement of Table 8.2. Such predictions use all estimated parameter functions, even including nonsignificant ones. Therefore, CARRY A – CARRY B is treated as having the value 0.550 implied by both the SOLUTION and the ESTIMATE aspects of our program. Alternatively, this nonsignificance could be used to justify redoing the analysis with carryovers omitted, getting new estimates of treatment effects and stage effects, and even estimating $\pi_1 - \pi_4$ = STAGE 1 – STAGE 4. In that case there would be a 3 df (numerator) F-test of stage effects comparable to that of the Type I analysis just seen.

The Type II expected mean square for subjects printed in our output is Var(Error) + 3.8095 Var(SUBJ) and the expected mean square for error is Var(Error). So we can subtract one mean square from the other (using less rounding than in Table 8.3) to get:

MS(Subjects) – MS(Error) = 2.2385 – .3236

$$= 1.9149$$

$$\approx Var(Error) + 3.8095 \, Var(SUBJ) - Var(Error)$$

$$= 3.8095 \, Var(SUBJ)$$

Therefore our estimate of $Var(SUBJ)$ is [MS(Subjects) –

MS(Error)]/3.8095 = 1.9149/3.8095 = 0.5027.

Testing These Data for Multigroup Sphericity and Performing Follow-Up Analyses

The methods of chapters 3 and 5 could be employed here to test each treatment-sequence group for sphericity (but too few subjects are available here as well), to test different groups' covariance matrices of estimated error components for inequality, and to perform an overall test of sphericity (discussed later) for the pooled covariance matrix of such components. Use of a saturated crossover design model with the same covariance structure as that for the repeated measurements model used in sphericity tests might be useful in performing conservative tests, just as in chapter 3, provided that the data appeared not to satisfy the sphericity assumption. If sphericity holds with the repeated measurements model and, thus, with the comparable saturated model as well, it also holds with Equation 8.1. This is because sphericity is a property of the observed scores rather than of elements contributing to them in a certain model.

Measuring Efficiencies and Variances in $\frac{\sigma^2}{n}$ Units of Estimates of Parameter Differences for the ABAB Versus BABA Switching Design

Our earlier method of computing variances in $\frac{\sigma^2}{n}$ units of estimates of differences between parameters can be employed here, with an extension to permit comparison of results from sum-to-zero and set-to-zero reparameterizations. Later, we discuss efficiency calculations separately. Table 8.4 shows the results of the former set of calculations, based on $n = 4$ subjects per sequence, s = 2 sequences, $p = 4$ stages, and $T = 2$ treatments:

TABLE 8.4

Dimensionless Variances of Estimated Parameter Functions for the ABAB Versus BABA Design

Estimator Variance of Effects in Multiples of $\dfrac{\sigma^2}{n}$ $= \Sigma\Sigma a_{gj}^2 = \dfrac{n(s.e.e.[\hat{\theta}])^2}{MS_{error}}$ (Set-to-Zero Model or Sum-to-Zero Model estimating difference between parameters)	Estimator Variance of Effects in Multiples of $\dfrac{\sigma^2}{n}$ $= \Sigma\Sigma w_{gj}^2$ (Sum-to-Zero Model estimating half the difference between parameters)	$s\Sigma\Sigma a_{gj}^2$ for (Set-to-Zero
1.0000	0.2500	2.000
2.7500	0.6875	5.500
4.0000	1.0000	8.000

Interpretation of this table requires an elaboration of earlier remarks about estimation procedures. The treatment effect difference for two treatments may be called $\tau_A - \tau_B$; and a corresponding centered treatment effect may be called $\tau^* = \tau_A^* = \tau_A - \bar{\tau} = 0.5(\tau_A - \tau_B)$. The latter has a counterpart of $-\tau^* = \tau_B^* = \tau_B - \bar{\tau} = -0.5(\tau_A - \tau_B)$, with $\tau_A^* + \tau_B^* = 0$. Note, however, that the difference of centered treatment effects is equal to the difference of uncentered effects: $\tau_A^* - \tau_B^* = \tau_A - \tau_B$. Set-to-zero analyses often focus on the estimation of quantities such as $\tau_A - \tau_B$. Sum-to-zero models often focus on the estimation of quantities such as $\tau^* = \tau_A^* = \tau_A - \bar{\tau} = 0.5(\tau_A - \tau_B)$. However, they sometimes emphasize the estimation of quantities such as $\tau_A - \tau_B$. Clearly the variance of an estimator differs depending on which quantity is estimated.

Given the previous paragraph, Table 8.4 takes into account the fact that SAS® GLM and Kershner and Federer (1981) each seemed to focus on estimation of the difference between parameters, employing set-to-zero reparameterization in each case. In contrast, Jones and Kenward (1989) seemed to employ sum-to-zero reparameterization and focus on estimation of half the parameter difference with this and some other examples. As mentioned in chapter 5, if it were necessary for clarity, different symbols could be used for the latter weights in order to distinguish them from the a_{gj} values we have been using for the former.

In this table variances of treatment effect and carryover effect estimates for the sum-to-zero model (with estimation of half the difference between parameters) exactly match Jones and Kenward's (1989) entries for Design 4.2.2 for treatment effects adjusted for carryover effects and carryover effects adjusted for treatment effects. Also the variances of set-to-zero model estimates match SAS® GLM results and the $s\Sigma\Sigma a_{gj}^2$ values for $s = 2$ and treatments or carryovers are exactly those given in Kershner and Federer's (1981) survey of two-treatment crossover designs.

Both sources show that the current design is much less sensitive than several other two-treatment, four-stage designs, and we see from Table 8.4 that, except for stage effect differences with a set-to-zero dimensionless variance of 1.0000, these dimensionless variances are discouragingly high compared with those in previous chapters. These results for treatment and carryover effects probably reflect in part the problem of variance inflation in this design to be discussed in the next section.

We can now compute efficiencies of estimating those parameter differences using our earlier formula:

$$E\hat{\theta} = \frac{\left(\dfrac{200}{r*}\right)}{\dfrac{n(s.e.e.[\hat{\theta}])^2}{MS_{Error}}} \tag{8.2}$$

with a denominator value from the second column of Table 8.4, with $r* = \dfrac{ps}{T} = 4$ for treatments or carryover and $r* = s = 2$ for stages.

Table 8.5 shows maximal efficiency for estimating stage effects but very small effiencies for estimating treatment and carryover effects.

TABLE 8.5
Calculation of Efficiencies of Estimators for Parameter
Differences for an ABAB Versus BABA Switching Design
From the Set-to-Zero Results of Table 8.4

Kind of Effects	$A = \sum\sum a_{kj}^2$ = Estimator Variance in multiples of $\dfrac{\sigma^2}{n}$	$B = 200/r*$	Efficiency = $E = B/A$
Stage 2 – Stage 4 or Stage 3 – Stage 4	1.0000	100.00	100.00
Treat A – Treat B	2.7500	50.00	18.18
Carry A – Carry B	4.0000	50.00	12.50

One way of interpreting the results in Table 8.5 is to say that the structure of this design makes it hard to separate treatment effects from carryover effects. For example, with the current switching design employing ABAB versus BABA patterns, we can easily see dependence between treatment and carryover effects: On any stage except Stage 1, Treatment A implies occurrence of Carryover B on the same stage, and Treatment B implies occurrence of Carryover A. This suggests that separating treatment and carryover effects will be difficult with this design. See Ratkowsky, Evans, and Alldredge (1993) for a detailed attempt to quantify the degree to which these effects can be separated in various experimental designs. Fortunately, if the model for the current design can properly be simplified to eliminate carryover effects, it is easy to show then that efficiency of estimating treatment effects becomes 100, the maximum possible. In such cases, the ABAB versus BABA design becomes quite attractive.

Method B: Using Contrasts in Analyzing Data From a Dual Balanced ABAB Versus BABA Design

A Computer Program for Generating Contrasts

This method is based on methods in Jones and Kenward (1989) for two-group dual designs. The basic idea is to find a contrast for each subject for each single parameter or parameter difference to be assessed. Typically each contrast is biased, but the mean difference between different sequence groups for a given contrast is unbiased. The distributional assumptions associated with the model of Equation 8.1 are sufficient but not necessary to justify the analysis method given next. It is enough to assume that each contrast is randomly selected from a population of normally distributed contrasts; if the contrasts for two sequence-treatment groups being compared have the same population variances, a t-statistic can be evaluated in the usual fashion. Otherwise, a so-called Satterthwaite correction provided by SAS® PROC TTEST can be employed.

Because a primarily SAS®-based book is desired, we compute contrasts here in an indirect way compared to that of Jones and Kenward. Ideally, we might not use SAS® for computing contrasts because SAS® has to approach those calculations indirectly and uses a main program that would be much too bulky if the sample size were large. See chapter 12 and Appendix 2 of this volume for an introduction to non-SAS® methods. However, with a fairly small number of subjects, the following procedure is useable:

First, we can find from output of the ABAB.SAS program in Table 8.2 what linear combinations of parameters are estimable. Second, for each subject we need to generate contrasts that are also estimates for each interesting estimable parameter function identified in the previous program. This is performed in a SAS® GLM program to be presented shortly. Finally, these contrasts are included in a later SAS® program in order to test significance for each of the interesting functions just given. This program called SAS® PROC TTEST, is not a GLM program, for it computes t-tests rather than directly employing the General Linear Model to perform analyses of variance or other forms of regression analysis calculating F ratios rather than the closely related t-tests of PROC TTEST.

Generating Contrasts to Estimate Certain Parameter Functions. Now we begin a new SAS® GLM program by writing a data step involving one subject from the first sequence and one from the second sequence, using input like that of Table 8.2. But, we assign scores of zero for all scores in the first sequence in order to make the output reflect only one subject's data. For the present data set, this yields an input section like the one shown in Table 8.6.

TABLE 8.6

First Input Section for a Program Generating Contrasts for Table 8.1 Data

---

```
input subj stage treat $ carry $ y @@; cards;
1 1 A 0    0     1 2 B A    0     1 3 A B    0     1 4 B A    0
5 1 B 0 12.5    5 2 A B 11.3     5 3 B A 10.6     5 4 A B 10.8
run;
```

With appropriate ancillary programming, this section of our program will yield contrasts for treatment, stage, and carryover effects for the first subject of Sequence 2, Subject 5, forming the data step called "data speak1" in our program. Similar work yields such contrasts for each other subject in that sequence. This yields 4 datasteps, ending in "data speak4" and each being followed by appropriate additional programming to compute one contrast for each estimable stage, treatment, or carryover effect.

To find contrasts for the 4 subjects in the first sequence, we do a similar set of 4 analyses with two-line data inputs having zero for every stage of a Sequence 2 subject, followed by programming needed for computing contrasts like those computed for Sequence 1 subjects. The end product of this programming is to produce Table 8.7.

TABLE 8.7
A Program Computing Contrasts Related
to the Hypothetical Speech Therapy Data of Table 8.1

```
* PROGRAM ABABCONT.SAS;
data speak1; input subj stage treat  $ carry y @@; cards;
1 1 A 0    0      1 2 B A    0      1 3 A B    0      1 4 B A    0
5 1 B 0 12.5      5 2 A B 11.3      5 3 B A 10.6      5 4 A B 10.8
run ; proc glm; class subj stage carry treat;
model y = subj treat stage carry/solution;
title 'ABAB vs BABA design data. ABABCONT.SAS with all factors.';
title2 'See Jones and Kenward, pp. 179–180, re efficiency and contrasts.';
title3 'Subjects 1 and 5 with zeroes on S1.';
data speak2; input subj stage treat  $ carry y @@; cards;
2 1 A 0    0      2 2 B A    0      2 3 A B    0      2 4 B A    0
6 1 B 0 14.1      6 2 A B 13.4      6 3 B A 12.7      6 4 A B 11.2
run ; proc glm; class subj stage carry treat;
model y = subj treat stage carry/solution;
title 'Subjects 2 and 6 with zeroes on S2.';
data speak3; input subj stage treat  $ carry y @@; cards;
3 1 A 0    0      3 2 B A    0      3 3 A B    0      3 4 B A    0
7 1 B 0 12.3      7 2 A B 12.6      7 3 B A 10.5      7 4 A B 9.1
run ; proc glm; class subj stage carry treat;
model y = subj treat stage carry/solution;
title 'Subjects 3 and 7 with zeroes on S3.';
data speak4; input subj stage treat  $ carry y @@; cards;
4 1 A 0  0      4 2 B A    0      4 3 A B    0      4 4 B A    0
8 1 B 0 13.6      8 2 A  B 11.3      8 3 B A 11.9      8 4 A B 10.7
run ; proc glm; class subj stage carry treat; model y = subj treat stage
carry/solution; title 'Subjects 4 and 8 with zeroes on S4.';
data speak5; input subj stage treat  $ carry y @@; cards;
1 1 A 0 14.0      1 2 B A 11.5      1 3 A B 12.8      1 4 B A 9.9
5 1 B 0    0      5 2 A B    0      5 3 B A    0      5 4 A B    0
run ; proc glm; class subj stage carry treat;
model y = subj treat stage carry/solution;
title 'S1 and S5 with zeroes on S5.';
data speak6; input subj stage treat  $ carry y @@; cards;
2 1 A 0 12.9      2 2 B A 11.1      2 3 A B 10.9      2 4 B A 8.9
6 1 B 0    0      6 2 A B    0      6 3 B A    0      6 4 A B    0
run; proc glm; class subj stage carry treat;
model y = subj treat stage carry/solution; title 'S2 and S6 with zeroes on S6.';
```

(Continued)

TABLE 8.7
(Continued)

```
data speak7; input subj stage treat  $ carry y @ @; cards;
3 1 A 0 15.6      3 2 B A 12.9      3 3 A B 12.1      3 4 B A 11.2
7 1 B 0    0      7 2 A B    0      7 3 B A    0      7 4 A B    0
run; proc glm; class subj stage carry treat;
model y = subj treat stage carry/solution;
title 'S3 and S7 with zeroes on S7.';
data speak8; input subj stage treat  $ carry y @ @; cards;
4 1 A 0 13.8      4 2 B A 11.4      4 3 A B 11.5      4 4 B A 9.8
8 1 B 0    0      8 2 A B    0      8 3 B A    0      8 4 A B    0
run ;
proc glm; class subj stage carry treat;
model y = subj treat stage carry/solution;
title 'S4 and S8 with zeroes on S8.'; run ;
```

A Computer Program for Using Previously Computed Contrasts in Significance Testing

The approach being used here is not original. However, it can be very convenient because it permits 4 t-tests to be conducted in a computer program with only one action line (a "proc", a "class" statement, and labeling of variables in a "var" statement) once a simple data step has been defined. The SOLUTION segments of the program just shown generate estimates such as TREAT A: -1.67500000 B and TREAT B: 0.00000000 B, which imply a (biased) contrast for TREAT A – TREAT B $= \tau_A - \tau_B$ of -1.675 for Subject 5 with "data speak1." Such biased estimates for treatments, stages, and first-order carryovers are noted in the output from this program and inserted in the t-test program shown next.

Our t-test procedure is set up to use differences between means of two groups; we want the total of means for our groups, these totals being unbiased, as it turns out. As the title lines of this program say, we have entered the negative of each Sequence Group 2 score in Table 8.8. This is consistent with the following argument: The arbitrary quantity, $X_1 - (-X_2)$, is surely equal to $X_1 + X_2$, justifying a t-test involving values of the former quantity as a way to assess significance of means of the latter quantity.

TABLE 8.8

A Program for Computing *t*-tests for Contrasts of Interest
in the Data Set of Table 8.1

```
* PROGRAM ababt_tst.sas;
data speak; input seq tauA_B pi2_4 pi3_4 laA_B @ @; cards;
1  2.250    .800    1.450    1.200    2  1.675    -.250    .100    1.900
1  2.450   1.100    1.000    2.000    2  1.600   -1.100   -.750    1.400
1  3.525    .850     .450    3.500    2  1.625   -1.750   -.700    1.800
1  2.750    .800     .850    2.300    2  2.150    -.300   -.600    1.700
run; proc ttest; class seq; var tauA_B pi2_4 pi3_4 laA_B;
title 'BEWARE: Sequence 2 estimates are the negative of true';
title2 'ones. This permits automatic calculation of t values.'; run ;
```

This program distinguishes group membership by which sequence is involved ("class seq;") and the different variables for which *t*-tests are required by a "var" command ("var tauA_B pi2_4 pi3_4 laA_B;").

Significance Test Results Based on the Aforementioned Program

The results of running this program are shown in Table 8.9.

TABLE 8.9

Summary of *t*-tests for Contrasts of Interest in the Data Set of Table 8.1

Contrast for:	Seq 1 Mean	Seq 2 Mean[+]	Mean Diff = Estimator	t	df [‡‡]
Treat A – Treat B	2.7440	1.7630	0.981	3.18*	6.0
Stage 2 – Stage 4	0.8875	–0.8500	1.738	4.76*	3.2
Stage 3 – Stage 4	0.9375	–0.4875	1.425	4.98**	6.0
Carry A – Carry B	2.2500	1.7000	0.550	1.12	3.3

Note. [†] Sequence 2 means are the negative of actual contrasts in order to facilitate use of *t*-tests on mean contrasts across all sequences and subjects. [‡] Fractional degrees of freedom appear when there is significant heterogeneity of variance for contrasts of the two sequence groups. * $p < 0.05$.   ** $p < 0.01$.

Table 8.9 shows significant treatment, Stage 2 – Stage 4, and Stage 3 – Stage 4 effects, suggesting that $\tau_A - \tau_B$, $\pi_2 - \pi_4$, and $\pi_3 - \pi_4$ are non-zero. However, there is not a significant carryover effect.

Comparison of Significance Tests With Methods A and B

The results just given are almost consistent with conclusions drawn from the Type II analysis of Table 8.3, which did not assess contrasts directly. The one discrepancy is that treatment effects earlier had been almost significant rather than clearly significant at the 0.05 level or better: When one compares the Type II F-values of Table 8.3 for the 1 df tests (treatment and carryover) to squared t-values based on Table 8.9, one finds $F = 4.33$ and $t^2 = 10.11$ for treatments, with $F = 0.93$ and $t^2 = 1.25$ for carryover. There is enough discrepancy between these two results to ask which method is preferable. We note first that exactly the same (OLS) parameter estimates are given with the two methods; only the estimates of variance differ. In cases of nonsphericity, Maxwell (1980) and Boik (1981) favored contrast effect t-tests with a separate estimate of variance of parameter differences for each contrast. See also Crowder and Hand (1990), who considered analysis of variance methods somewhat like that here to be based on estimating variance of an estimator from the average of variances of estimators of all possible differences between pairs of effects such as Stage 1 – Stage 2, Stage 1 – Stage 3, Stage 1 – Stage 4, Stage 2 – Stage 3, and so on. They view Rouanet and Lepine (1970) as acceptant of this approach.

In the present situation where sphericity appears to hold, there is little theoretical reason to prefer one method over the other. Method B (the contrast method) cannot be used unless there are replications of each different sequence. With this replication in dual balanced designs such as the present one, we advocate use of the Method B because of its simplicity. This is especially appropriate if the methods of Appendix 2 are employed in place of the present somewhat unwieldy SAS® procedure for generating contrasts.

This table does not provide an omnibus test for assessing differences among more than two stages. However, a reasonable multivariate test procedure using the repeated measurments options in SAS® is available and will now be presented.

Method C: A Multivariate Test Procedure for Stage Effects

We now perform a familiar SAS® GLM repeated measurements analysis whose primary purpose is to provide a global test of stage effects without assuming sphericity. Table 8.10 presents a program intended to do this for Stages 2 through 4, ignoring Stage 1 because of previously noted problems in comparing a stage without carryover to stages that all have the same carryover, on the average (see Table 8.10).

TABLE 8.10

A Repeated Measurement Program for a Multivariate Analysis
of Possible Stage Effects in Hypothetical Data
From an ABAB Versus BABA Reversal Design

```
* PROGRAM ABABREP3.SAS;
data speak; input seq y1 y2 y3 y4; cards;
1 14.0 11.5 12.8  9.9
1 12.9 11.1 10.9  8.9
1 15.6 12.9 12.1 11.2
1 13.8 11.4 11.5  9.8
2 12.5 11.3 10.6 10.8
2 14.1 13.4 12.7 11.2
2 12.3 12.6 10.5  9.1
2 13.6 11.3 11.9 10.7
run; proc glm; class seq; model y2-y4 = seq/nouni; repeated stage/printe;
title 'ABAB vs BABA repeated measures ANOVA for 3 stages:
    ABABREP3.SAS'; run;
```

This program compares only Stages 2 through 4; if one could justify a comparison of performance on all four stages, one would simply change the "model" statement to include "y1–y4" rather than the present "y2–y4". An overall sphericity test from this analysis suggests that multivariate testing of stage effects is not necessary: The χ^2 statistic associated with Mauchly's criterion when applied to orthogonal components is only 0.41, which with 2 df has a significance level of 0.82, far from conventional standards. Furthermore, the Geisser-Greenhouse (G-G) and Huynh-Feldt (H-F) ε values are 0.9276 and 1.5490, suggesting no need to correct for nonsphericity.

The multivariate test of effects in this program that is most relevant to the model of (8.1) is the test of stage effects. Regardless of which of three underlying statistics is computed, it leads to $F = 13.73$ for 2 and 12 df, with $p < 0.01$, confirming the Type II assessment of stage efffects in Table 8.3, but with somewhat less significance than before. Presumably this reflects greater sensitivity because of the exclusion of treatment and carryover effects from the error mean square in Table 8.3.

ANALYZING DATA FROM A MORE GENERAL
DESIGN: $A^{m1}B^{m2}A^{m3}B^{m4}$ VERSUS $B^{m1}A^{m2}B^{m3}A^{m4}$

Method D: Contrast Analysis Method for a Specific Design

Hypothetical Data and a Computer Program
for Generating Contrasts

Let us modify the dataset in Table 8.1 to be a bit more similar to data from Ingham and Andrews (1973), but to use $m = 4$ for every stage rather than the varied values already noted for that study. To keep our programs brief, only two subjects will be used in each sequence such as $A^4B^4A^4B^4$. The contrasts method (Method B) will be adapted for use with the current design; it can easily be extended to an $A^{m1}B^{m2}A^{m3}B^{m4}$ versus $B^{m1}A^{m2}B^{m3}A^{m4}$ design with different values of m_1, m_2, m_3, and m_4. Table 8.11 shows possible data for this experiment.

TABLE 8.11

Hypothetical Data From an $A^4B^4A^4B^4$ Versus $B^4A^4B^4A^4$
Design With Two Subjects per Sequence

Sequence	Sequence 1				Sequence 2			
Subject	S1	S2	Mean		S3	S4	Mean	Grand Mean
Stage and Treatment				Stage and Treatment				
1 A	14.0	12.9	13.45	1 B	12.5	14.1	13.30	13.38
2 A	14.2	13.0	13.60	2 B	11.9	13.6	12.75	13.18
3 A	12.9	12.2	12.55	3 B	11.4	13.6	12.50	12.52
4 A	13.8	12.1	12.95	4 B	11.2	13.9	12.55	12.75
Phase Mean	13.72	12.55	13.14	Phase Mean	11.75	13.80	12.78	12.96
5 B	11.5	11.1	11.30	5 A	11.3	13.4	12.35	11.82
6 B	11.1	10.9	11.00	6 A	13.1	14.1	13.60	12.30
7 B	11.7	10.6	11.15	7 A	11.6	13.7	12.65	11.90
8 B	11.6	10.8	11.20	8 A	12.2	14.0	13.10	12.15
							(Continued)	

TABLE 8.11
(Continued)

Sequence	Sequence 1			Sequence 2			
Subject	S1	S2	Mean	S3	S4	Mean	Grand Mean
Stage and Treatment				Stage and Treatment			
Phase Mean	11.48	10.85	11.16	Phase Mean	12.05	13.80	12.92	12.04
9 A	12.8	10.9	11.85	9 B	10.6	12.7	11.65	11.75
10 A	13.5	12.2	12.85	10 B	9.8	12.9	11.35	12.10
11 A	13.7	11.3	12.50	11 B	10.2	13.0	11.60	12.05
12 A	13.0	10.9	11.95	12 B	10.6	13.2	11.90	11.92
Phase Mean	13.25	11.32	12.29	Phase Mean	10.30	12.95	11.62	11.96
13 B	9.9	8.9	9.40	13 A	10.8	11.2	11.00	10.20
14 B	10.1	9.3	9.70	14 A	11.1	12.8	11.95	10.82
15 B	10.6	9.7	10.15	15 A	11.5	10.7	11.10	10.62
16 B	10.4	9.5	9.95	16 A	11.3	11.2	11.25	10.60
Phase Mean	10.25	9.35	9.80	Phase Mean	11.18	11.48	11.32	10.56
Subject Mean	12.18	11.02	11.60	Subject Mean	11.32	13.01	12.16	11.88
Treatment Mean	A (Token Reward)			B (Token Reward & Penalty) 11.34			
	12.42						

The Model on Which This Analysis is Based

Now we use the fact that four patterns of successive treatment pairs occur within a subject: AA, AB, BA, and BB. Carryovers have been coded carry = 1 for a carryover from A to A (λ_{AA}), 2 for going from A to B (λ_{AB}), 3 for B to A (λ_{BA}), and 4 for B to B (λ_{BB}) in order to allow for such possibilities as that carryover is different from A to A (no change in treatment from previous stage to current stage) than from A to B (change). As before, the carryover on Stage 1 is always coded as 0. Now the model for our observations is:

$$Y_{ijk} = \mu + s_i + \pi_j + \tau_k + \lambda_{k'k} + e_{ijk} \qquad (8.3)$$

where all parameters are defined as for Equation 8.1 except that we have a parameter $\lambda_{k'k}$ which is the carryover effect from a previous treatment k' to the current treatment k.

A Computational Strategy for Finding and Using Contrasts

First, we must run a SAS® GLM program for a model with sequence effects but no intercept μ in order to be able to learn what linear combinations of other parameters are estimable. This changes (8.3) to:

$$Y_{gijk} = \alpha_g + s_i + \pi_j + \tau_k + \lambda_{k'k} + e_{ijk} \qquad (8.4)$$

where α_g specifies a sequence g effect and all other symbols are interpretable from earlier models. Although (8.3) is our prime interest and would give reasonable results about estimability, this approach is better because it coordinates theory and the separate contrast formulas for subjects in different sequence groups. Rather than performing an analysis of variance like that of Table 8.2 before calculating contrasts, we use a related analysis of variance program solely for the purpose of determining what is estimable.

Checking Estimability With a Sequence Effects Model Program With No Intercept. Table 8.12 is the SAS® GLM program needed to check estimability in the situation just described; related text coordinates its contents with theory for the current dataset (see Table 8.12).

TABLE 8.12

Determining Estimability of Linear Combinations of Parameters
of Equation 8.4

```
* PROGRAM ABABM_NO.SAS
data speak2; input subj stage treat $ carry y seq  @@; cards;
1   1 A 0 14.0 1      1   2 A 1 14.2 1      1   3 A 1 12.9 1      1   4 A 1 13.8 1
1   5 B 2 11.5 1      1   6 B 4 11.1 1      1   7 B 4 11.7 1      1   8 B 4 11.6 1
1   9 A 3 12.8 1      1  10 A 1 13.5 1      1  11 A 1 13.7 1      1  12 A 1 13.0 1
1  13 B 2  9.9 1      1  14 B 4 10.1 1      1  15 B 4 10.6 1      1  16 B 4 10.4 1
2   1 A 0 12.9 1      2   2 A 1 13.0 1      2   3 A 1 12.2 1      2   4 A 1 12.1 1
2   5 B 2 11.1 1      2   6 B 4 10.9 1      2   7 B 4 10.6 1      2   8 B 4 10.8 1
                                                              (Continued)
```

TABLE 8.12
(Continued)

```
2  9 A 3 10.9 1    2 10 A 1 12.2 1    2 11 A 1 11.3 1    2 12 A 1  10.9 1
2 13 B 2  8.9 1    2 14 B 4  9.3 1    2 15 B 4  9.7 1    2 16 B 4   9.5 1
3  1 B 0 12.5 2    3  2 B 4 11.9 2    3  3 B 4 11.4 2    3  4 B 4  11.2 2
3  5 A 3 11.3 2    3  6 A 1 13.1 2    3  7 A 1 11.6 2    3  8 A 1  12.2 2
3  9 B 2 10.6 2    3 10 B 4  9.8 2    3 11 B 4 10.2 2    3 12 B 4  10.6 2
3 13 A 3 10.8 2    3 14 A 1 11.1 2    3 15 A 1 11.5 2    3 16 A 1  11.3 2
4  1 B 0 14.1 2    4  2 B 4 13.6 2    4  3 B 4 13.6 2    4  4 B 4  13.9 2
4  5 A 3 13.4 2    4  6 A 1 14.1 2    4  7 A 1 13.7 2    4  8 A 1  14.0 2
4  9 B 2 12.7 2    4 10 B 4 12.9 2    4 11 B 4 13.0 2    4 12 B 4  13.2 2
4 13 A 3 11.2 2    4 14 A 1 12.8 2    4 15 A 1 10.7 2    4 16 A 1  11.2 2
run; proc glm; class subj stage carry treat seq;
model y = seq subj treat stage carry/e noint;
title 'ABABM_NO.SAS – no intercept model.'; run;
```

Because of the E option in its MODEL command, this program provides a listing of the General Form of Estimable Functions. The only surprises appear in the sections on STAGE and CARRY:

	Effect	Coefficients
STAGE	5	L13
	9	L17
	13	L21
	16	L1+L2–L9–L10–L11–L12–L13–L14–L15–L16
		–L17–L18–L19–L20–L21–L22–L23
CARRY	0	L9
	1	L26
	2	L27
	3	L13+L17+L21–L27
	4	L1+L2–L9–L13–L17–L21–L26

First, consider the available information from setting L13 = 1 and all other coefficients = 0, all L13 values of the total program output being present in the previous listings. We find that STAGE 5 – STAGE 16 + CARRY 3 – CARRY 4 is estimable. Similarly, setting L17 = 1 and all others = 0 shows that STAGE 9 – STAGE 16 + CARRY 3 – CARRY 4 is estimable. Also, setting L21 = 1 and all others = 0 shows that STAGE 13 – STAGE 16 + CARRY 3 – CARRY 4 is estimable.

Because estimating combinations of stage and carryover effects is not satisfying, we settle for estimating two linear functions of these three estimable quantities. Algebraically, the difference between the first and third estimable quantities is STAGE 5 – STAGE 13. Similarly, the difference between the second and third estimable quantities is STAGE 9 – STAGE 13. Therefore, those two differences are also estimable and will be assessed by appropriate contrasts and t-tests.

Second, consider the case in which L26 = 1 and all else = 0. The previous listings imply that for the current model CARRY 1 – CARRY 4 is estimable. Similarly, if L27 = 1 and all else = 0, we see that CARRY 2 – CARRY 3 is estimable. Therefore, those two quantities will be assessed by appropriate contrasts and t-tests.

Notice that Type I and III ANOVAs are performed with the previous program. We do not discuss them now because of our preference for t-tests based on contrasts.

Computing Contrasts for the Present Data Set. Next, for each subject we need to generate contrasts that are also estimates for each interesting estimable parameter function identified in the previous program. This is performed in the SAS® GLM program of Table 8.13. Just as in an earlier ABAB versus BABA design example, Table 8.7, one ANOVA is run for each subject. In order to trick SAS®, we have each separate ANOVA subprogram analyze the 16 scores for one subject in one sequence group compared to 16 artificial zero scores for a subject in the other sequence group. This permits the SOLUTION option for the MODEL command to compute our desired contrasts (see Table 8.13).

TABLE 8.13

A Program Computing Contrasts Related to the
Hypothetical Speech Therapy Data of Table 8.11

```
* PROGRAM ING_CONT.SAS;
data nspeak1; input subj stage treat $ carry y @@; cards;
1   1 A 0   0      1   2 A 1   0      1   3 A 1   0      1   4 A 1   0
1   5 B 2   0      1   6 B 4   0      1   7 B 4   0      1   8 B 4   0
1   9 A 3   0      1  10 A 1   0      1  11 A 1   0      1  12 A 1   0
1  13 B 2   0      1  14 B 4   0      1  15 B 4   0      1  16 B 4   0
3   1 B 0  12.5    3   2 B 4  11.9    3   3 B 4  11.4    3   4 B 4  11.2
3   5 A 3  11.3    3   6 A 1  13.1    3   7 A 1  11.6    3   8 A 1  12.2
3   9 B 2  10.6    3  10 B 4   9.8    3  11 B 4  10.2    3  12 B 4  10.6
3  13 A 3  10.8    3  14 A 1  11.1    3  15 A 1  11.5    3  16 A 1  11.3
run; proc glm; class subj stage carry treat;
model y = subj treat stage carry/solution;
title 'A4B4A4B4 vs. B4A4B4A4 design data. ING_CONT.SAS for contrasts.';
```
                                                        (Continued)

TABLE 8.13
(Continued)

---

title2 'Subjects 1 and 3 with zeroes on S1';
data nspeak2; input subj stage treat $ carry y @@; cards;

2	1 A 0	0	2	2 A 1	0	2	3 A 1	0	2	4 A 1	0
2	5 B 2	0	2	6 B 4	0	2	7 B 4	0	2	8 B 4	0
2	9 A 3	0	2	10 A 1	0	2	11 A 1	0	2	12 A 1	0
2	13 B 2	0	2	14 B 4	0	2	15 B 4	0	2	16 B 4	0
4	1 B 0	14.1	4	2 B 4	13.6	4	3 B 4	13.6	4	4 B 4	13.9
4	5 A 3	13.4	4	6 A 1	14.1	4	7 A 1	13.7	4	8 A 1	14.0
4	9 B 2	12.7	4	10 B 4	12.9	4	11 B 4	13.0	4	12 B 4	13.2
4	13 A 3	11.2	4	14 A 1	12.8	4	15 A 1	10.7	4	16 A 1	11.2

run ; proc glm; class subj stage carry treat;
model y = subj treat stage carry/solution;, ,
title 'A4B4A4B4 vs. B4A4B4A4 design data. ING_CONT.SAS for con-'
trasts.';
title2 'Subjects 2 and 4 with zeroes on S2'; run;
data nspeak3; input subj stage treat $ carry y @@; cards;

1	1 A 0	14.0	1	2 A 1	14.2	1	3 A 1	12.9	1	4 A 1	13.8
1	5 B 2	11.5	1	6 B 4	11.1	1	7 B 4	11.7	1	8 B 4	11.6
1	9 A 3	12.8	1	10 A 1	13.5	1	11 A 1	13.7	1	12 A 1	13.0
1	13 B 2	9.9	1	14 B 4	10.1	1	15 B 4	10.6	1	16 B 4	10.6
3	1 B 0	0	3	2 B 4	0	3	3 B 4	0	3	4 B 4	0
3	5 A 3	0	3	6 A 1	0	3	7 A 1	0	3	8 A 1	0
3	9 B 2	0	3	10 B 4	0	3	11 B 4	0	3	12 B 4	0
3	13 A 3	0	3	14 A 1	0	3	15 A 1	0	3	16 A 1	0

run ; proc glm; class subj stage carry treat;
model y = subj treat stage carry/solution;
title 'A4B4A4B4 vs. B4A4B4A4 design data. ING_CONT.SAS for contrasts.';
title2 'Subjects 1 and 3 with zeroes on S3'; run;
data nspeak4; input subj stage treat $ carry y @@; cards;

2	1 A 0	12.9	2	2 A 1	13.0	2	3 A 1	12.2	2	4 A 1	12.1
2	5 B 2	11.1	2	6 B 4	10.9	2	7 B 4	10.6	2	8 B 4	10.8
2	9 A 3	10.9	2	10 A 1	12.2	2	11 A 1	11.3	2	12 A 1	10.9
2	13 B 2	8.9	2	14 B 4	9.3	2	15 B 4	9.7	2	16 B 4	9.5
4	1 B 0	0	4	2 B 4	0	4	3 B 4	0	4	4 B 4	0
4	5 A 3	0	4	6 A 1	0	4	7 A 1	0	4	8 A 1	0
4	9 B 2	0	4	10 B 4	0	4	11 B 4	0	4	12 B 4	0
4	13 A 3	0	4	14 A 1	0	4	15 A 1	0	4	16 A 1	0

run ; proc glm; class subj stage carry treat;
model y = subj treat stage carry/solution;
title 'A4B4A4B4 vs. B4A4B4A4 design data. ING_CONT.SAS for contrasts.';
title2 'Subjects 2 and 4 with zeroes on S4'; run ;

Table 8.13 differs from Table 8.7 mainly in the presence of 16 observations per subject rather than 4, making a great deal of data available for estimating contrasts for each subject of the current experiment.

Performing t-Tests With Contrasts for the Present Data Set

Most contrasts needed for these *t*-tests come directly from the "Estimate" Column immediately after the *F*-tests for a specific ANOVA subprogram. For example, TREAT A – TREAT B for Subject 1 in Sequence 1 comes from the third subprogram and has the rounded value $1.855 - 0 = 1.855$. However, STAGE 5 – STAGE 13 = $-0.17196970 - (-0.97196970) = 0.800$ and STAGE 9 – STAGE 13 = $0.47803030 - (-0.97196970) = 1.450$ for that subject because of previous information about the General Form of Estimable Functions. Similarly, for that subject we estimate CARRY 1 – CARRY 4 = $-0.57121212 - 0 = -0.571$, estimating $\lambda_{AA} - \lambda_{BB}$, and CARRY 2 – CARRY 3 = (CARRY 2 – CARRY 4) – (CARRY 3 – CARRY 4) = $0.67272727 - 0 = 0.673$, estimating $\lambda_{AB} - \lambda_{BA}$.

Finally, under the assumption of random sampling from each population of contrasts employed, these contrasts are included in a SAS® PROC TTEST program in order to test significance for each interesting function just shown. The program in Table 8.13 collects estimates for each subject in its DATA step, labeling estimates of treatment effect differences with tau_AB for $\tau_A - \tau_B$, stage differences as in pi2_16 for $\pi_2 - \pi_{16}$, and carryover differences as in lAA_BB for $\lambda_{AA} - \lambda_{BB}$. Otherwise, this program takes the same basic approach to computation of *t*-tests as in our Method B example (see Table 8.14).

Table 8.15 presents the results of the *t*-tests just performed, showing a significant treatment and an almost significant Stage 6 – Stage 16 effect difference. Carryover and other stage differences are not significant. Because we are testing hypotheses about contrasts between parameters, no assumption of sphericity needs to be made or tested. Notice that estimators appear in this table, with $\hat{\tau}_A - \hat{\tau}_B = 0.706$ and $\hat{\pi}_6 - \hat{\pi}_{16} = 1.650$ being the values for those effects that approach significance.

One might want to perform an omnibus *F*-test for stage effects like that programmed in Table 8.10. Instead of comparing 16 stages, however, we are forced by the estimability information leading to the *t*-tests to compare no more than 12 stages at a time: all but Stages 1, 5, 9, and 13. Hence, we can test H: μ_j = constant for all *j* except 1, 5, 9, and 13; equivalently, we can test H: π_j = constant for all *j* except 1, 5, 9, and 13. Univariate and multivariate tests of this hypothesis can both be per-

TABLE 8.14
A Program for Computing *t*-tests for Contrasts of Interest
in the Data Set of Table 8.11

```
ıg_t-tst.sas; data nspeak;
B pi2_16 pi3_16 pi4_16 pi5_13 pi6_16 pi7_16 pi8_16
pi11_16 pi12_16 pi14_16 pi15_16 lAA_BB lAB_BA; cards;
   1.800        1.150        1.600        0.800        0.250        0.550
   1.450        1.550        1.200       -0.250        0.000       -0.571
   1.750        1.350        1.300        1.100        0.700        0.550
   1.350        0.900        0.700       -0.100        0.100       -1.058
  -0.300       -0.050        0.050       -0.250       -0.900       -0.150
   0.750        0.550        0.350        0.100       -0.100       -1.741
  -1.200       -1.200       -1.350       -1.100       -1.450       -1.250
  -0.850       -0.900       -1.000       -0.800        0.250       -0.835
class seq; var tau_AB pi2_16 pi3_16 pi4_16 pi5_13 pi6_16
i9_13 pi10_16 pi11_16 pi12_16 pi14_16 pi15_16 lAA_BB lAB_BA;
 Sequence 2 estimates are the negative of true';
ıs permits automatic calculation of t values.'; run ;
```

TABLE 8.15

Summary of t-tests for Contrasts of Interest in the Data Set Just Given

Sequence 1 Mean	Sequence 2 Mean†	Mean Diff = Estimator
1.9105	1.2045	0.706
1.7750	-0.7500	2.525
1.2500	-0.6250	1.875
1.4500	-0.6500	2.100
0.9500	-0.6750	1.625
0.4750	-1.1750	1.650
0.5500	-0.7000	1.250
0.5750	-0.9250	1.500
1.2250	-0.3250	1.550
1.4000	-0.0500	1.450
1.2250	-0.1750	1.400
0.9500	-0.3250	1.275
-0.1750	-0.3500	0.175
0.0500	0.0750	-0.025
-0.8145	-1.2880	0.4735
1.0140	1.0730	-0.059

re the negative of actual contrasts in order to facilitate use of t-tests on mean contrasts across all sequence:
vhen there is significant (p < 0.10) heterogeneity of variance for contrasts of the two sequence groups. * p
d deviation for Sequence Group 1 is zero.

formed by a SAS® GLM program with REPEATED option similar to that of Table 8.10 but modeling data for all but Stages 1, 5, 9, and 13 rather than for Stages 2, 3 and 4 as in that table.

Efficiency of Estimating Stage, Treatment, and Carryover Effects in an $A^4B^4A^4B^4$ Versus $B^4A^4B^4A^4$ Design

Table 8.16 presents the results of our efficiency analysis for the current design. Computational details need not be illustrated because no new principles are invoked. Regrettably, the efficiency of this design for anything except estimation of stage effect differences is even lower than with the ABAB versus BABA design whose efficiencies were reported in Table 8.5.

TABLE 8.16
Dimensionless Variances of Estimators and Their Efficiency
With an $A^4B^4A^4B^4$ Versus $B^4A^4B^4A^4$ Design
and the Model of Equation 8.3

Kind of Effects	$\sum \sum a_{gj}^2 =$ Estimator Variance in multiples of $\dfrac{\sigma^2}{n}$	Efficiency = E
Stage 2 – Stage 16 or other estimable stage difference	1.00	100.00
Treat A – Treat B	2.14	5.84
Carry AA – Carry BB	2.30	5.43
Carry AB – Carry BA	2.91	4.30

FINAL THOUGHTS

An alternate approach to the analysis of data from reversal designs with more than one successive stage on a single treatment would be patterned after Wallenstein and Fisher's (1977) approach to the $A^m B^m$ versus $B^m A^m$ design, treating an A^m or B^m unit as an A or B phase and the m stages within a phase as times, with phases and times becoming a 2-way factorial structure within subjects. We prefer the present approach because of possible stage effects throughout the entire experiment rather than simply within phases.

THINGS TO REMEMBER

Major Analysis Options for Reversal (Switching) Designs

1. For data from a replicated ABAB versus BABA design one option is to perform an ANOVA based on a model including subject, treatment, stage, carryover, and error effects and assuming a spherical covariance structure.

2. Because the current experimental design is a dual-balanced one, it is possible to use a different analysis method that does not assume sphericity of the raw scores. First, one computes contrasts for each subject for appropriate parameters, such as treatment effect difference $\tau_A - \tau_B$ and carryover effect difference $\lambda_A - \lambda_B$. Then, one computes mean contrasts and t-values across treatment-sequence groups in order to establish the apparent size and statistical significance of each statistic. For a family of more than two parameters such as for four stages, an overall test using contrasts is not feasible. However, a univariate (under sphericity) or multivariate overall test comparing all or almost all of the stages may be possible under appropriate assumptions.

3. Methods in Points 1 and 2 are easily adapted to other reversal designs such as $A^4 B^4 A^4 B^4$ versus $B^4 A^4 B^4 A^4$.

Interpreting Results of Computational Methods Not Previously Discussed

1. A SAS® PROC GLM program to generate contrasts for each individual subject in a dual-balanced experiment leads to one contrast for each subject for each parameter or parameter difference to be estimated (e.g., $\tau_A - \tau_B$, $\pi_2 - \pi_4$, $\pi_3 - \pi_4$, and $\lambda_A - \lambda_B$ for the ABAB versus BABA design). The investigator needs to be able to write an appropriate program to generate such contrasts and another to compute t-tests for

assessing the significance of each such effect. A sign change in one set of estimates is essential to proper significance testing.

2. Determination of what effects can be estimated may require use of a model and computer program without an intercept, as in (8.4) and Table 8.12, where this permits separate estimation of sequence effects rather than of an intercept plus a difference between sequence effects. A "noint" option in the "model" statement of this table is used for this purpose. Note from Appendix 2 that the inclusion of sequence effects in this model is an act of convenience needed to facilitate data analysis despite not being needed for the psychological understanding of the data.

EXERCISES

1. Run the SAS® programs in this chapter. Do you obtain the same results reported here?

2. (a) Drop some data from Tables 8.11 and 8.12 to make an $A^4B^2A^2B^4$ versus $B^4A^2B^2A^4$ design. Do anything else that needs to be done in the program of Table 8.12 before it can be run for the new design. (b) Redo Table 8.13 for this new design, taking into account the result of running the revised Table 8.12 program. (c) Use output from the revised Table 8.13 to generate a t-test program like that of Table 8.14 for the new design. (d) Run this t-test program and interpret its output.

3. For ethical reasons, one hesitates to withhold a superior treatment method from subjects in order to show how well it works. On the other hand, what seems initially to be a preferable method sometimes fails to give good results in the long run. Would you think that a $A^{m1}B^{m2}A^{m3}B^{m4}$ versus $B^{m1}A^{m2}B^{m3}A^{m4}$ design is better or worse than a between-subjects design with one group of subjects receiving Treatment A throughout and another group receiving Treatment B throughout? Why? Does your answer depend on the specific response to be influenced or on the specific treatments to be employed? Explain.

9

Data Analysis for Multiple-Baseline Designs

INTRODUCTION

This chapter looks at simple versions of a so-called *multiple-baseline design*, a design in which initial (baseline) performance under one treatment is examined before possible introduction of a second treatment. What makes such a design a multiple-baseline design is that different subjects receive different amounts of experience in the baseline condition. Then they go on to receive a different treatment or level of the experimental variable that changes from treatment to treatment.

We have already seen that sometimes clinical psychologists or speech therapists trying to evaluate the effectiveness of introducing a new method of therapy perform an experiment in which some subjects switch from an old method (Treatment A) to a new method (Treatment B). For example, Treatment A may be no change from what each patient has been experiencing before seeking help in a clinic. Treatment B may be a behavior modification therapy. Clients may be tested on at least three stages during the clinical experiment, with different subjects or groups of subjects having different patterns of treatments. All subjects begin with Treatment A but vary in the number of stages on A before possibly going on to Treatment B.

Every subject starts with Treatment A. In a multiple-baseline experiment across subjects such as the one to be described, a subject never switches more than once from A to B. The different points of switch from A to B define the length of the baseline measurement prior to that switch. These different lengths of baseline testing are intended to show whether Treatment B works the same regardless of when it begins. If the new treatment is successful with different subjects and different lengths of baseline testing, it seems reasonable to think that the treatment might be effective with new patients as well.

METHOD A: ANALYZING DATA FROM A MULTIPLE-BASELINE EXPERIMENT INTERPRETED BY A CROSSOVER DESIGN MODEL

A Three-Baseline, Three Sequence Unreplicated Design

Consider the design in Table 9.1.

TABLE 9.1
A Three-Baseline, Three-Sequence Unreplicated Experimental Design

	Stage 1	Stage 2	Stage 3
Subject 1	A	A	A
Subject 2	A	A	B
Subject 3	A	B	B

Subject 1 has nothing but a baseline measurement for Treatment A performance. Subject 2 has two stages of baseline for A, followed by a switch to B. Subject 3 has one stage of baseline for A, followed by two stages of measurement with B. (One could use more than one subject with each treatment sequence, making three groups of subjects. However, multiple baseline studies often employ only a single subject per sequence.) What should we try to learn from data obtained with this design?

1. We would like to assess any differential treatment effect (i.e., the performance difference due to receiving Treatment B rather than A).

2. We would like to test for a differential practice effect, the performance difference due to being in one stage rather than some other stage.

3. We would like to test for a differential carryover effect such as the difference in current performance due to receiving Treatment A or Treatment B in the preceding stage. For example, in the previous treatment plan, how does Subject 2 perform on Stage 3 compared to Subject 3 (AAB versus ABB), with a carryover from A on Stage 3 in one case and a carryover from B in the other? For now, we assume that this is a *classical carryover* (i.e., a delayed effect of the prior treatment), so that

we would expect the same carryover from A on the second stage of an AA sequence as on the second stage of an AB sequence.

A Model for Behavior in This Experiment

Here is a model involving these three kinds of effects: For i = subject, j = stage, k = treatment, and k' = prior treatment, let

$$Y_{ijk} = \mu + s_i + \pi_j + \tau_k + \lambda_{k'} + e_{ijk} \tag{9.1}$$

The parameters in Equation 9.1 have the following interpretations: μ is an arbitrary constant, s_i is the random effect of Subject i and is i.i.d. $N(0,\sigma_s^2)$, π_j is the effect of Stage j, τ_k is the effect of Treatment k, $\lambda_{k'}$ is the classical carryover from Treatment k' on one stage to any treatment on the next stage, and e_{ijk} is the random error for Y_{ijk}. These error components are normally distributed with a mean of zero. In an approach similar to that for earlier designs, we assume that subject effects are independent of each other and that error components e_{ijk} for each subject have the following covariance matrix:

$$\Sigma_e = \begin{pmatrix} \lambda + 2\gamma_1^* & \gamma_1^* + \gamma_2^* & \gamma_1^* + \gamma_3^* \\ \gamma_1^* + \gamma_2^* & \lambda + 2\gamma_2^* & \gamma_2^* + \gamma_3^* \\ \gamma_1^* + \gamma_3^* & \gamma_2^* + \gamma_3^* & \lambda + 2\gamma_3^* \end{pmatrix}$$

Next, we add assumptions of independence of error scores for different subjects, implying $Cov(e_{ijk}, e_{i'j'k'}) = 0$ for $i \neq i'$ regardless of whether different stages or treatments are involved. Also, we assume $Cov(s_i, e_{ijk}) = 0$, regardless of whether $i = i'$. Given these assumptions, we can obtain the following covariance matrix for all observations Y_{ijk} in any single treatment-sequence group:

$$\Sigma_Y = \begin{pmatrix} \lambda + 2\gamma_1 & \gamma_1 + \gamma_2 & \gamma_1 + \gamma_3 \\ \gamma_1 + \gamma_2 & \lambda + 2\gamma_2 & \gamma_2 + \gamma_3 \\ \gamma_1 + \gamma_3 & \gamma_2 + \gamma_3 & \lambda + 2\gamma_3 \end{pmatrix} \text{ where } \gamma_j = \gamma_j^* + 0.5\sigma_s^2$$

The pattern in Σ_Y is that of Type H covariance structure, ensuring that sphericity holds for every treatment-sequence group.

We are dealing with one of the simplest multiple-baseline designs that will permit assessment of the carryover effects hypothesized here: λ_A from Treatment A on one stage and λ_B from Treatment B on one stage. With this model, the size of the carryover effect does not depend on which treatment occurs in the new (current) stage.

Hypothetical Data From This Experiment

Here is a possible data set for the design just presented. Scores and treatments are shown for each subject on each stage (see Table 9.2).

TABLE 9.2

Observed Scores and Means for a Hypothetical Multiple-Baseline Study

Stage 1	Score (Y) and Treatment			
	Stage 1	Stage 2	Stage 3	Subject Means
Subject 1	91 (A)	96 (A)	102 (A)	96.33
Subject 2	104 (A)	101 (A)	41 (B)	82.00
Subject 3	99 (A)	39 (B)	53 (B)	63.67
Stage Means	98.00	78.67	65.33	80.67
Treatment Means	98.83 (A)	44.33(B)		

These data show higher means for Treatment A than B, for Stage 1 than 2 or 3, and for Subjects 1 and 2 than for Subject 3. However, these means are hard to interpret. For example, the higher means for Stages 1 and 2 might be due to Treatment A appearing more often on those stages than on Stage 3, so that we are seeing treatment effects generating apparent stage effects that are not real. So, we need a clever data analysis method (or to be British about this, a cunning method) that can separate out the possible effects in our model.

A Relevant Computer Program

Here is a SAS® GLM program that yields an appropriate analysis of the above data for this hypothetical experiment (Table 9.3). Significance tests for possible random subject effects and fixed effects of stages, treatments, and carryovers are reported, together with estimation of the sizes of each estimable fixed effect difference. In addition the inclusion of the "RANDOM SUBJ" statement and the E2 option of the "MODEL" statement combine to let us know the expected value for each mean squares and what functions of parameters to estimate.

TABLE 9.3

A Program for Analyzing AAA Versus AAB Versus ABB Data

---

* Program THREEMULT.SAS—Unreplicated AAA Versus AAB Versus ABB design;
DATA THREEMU; INPUT SUBJ STAGE TREAT $ CARRY $ Y @@;
CARDS ;

1 1 A 0	91	1 2 A A	96	1 3 A A	102
2 1 A 0	104	2 2 A A	101	2 3 B A	41
3 1 A 0	99	3 2 B A	39	3 3 B B	53

RUN; PROC GLM; CLASS SUBJ STAGE TREAT CARRY;
MODEL Y = SUBJ STAGE TREAT CARRY/SS1 E2 SS3 SS4 SOLUTION;
ESTIMATE 'STAGE 2 – STAGE 3' STAGE 0 1 –1;
ESTIMATE 'TREAT A – TREAT B' TREAT 1 –1;
ESTIMATE 'CARRY A – CARRY B' 0 1 –1; RANDOM SUBJ;
TITLE 'ANALYSIS OF UNREPLICATED AAA VS. AAB VS. ABB DATA.'; RUN;

Significance Test Results Based on the Previous Program

This program yields the following analysis of variance table for Type III analysis as well as a different one for a Type I analysis (not shown; see Table 9.4):

TABLE 9.4

ANOVA Results for Unreplicated Three-Sequence Multiple-Baseline Data
(These are simultaneously Type II, III, and IV results)

Source	Sum of Squares	df	Mean Square	F
Subjects	69.64	2	34.82	2.36
Stages 2:3	23.08	1	23.08	1.56
Treatments	2,860.17	1	2,860.17	193.91**
Carryovers	49.00	1	49.00	3.32
Error	29.50	2	14.75	—

Note. ** $p < 0.01$.

Table 9.4 shows that the only significant effects are treatment effects. One notable fact in this table is that, even though there were three stages in the experiment, there is only one degree of freedom for them. The familiar reason for this is that we can only compare stage effects for Stages 2 and 3; Stage 1 can have no carryover effects, making its average reflect only stage effects and treatment effects, whereas other stage averages reflect all three kinds of effects. It is also true that the differences in means for Stages 2 and 3 include treatment and carryover effects. However, it is possible to disentangle the three kinds of effects in that case.

Note that Types II, III, and IV all yield the entries in Table 9.4. But, had we included an E1 option in the MODEL statement of Table 9.3, we would have found that most of the expected mean squares for effects analyzed in this table have simpler elements for their quadratic forms, Q( ), with types other than Type I, just as was true in earlier chapters. Therefore, we do not present Type I results in Table 9.4. Any stage effects with a Type I analysis in the order listed here would quite possibly be contaminated by population treatment effects that could have produced the significant treatment effects in the Type II analysis. And a significant Type I F for treatments could reflect in part some population carryover effects even though both Type I and Type II F-values for carryover would be identical and nonsignificant here.

One feature of Table 9.4 deserves special mention: The number of degrees of freedom for error is only two. Because Draper and Joiner (1984) gave evidence that ANOVA's or t-tests with only one degree of freedom for error are not legitimate, the present design is the simplest three-sequence multiple baseline design that can be reasonably employed. Ordinarily, we would prefer to have a replicated version of this design in order to increase the power of our significance tests.

Estimation of Effects

Finally, these effect differences of interest: $\pi_2 - \pi_3$, $\tau_A - \tau_B$, and $\lambda_A - \lambda_B$ are seen from E2 output to be estimable. In particular, we can estimate the size of the only significant effect: the treatment effect difference, $\tau_A - \tau_B$. With the SOLUTION output, we find TREAT A yielding an estimate of 65.50 B and TREAT B yielding 0.00 B, where the B entries indicate bias. However, the difference between these estimates, 65.50, is an unbiased estimate of $\tau_A - \tau_B$. Exactly the same estimate comes with the ESTIMATE output.

METHOD B: COMPUTING EFFICIENCIES AND VARIANCES OF ESTIMATORS (IN $\frac{\sigma^2}{n}$ UNITS) FOR THE CURRENT EXAMPLE

We remind ourselves that we are looking for the following quantity for each estimable parameter difference of interest in the present chapter:

$$Variance\ of\ Estimator\ in\ \frac{\sigma^2}{n}\ units = \Sigma\ \Sigma\ \alpha_{gj}^2 = \frac{n(s.e.e.[\hat{\theta}])^2}{MS_{error}} \qquad (9.2)$$

We also want to compute efficiencies of estimating those parameter differences using our earlier formula:

$$E\hat{\theta} = \frac{\left(\dfrac{200}{r*}\right)}{\dfrac{n(s.e.e.[\hat{\theta}])^2}{MS_{Error}}} \qquad (9.3)$$

This multiple baseline design has $n = 1$ subjects per sequence, $p = 3$ stages, s = 3 sequences, and $T = 2$ treatments. The dimensionless replication values are $r* = \frac{ps}{T} = 4.5$ for treatments or carryover and $r* = s = 3$ for stages. The standard errors of estimate for parameter differences computed with the Table 9.3 program are shown in Table 9.5, together with computation of the dimensionless variances and efficiencies of the current design for estimating various differences among parameter values.

As usual, this table shows smaller dimensionless variances for estimates of stage-effect differences and higher values for carryover-effect differences than for treatment-effect differences. The opposite trend holds for efficiencies, with the opposite rank ordering appearing. The efficiency values are quite low except in the case of the difference between Stage 2 and Stage 3 effects. Even its E value of 61.54 is disappointing in view of the fact that efficiency for estimating stage effect differences is often a maximal possible of 100.

TABLE 9.5
Calculation of Efficiencies and Dimensionless Variances
for Estimators with Output of Program in Table 9.3

A = Standard Error of Estimate = s.e.e.	B = A^2 = Variance of Estimate = A^2	C = 1B/MSerror = nB/D= $\Sigma\Sigma a_{gj}^2$ = Estimator Variance in multiples of $\dfrac{\sigma^2}{n}$	r*	Efficier $\dfrac{200}{r*\Sigma\Sigma}$
3	3.99739499	15.97916671	1.0833	3	61.54
B	4.70372193	22.12499999	1.5000	4.5	29.63
B	5.76085931	33.18749999	2.2500	4.5	19.75
	D = 14.75				

RELATED MULTIPLE-BASELINE DESIGNS

Method C: Analyzing Data From a Replicated Multiple-Baseline Design

Suppose that at least one treatment order is experienced by two or more subjects. For example, each order such as the AAA order in the original design of this chapter might be employed for five subjects. Obviously, this change in design will require an increase in the number of lines of input. As usual, we do not test for sequence effects. (For an exception, see Milliken and Johnson's work with a six-sequence, three-treatment crossover design (1984), where the use of every treatment the same number of times in each sequence makes the expected values of means for different sequences differ only with respect to carryover values.) However, we will include a SEQ (for sequence column) in the INPUT statement for use in Method D (next).

Table 9.6 is a new within-subjects program that includes the original data and much computer input of Tables 9.2 and/or 9.3 plus new data for four other subjects from each of the sequences AAA, AAB, and ABB. Information from the original Subject 1 now applies to Subject 1 of Treatment Sequence 1. Similarly, information from the original Subjects 2 and 3 now applies to Treatment Sequence 2, Subject 6, and Treatment Sequence 3, Subject 11.

TABLE 9.6
Program of Table 9.3 Expanded to Include Five Subjects
for Each of Three Sequences

---

* Program MUL35.SAS—AAA versus AAB versus ABB with 5Ss per sequence;
DATA MUL35; INPUT SEQ SUBJ STAGE TREAT $ CARRY Y @@;
CARDS;

1	1	1	A	0	91		1	1	2	A	A	96		1	1 3 A A 102
1	2	1	A	0	94		1	2	2	A	A	97		1	2 3 A A 100
1	3	1	A	0	90		1	3	2	A	A	96		1	3 3 A A 105
1	4	1	A	0	92		1	4	2	A	A	93		1	4 3 A A 99
1	5	1	A	0	91		1	5	2	A	A	98		1	5 3 A A 104

(Continued)

TABLE 9.6
(Continued)

2	6	1	A	0	104	2	6	2	A	A	101	2	6	3	B	A	41
2	7	1	A	0	110	2	7	2	A	A	108	2	7	3	B	A	57
2	8	1	A	0	103	2	8	2	A	A	105	2	8	3	B	A	47
2	9	1	A	0	107	2	9	2	A	A	109	2	9	3	B	A	44
2	10	1	A	0	96	2	10	2	A	A	104	2	10	3	B	A	39
3	11	1	A	0	99	3	11	2	B	A	39	3	11	3	B	B	53
3	12	1	A	0	89	3	12	2	B	A	36	3	12	3	B	B	59
3	13	1	A	0	94	3	13	2	B	A	37	3	13	3	B	B	55
3	14	1	A	0	96	3	14	2	B	A	39	3	14	3	B	B	50
3	15	1	A	0	93	3	15	2	B	A	35	3	15	3	B	B	56

RUN: PROC GLM; CLASS SUBJ STAGE TREAT CARRY;
MODEL Y = SUBJ STAGE TREAT CARRY/SOLUTION SS1 E2 SS3 SS4;
RANDOM SUBJ; ESTIMATE 'STAGE 2 – STAGE 3' STAGE 0 1 –1;
ESTIMATE 'TREAT A – TREAT B' TREAT 1 –1;
ESTIMATE 'CARRY A – CARRY B' CARRY 0 1 –1; RUN ;

Note that all data points appear in Table 9.6; no separate table of the complete data set is provided. Results of the current analysis appear in Table 9.7.

TABLE 9.7
ANOVA Results for Replicated Three-Sequence Multiple-Baseline Experiment

Source	Sum of Squares	df	Mean Square	F
Subjects	944.70	14	67.48	6.09****
Stages 2:3	84.68	1	84.68	7.64*
Treatments	13,483.20	1	13,483.20	1,216.32****
Carryovers	457.61	1	457.61	41.28****
Error	288.22	26	11.08	—

Note. *$p < 0.05$.   ****$p < 0.0001$.

Table 9.7 shows that all tests were significant; actually Type II through IV analyses yield identical significant results. Except for subjects and stages, Type I sums of squares are identical to the others. However, expected mean squares and other estimability information obtainable with an E1 command could make it clear that Type I is less appropriate than the other analyses.

Estimation procedures based on the SOLUTION option of Table 9.7 are obvious. We do not recalculate efficiency values from Table 9.5 because the only effect of replication on the current analysis is to reduce the variability of estimates inversely with respect to n. Variances in multiples of $\frac{\sigma^2}{n}$ and efficiency values from Table 9.5 also apply to the present replicated design.

Method D: Checking Multisample Sphericity Using the "REPEATED" Option in "PROC GLM"

Table 8 presents a program for performing most of the testing of the multisample sphericity assumption for our replicated multiple baseline example. Much of this program is involved in reorganization of the data step of Table 9.6 to make it useable in a SAS® GLM program using a REPEATED option and requiring less repetition of information than employed in other GLM programs (see Table 9.8).

TABLE 9.8

A Repeated Measurements Analysis Program for Data
From a Replicated Multiple Baseline Experiment

```
* PROGRAM MUL35REP.SAS  – REPEATED MEASUREMENTS;
* Part 1 Splitting data  into separate different treatment-sequence group files;
DATA GROUP1 GROUP2 GROUP3; INPUT SEQ SUBJ STAGE TREAT $
   Y @@;
IF SEQ = 1 THEN OUTPUT GROUP1; IF SEQ = 2 THEN OUTPUT
GROUP2;
IF SEQ = 3 THEN OUTPUT GROUP3; CARDS;
```

(Continued)

TABLE 9.8
(Continued)

1	1	1	A	91		1	1	2	A	96		1	1	3	A	102
1	2	1	A	94		1	2	2	A	97		1	2	3	A	100
1	3	1	A	90		1	3	2	A	96		1	3	3	A	105
1	4	1	A	92		1	4	2	A	93		1	4	3	A	99
1	5	1	A	91		1	5	2	A	98		1	5	3	A	104
2	6	1	A	104		2	6	2	A	101		2	6	3	B	41
2	7	1	A	110		2	7	2	A	108		2	7	3	B	57
2	8	1	A	103		2	8	2	A	105		2	8	3	B	47
2	9	1	A	107		2	9	2	A	109		2	9	3	B	44
2	10	1	A	96		2	10	2	A	104		2	10	3	B	39
3	11	1	A	99		3	11	2	B	39		3	11	3	B	53
3	12	1	A	89		3	12	2	B	36		3	12	3	B	59
3	13	1	A	94		3	13	2	B	37		3	13	3	B	55
3	14	1	A	96		3	14	2	B	39		3	14	3	B	50
3	15	1	A	93		3	15	2	B	35		3	15	3	B	56

RUN; * Part 2 Revamping Group 1 data and using it with repeated measurements option;

PROC TRANSPOSE DATA = GROUP1 OUT = NE1(RENAME = (_1 = Y1 _2 = Y2 _3 = Y3)); BY SEQ SUBJ; ID STAGE; PROC GLM DATA = NE1; MODEL Y1-Y3 = / NOUNI; REPEATED STAGE POLYNOMIAL/PRINTE SUMMARY;

TITLE 'REPEATED MEASUREMENTS ANALYSIS FOR SEQUENCE 1.';

* Part 3 Revamping Group 2 data for use with repeated measurements option;

PROC TRANSPOSE DATA = GROUP2 OUT = NE2(RENAME = (_1 = Y1 _2 = Y2 _3 = Y3)); BY SEQ SUBJ; ID STAGE; PROC GLM DATA = NE2; MODEL Y1-Y3 = /NOUNI; REPEATED STAGE POLYNOMIAL/PRINTE SUMMARY;

TITLE 'REPEATED MEASUREMENTS ANALYSIS FOR SEQUENCE 2.';

* Part 4 Revamping Group 3 data for use with repeated measurements option;

PROC TRANSPOSE DATA = GROUP3 OUT = NE3(RENAME = (_1 = Y1

(Continued)

TABLE 9.8

(Continued)

_2 = Y2 _3 = Y3)); BY SEQ SUBJ; ID STAGE; PROC GLM DATA = NE3;
MODEL Y1–Y3 = /NOUNI;   REPEATED STAGE POLYNOMIAL/ PRINTE
SUMMARY; TITLE 'REPEATED MEASUREMENTS ANALYSIS FOR
SEQUENCE 3.';

* Part 5 Combining data sets for the 3 groups for use in an overall analysis;
PROC APPEND BASE = NE1 DATA = NE2; PROC APPEND BASE = NE1
DATA = NE3; PROC GLM DATA = NE1; CLASS SEQ; MODEL Y1–Y3 =
SEQ / NOUNI; REPEATED STAGE POLYNOMIAL/PRINTE SUMMARY;
TITLE 'REPEATED MEASUREMENT ANALYSIS AND DATA
SUMMARY FOR 3 GROUPS.'; PROC PRINT DATA = NE1; RUN;

This table starts with the same data input as in Table 9.6 except that "CARRY" is deleted from the "INPUT" statement. As Part 1 indicates, an initial purpose of the program is to take existing data and split it into separate files for the three treatment-sequence groups. Part 2 uses an approach from a SAS® manual (SAS Institute Inc., 1989d) to transpose Group 1 data into a format having only one subject identifier per subject, with three observations (Y_1, Y_2, and Y_3) for each subject in order to facilitate use of the "REPEATED" option in "PROC GLM". Then a repeated measurements analysis is performed on the orthogonal polynomial contrasts of Group 1 data. Parts 3 and 4 perform similar tasks for Group 2 and Group 3 data. Part 5 recombines the transposed data for the three groups and performs a final repeated measurements analysis.

As mentioned in chapter 5, two criteria need to be met if multisample sphericity is present: (1) Data from each group must come from a population whose covariance matrix has a Type H structure, thus having sphericity in each group. (2) Data from each group must have the same population covariance group. We now report on three indications of the degree to which these assumptions are met. First, we finally have a hypothetical data set large enough that we can perform separate Mauchly tests of sphericity for each treatment-sequence group. The $\chi^2(2)$ approximations for the relevant Mauchly tests for the three treatment-sequence groups are 2.74 ($p = 0.25$), 0.52 ($p = 0.77$), and 4.56 ($p = 0.10$), respectively. Except perhaps for group 3, this gives no reason to doubt the presence of sphericity in the three populations in question.

Second, the comparable $\chi^2(2)$ approximation for the three groups combined is 3.07 with $p = 0.22$, again a result consistent with multisample sphericity.

Finally, we need to test for equality of the covariance matrices for the three groups. This requires us to perform procedures already illustrated in chapter 5. We work with SAS® output of so-called Error SS&CP matrices for each sequence group, dealing in each case with polynomial contrasts of stage scores. Such a matrix is equal to $(n_g - 1)C' \hat{\Sigma}_g C$, where $n_g = 5$ for each group g, C is a p by $p - 1$ matrix with $p = 4$ stages, and $\hat{\Sigma}_g$ is the estimated covariance matrix for Group g across the different stages. As in chapter 5, we let $\chi^2 = (1 - E_1)M$ with

$$M = \sum_{g=1}^{G}(n_g - 1)[\ln(|C'\hat{\Sigma}_{pooled}C|/|C'\hat{\Sigma}_g C|)]. \text{ Here}$$

$$E_1 = \frac{2p^2 + 3p - 1}{6(p+1)(G-1)}\left(\sum_{g=1}^{G}\frac{1}{n_g - 1} - \frac{1}{\sum_{g=1}^{G}(n_g - 1)}\right)$$

and $df = \dfrac{p(p+1)(G-1)}{2}$.

Because $n_g - 1 = 4$ for each group, the Error SS&CP matrices in our program's output tell us that:

$$4C_1'\hat{\Sigma}C_1 = \begin{pmatrix} 29.60 & -1.50 \\ -1.50 & 3.87 \end{pmatrix}, \quad 4C_2'\hat{\Sigma}C_2 = \begin{pmatrix} 39.60 & 17.21 \\ 17.21 & 56.80 \end{pmatrix}$$

$$4C_3'\hat{\Sigma}C_3 = \begin{pmatrix} 90.60 & 20.55 \\ 20.55 & 10.87 \end{pmatrix} \quad \text{and} \quad 4C_{pooled}'\hat{\Sigma}C_{pooled} = \begin{pmatrix} 159.80 & 36.26 \\ 36.26 & 71.53 \end{pmatrix}$$

yielding $\chi^2 = (1 - E_1)M = (1 - 0.3611)36.14 = 23.09$ with $df = 12$ and $p < 0.05$. This suggests that different treatment-sequence groups do not have the same population covariance matrix. In the light of this test and the possible nonsphericity found for group 3 data, the assumption of multigroup sphericity is questionable.

At this point, an investigator might well consider use of a saturated crossover design model analogous to the one used in chapter 3, with the possibility of ensuing conservative tests such as those performed there.

But, there is also the possibility of one or more Type I errors having occurred in the sphericity tests just discussed, negating further testing.

Dual-Balanced Designs

We could obtain the mirror image of each subject's sequence of experiences in Table 9.1, reversing each original treatment sequence to form a mirrored sequence. This means that the AAA, AAB, and ABB sequences of that table would now be supplemented by BBB, BBA, and BAA sequences for Subjects 4 through 6, respectively, or for new sequences 4 through 6 in Table 9.6. Such designs permit testing of models with new possibilities of types of carryover effect. Further discussion of these mirror image (dual-balanced) multiple baseline designs is deferred until chapter 10.

Longer Series of Experimental Treatments (More Stages)

The experimenter could add a certain constant number of stages to each subject, using the last treatment that subject received. For example, here is a 6-trial variant of the design (Table 9.9A).

TABLE 9.9A
A More Lengthy Multiple-Baseline Experiment

	Stage 1	Stage 2	Stage 3	Stage 4	Stage 5	Stage 6
Subject 4	A	B	B	B	B	B
Subject 5	A	A	B	B	B	B
Subject 6	A	A	A	B	B	B

The model for this experiment would be the same as before, and the only required change in the original SAS® GLM program would be to include appropriate input for each of the 18 data points that would be obtained.

Additional Sequences of Treatments for a Long Experiment

It is possible to use a new design such as that just given and add more subjects, each with a new treatment sequence. For example (Table 9.9B), we could add:

TABLE 9.9B
Additional Treatment Sequences for a More Lengthy Experiment

	Stage 1	Stage 2	Stage 3	Stage 4	Stage 5	Stage 6
Subject 4	A	A	A	A	B	B
Subject 5	A	A	A	A	A	B
Subject 6	A	A	A	A	A	A

to that design. When the design is that of Tables 9.9A and 9.9B combined, we are comparing subjects whose last experience with A is on Stage 1, 2, 3, 4, 5, or 6, depending on which of the six subjects we are studying. Our original model, Equation 9.1, also applies to the new design. The SAS® PROC GLM program merely needs to include appropriate input for each of the 36 data points that would be obtained in the large design combining Tables 9.9A and 9.9B. The contents of each data line would be very similar to existing lines in the program.

FINAL THOUGHTS

The content of some psychological research makes multiple baseline designs very attractive there. In addition, analysis of data resulting from them is relatively straightforward. However, the efficiency of our AAA versus AAB versus ABB design is not very high. This means that a relatively large number of subjects must be employed with this design if it is to have a reasonably standard error of estimate for the difference between treatment effect paramters, for example.

THINGS TO REMEMBER

Major Analysis Options

1. Analysis of data from an unreplicated multiple baseline study with, for example, AAA versus AAB versus ABB sequences uses a familiar SAS® PROC GLM approach with a model including random subject and fixed stage, treatment, and carryover effects. Carryover continues to be modeled as classical, reflecting only the delayed effects of the immediately prior treatment.

2. Analysis of data from a replicated multiple-baseline study with the same sequences as those in #1 requires only the addition of additional information for new subjects.

3. Repeated measurements ANOVAs supplement the analysis in #2, testing for sphericity in each treatment-sequence group and in the three groups when pooled. If the assumption of multigroup sphericity appears to fail, a conservative analysis based on a saturated crossover model may be desirable.

Interpreting Results of Computational Methods Not Previously Discussed

1. For the first time, we have a computational example with enough subjects per treatment group to permit testing of the sphericity assumption separately for each group. Significance of one or more such tests suggests that routine ANOVA procedures are inappropriate. However, the tendency of such tests (mentioned in chap. 3) to exhibit significance in the presence of small departures from sphericity suggest caution, especially when several separate sphericity tests are being conducted.

2. Retyping of data files or computer programs can be minimized by using "PROC TRANSPOSE" and "PROC APPEND" to rearrange data not originally in SAS®'s form for repeated measurements analysis and also to combine data from different groups into a single set for an overall analysis.

EXERCISES

1. Run the programs in this chapter. Do you obtain the same results as reported above?

2. Develop a saturated model for the data of Table 9.6. Test the model by the methods of chapter 3, performing conservative tests where meaningful. Be sure to take care to examine expected mean squares to see whether the tests you perform can be justified.

10

Data Analysis for Dual-Balanced Multiple-Baseline Designs

INTRODUCTION

This chapter deals with a new category of multiple-baseline designs having the advantage of permitting assessment of a broader class of carryover effects than hitherto discussed. A further feature of this chapter is the relating of carryover effects to psychological phenomena first observed in studies of motivation and reward.

Every now and then psychologists discover something that everyone already knows, sort of. In the context of multiple-baseline experimental designs, this chapter considers such an example. We all believe that our expectations are guided by our experience and perhaps by the experience of other people whom we observe. So we sometimes talk of rising expectations in Third World countries that either are showing economic development or are seeing television or newspaper reports of rising standards of living in other countries. We also are aware that broken promises in personal affairs or broken contracts in business relations can greatly change expectations in those realms. Psychologists may study these phenomena in real life but often prefer to examine them in laboratory settings where other variables can be carefully controlled. Somewhat surprisingly, they also like to test them with nonhumans. This is partly because they think other animals are basically very much like humans both in psychology and biology. Perhaps, too, psychologists want to see what happens with organisms who apparently do not use language to mediate their behavior.

The second advantage of using animals for research on expectation is also a disadvantage. Especially to a behavioristic psychologist, expectations seem ethereal, mental, or even spiritual rather than biological. So a behaviorist may be troubled by other psychologists who speak of expectation in animals or even perhaps in people. Yet the studies to be considered here were considered very important by behaviorists as well as other psychologists. At first we will use nonbehavioral terminology, but later we will try to make peace with a behaviorist's concerns.

Crespi (1942, 1944) and Zeaman (1949) are among the many investigators who have found that rats running repeatedly through a straight tunnel (called a runway) to obtain food will run faster if previous runs have been rewarded with large amounts of food than with small amounts of food. These authors went on to show that rats with a history of large amounts of food reward who are shifted to a series of tests in which a run is followed by a small reward changed their behavior, running slowly thereafter. A shift from small reward to large reward produces the opposite effect, faster running than before. Doesn't this sound like common sense? Aren't these rats simply adjusting their running speed to reflect their changes in expectation of amount of reward? Don't we also expect most people to work harder for large reward than for small reward?

But these authors obtained a further finding that might not be predicted by every ordinary intelligent human being or even by every ordinary psychologist: Just after a shift from large reward to small reward, rats temporarily ran even slower than a control group of rats originally trained with small reward. Crespi called this phenomenon a *depression effect* because it was like a temporary feeling of depression after something goes wrong in our lives.

Crespi and Zeaman also observed an opposite effect: They reported that, just after the shift from low to high amounts of reward amounts, their rats temporarily ran even faster than a control group of rats originally trained with high reward. Crespi called this an *elation effect* because it was like human enthusiasm, excitement, or elation after an unexpected success such as winning a million dollar lottery. The brevity of an elation or depression effect may be considered to reflect its emotional quality; after more experience with a new amount of reward, the animals settled down to run at the speed normally used with that reward level. A more behavioristic terminology might call elation a positive contrast effect and depression a negative contrast effect. In reviewing these findings, Hall (1966) concluded that follow-up studies confirmed the phenomenon of depression effects (negative contrast effects) but usually not of elation effects (positive contrast effects).

A HYPOTHETICAL DUAL-BALANCED MULTIPLE-BASELINE EXPERIMENT ON ELATION VERSUS DEPRESSION EFFECTS

Method A: Analyzing Data From Such Designs

Orientation

Let us expand the design of earlier elation versus depression effects experiments while keeping their basic idea. We now define Treatment A as giving a large reward to a rat for running through a straight alley. Also Treatment B is the new term given a small reward for the same response. We can form another interesting kind of multiple-baseline design by using several treatment sequences rather than only the Large–Small and Small–Large sequences of the original studies.   Because this is still to be a multiple-baseline experiment, a subject must never switch more than once from A to B or B to A.

A Specific Design

Consider the design shown in Table 10.1.

TABLE 10.1
A Six-Sequence Dual-Balanced Multiple Baseline Design

	Stage 1	Stage 2	Stage 3
Subject 1	A	A	A
Subject 2	A	A	B
Subject 3	A	B	B
Subject 4	B	B	B
Subject 5	B	B	A
Subject 6	B	A	A

Subject 1 has nothing but a baseline measurement for Treatment A performance, but Subject 2 has two stages of baseline for A, followed by a switch to B. Subject 3 has one stage of baseline for A, followed by two stages of measurement with B.   Subjects 4 through 6 are similar but begin with Treatment B. As in earlier designs, one could use more than one subject with each treatment sequence if desired, making six groups of subjects.

Because Subjects 4 through 6 have treatment patterns like Subjects 1 through 3 but with B replacing A and vice versa, we say that Table 10.1

is a dual-balanced design comparable to those of chapter 8. Unfortunately, because there are more than two treatment-sequence patterns and because Table 10.1 has no replication within sequence groups, we cannot perform *t*-tests of contrasts analogous to those in chapter 8.

What Might We Be Able to Tell From Data Obtained With This Design?

1. We would like to assess treatment effect, the performance difference due to receiving Treatment A rather than B.

2. We would like to test for a practice effect, the performance difference due to being in one stage rather than some other stage.

3. We would like to compare specialized carryover effects such as those associated with performance differences on the second part of an AA pair and of a BA pair. With this six-group design it turns out that we can compare four different carryovers rather than only two as in the three-sequence multiple-baseline designs of chapter 9. We will see that, for the current experimental problem on effects of changing reward sizes, one of these carryover effects is an elation effect and one is a depression effect.

4. Less important, we would like to test for subject effects of the different subjects in the experiment.

A Model for Data From This Experiment

Let us use the label Y_{ijk} for our dependent variable, response speed, where i = subject, j = stage, k = treatment, and k' = prior treatment. Here is a model permitting the assessment of the four kinds of effects just mentioned:

$$Y_{ijk} = \mu + s_i + \pi_j + \tau_k + \lambda_{k'k} + e_{ijk} \tag{10.1}$$

The parameters in Equation 10.1 have the following interpretations: μ is an arbitrary constant, s_i is the random effect of Subject i and is i.i.d. $N(0, \sigma_s^2)$, π_j is the effect of Stage j, γ_k is the effect of Treatment k, $\lambda_{k'k}$ is the carryover from Treatment k' on one stage to Treatment k on the next stage, and e_{ijk} is the random error for Y_{ijk}. As usual, errors for any subject are independent of all other subject effects and independent of errors for all other subjects. For each subject, errors are assumed to be normally distributed with mean zero and the same Type H covariance structure. These assumptions ensure that the Y_{ijk} have a common Type H covariance structure and, thus, multisample sphericity. Notice that using two subscripts on our carryover symbols permits four carryover effects to be hypothesized here, rather than the two of most of our previous two-treatment models:

λ_{AA} from Treatment A on one stage to Treatment A on the next,

λ_{AB} from Treatment A on one stage to Treatment B on the next,

λ_{BA} from Treatment B on one stage to Treatment A on the next, and

λ_{BB} from Treatment B on one stage to Treatment B on the next stage.

These carryovers may be called *transitional carryovers* because they assess the effects of change from a treatment on one stage to another treatment on the next stage. Although dual balance may not be necessary to gain this flexibility, a variety of treatment orders with all four pairs of successive treatments (AA, AB, BA, and BB) is essential to use of a model with these four carryovers.

Hypothetical Data for This Dual-Balanced Baseline Design

Here is a possible data set for the design just presented.

TABLE 10.2

Hypothetical Data for an Experiment Employing an Unreplicated
Six-Sequence Design Assessing Effects of Reward Size
(Response speeds are reported in arbitrary units.)

Subject = Sequence	Stage 1	Stage 2	Stage 3	Subject Mean
Subject 1	20.46 (A)	19.97 (A)	19.28 (A)	19.90
Subject 2	19.68 (A)	20.90 (A)	5.99 (B)	15.52
Subject 3	21.73 (A)	7.68 (B)	12.42 (B)	13.94
Subject 4	11.74 (B)	10.84 (B)	12.49 (B)	11.69
Subject 5	10.96 (B)	11.29 (B)	25.72 (A)	15.99
Subject 6	10.40 (B)	24.78 (A)	20.98 (A)	18.72
Stage Mean	15.83	15.91	16.15	15.96
Treatment Mean	21.50 (A)		10.42 (B)	

These data show higher means for Treatment A than B and for Stage 3 than for 1 or 2. There are also differences in means for the different subjects of the experiment. However, it is evident that we cannot tell from the means alone how much treatment effects may differ from each other. The same thing is true for stage effects and for carryover effects.

Analysis of Data

An Appropriate SAS® GLM Program. Here is a SAS® GLM program that yields appropriate results for this kind of multiple baseline design (see Table 10.3).

TABLE 10.3

A Program to Analyze the Reward-Size Effects Data

in Table 10.2

```
* PROGRAM MULTBAS.SAS;
DATA MULTBAS; INPUT SUBJ STAGE TREAT $ CARRY $ Y @@;
CARDS ;
1 1 A 0 20.46        1 2 A AA 19.97      1 3 A AA 19.28
2 1 A 0 19.68        2 2 A AA 20.90      2 3 B AB  5.99
3 1 A 0 21.73        3 2 B AB  7.68      3 3 B BB 12.42
4 1 B 0 11.74        4 2 B BB 10.84      4 3 B BB 12.49
5 1 B 0 10.96        5 2 B BB 11.29      5 3 A BA 25.72
6 1 B 0 10.40        6 2 A BA 24.78      6 3 A AA 20.98
RUN ; PROC GLM; CLASS SUBJ STAGE TREAT CARRY;
MODEL Y = SUBJ STAGE TREAT CARRY/E SS1 E2 SS3 SS4 SOLUTION;
RANDOM SUBJ; ESTIMATE 'CA_BA – CA_AA' CARRY 0 –1 0 – 1 0;
ESTIMATE 'STAGE 2 – STAGE 3'  STAGE 0 1 –1;
ESTIMATE 'TREAT A – TREAT B' TREAT 1 –1;
ESTIMATE 'CA_AA – CA_BB' CARRY 0 1 0 0 –1;
ESTIMATE 'CA_AB – CA_BB' CARRY 0 0 1 0 –1;
ESTIMATE 'CA_BA – CA_BB' CARRY 0 0 0 1 –1;
TITLE 'ANALYSIS FOR A 6 SEQ  MULTIPLE BASELINE STUDY';
RUN ;
```

CARRY values of AA, AB, BA, and BB refer to λ_{AA}, λ_{AB}, λ_{BA}, and λ_{BB}, as expected.

Results of Data Analysis

ANOVA. Table 10.4 gives Type II analysis output based on the program shown in Table 10.3.

TABLE 10.4

Type II ANOVA Results for a Multiple-Baseline Experiment
on Effects of Reward Size

Source	Sum of Squares	df	Mean Square	F
Subjects	5.76	5	1.15	2.30
Stages 2:3	0.17	1	0.17	0.34
Treatments	72.36	1	72.36	144.76****
Carryovers	21.97	3	7.32	14.65**
Error	3.00	6	0.50	—

Note. ** $p < 0.01$. **** $p < 0.0001$.

This table shows that the only significant effects are treatment effects and carryover effects. Note that there is only one degree of freedom for stages. The reason for this is familiar from earlier designs: In view of the E2 estimability tables (not shown), we can only compare stage effects for Stages 2 and 3; Stage 1 has no carryover effects, making the Stage 1 average reflect only a Stage 1 effect and an average of treatment effects whereas other stage averages reflect all three kinds of effects.

Estimation of Effects. Again because of results shown in the E2 estimability tables, we know that we can estimate the size of relevant effect differences other than STAGE 1 – STAGE 3 from program output. The SOLUTION estimates described next are consistent with the ESTIMATE command output from this program. We find TREAT A yielding an estimate of 10.01 B and TREAT B yielding 0.00 B, where the B entries indicate bias. The difference between these estimates, 10.01, is an unbiased estimate of $\tau_A - \tau_B$. This means that, after taking into account all other effects, the best estimate of the difference between running speeds under high and low reward is 10.01. Similarly, CARRY AA – CARRY BB = 0.004 – 0.00 = 0.004 is the estimate of $\lambda_{AA} - \lambda_{BB}$. This suggests that there is almost no difference between the carryover in moving from A to A (large reward to large reward) and the carryover in moving from B to B (small reward to small reward). Also CARRY AB – CARRY BB = –4.46 – 0.00 = –4.46 is the estimate of $\lambda_{AB} - \lambda_{BB}$. This is the difference between the carryover in moving from A to B (large reward to small reward) and the carryover in moving from B to B (small reward to small reward). Notice that this negative number is what was called a depression effect earlier in this chapter.

Finally CARRY BA – CARRY AA = 4.22 is the estimate of $\lambda_{BA} - \lambda_{AA}$. This is the difference between the carryover in moving from B to A (small reward to large reward) and the carryover in moving from A to A (large reward to large reward). Correspondingly, this positive number is what was earlier called an elation effect. So these data suggest a fairly large elation effect and a fairly large depression effect in the opposite direction.

Because there is no treatment before Stage 1, we do not expect a carryover value for that stage even though our computer program coded CARRY as 0 for that stage. It is no surprise, therefore, that when we use the E and E2 commands we find no linear combination of CARRY 0 and other carries to be estimable unless we allow another effect (STAGE 1) to be involved as well.

This is one of the simplest multiple baseline designs that will permit assessment both of stage of practice and of the carryover effects hypothesized here: λ_{AA}, λ_{AB}, λ_{BA}, and λ_{BB}. Having some subjects begin with Treatment A and other subjects begin with Treatment B seems to be necessary for this purpose. However, if one can assume no stage of practice effects, a simpler design could be used.

Method B: Calculating Efficiencies and Variances (in $\frac{\sigma^2}{n}$ Terms) of Estimated Parameter Differences for the Current Multiple-Baseline Design

This dual-balanced multiple-baseline design has $n = 1$ subjects per sequence, $p = 3$ stages, $s = 6$ sequences, and $T = 2$ treatments. Based on methods from earlier chapters, Table 10.5 shows efficiencies and dimensionless variances of parameter differences for the dual-balanced multiple baseline design and model of Table 10.3. In addition, results are given for the present design but with a simpler model assuming only two classical carryovers (λ_A and λ_B) rather than the four transitional carryovers just shown. Table 10.5 also displays comparable statistics from Table 9.5 for a three-group three-stage multiple-baseline design using a classical carryover model. The formulas employed come from chapter 5, with the only slight surprise being different r^* values for treatments and carryovers with the transitional carryover model. This is

TABLE 10.5

A Comparison of Efficiencies and Estimator Variance Values (in $\frac{\sigma^2}{n}$ units) for Two Multiple Baseline Designs and Two Kinds of Carryover Effects

Model	AAA, AAB, or ABB in chapter 9, Equation 9.1 (Classical carryover model)		AAA, AAB, ABB, BBB, BBA, or BAA in chapter 10, Equation 10.1 (Transitional carryover model)		AAA, AAB, ʌ BBA, or BAA (Classical carry
	Estimator Variance in multiples of $\frac{\sigma^2}{n}$	Efficiency = E with r* = 3 for stages and 4.5 for treatments and for carryover	Estimator Variance in multiples of $\frac{\sigma^2}{n}$	Efficiency = E with r* = 6 for stages, 9 for treatments, and 4.50 for carryover	Estimator Variance in multiples of $\frac{\sigma^2}{n}$
ᴇ 3	1.0833	61.54	0.3333	100.00	0.3333
B	1.5000	29.63	1.3846	16.05	0.3846
/ B	2.2500	19.75	na	na	0.6154
ɪrry BB	na	na	1.6154	27.51	na
ʀy BB	na	na	1.3154	33.79	na
ɪrry BB	na	na	2.7000	16.46	na

applicable.

a consequence of modeling four carryovers but only two treatment effects in that example (see Table 10.5).

The first and third sections of this table show that, when the classical model is used, the dual-balanced multiple-baseline design is more sensitive than its cousin, having consistently higher efficiencies and smaller dimensionless variances for its estimators.   Comparison of Sections 2 and 3 shows that when the design is held constant and the model changes, use of more carryover parameters reduces the sensitivity of the dual-balanced design in its assessment of treatment effects (affecting both dimensionless variance of estimates and efficiency) but has no effect on the efficiency or relevant variance for estimates of stage effects. Clearly each of these approaches has certain advantages over the other. A more complex carryover model may be attractive in describing behavior best modeled by it. However, this advantage is traded for lowered sensitivity for assessing the treatment effects.

RELATED DESIGNS

This section more or less duplicates the comparable section of chapter 9. It may be ignored if you have already been working with the replicated three-sequence multiple-baseline design of that chapter.

A Replicated Dual-Balanced Multiple-Baseline Design

The Design Itself

Suppose that at least one treatment order is represented by two or more subjects. For example, each order such as the AAA order in the original design of this chapter might involve four subjects. (Usually the number of subjects would be equal for each of the original treatment orders or sequences, but this does not have to be true to permit a reasonable data analysis to occur.) The statistical model for this design changes very slightly from that for the unreplicated design to:

$$Y_{gijk} = \mu + s_i + \pi_j + \tau_k + \lambda_{k'k} + e_{gijk} \qquad (10.2)$$

where g identifies a certain treatment-sequence group, there is no fixed effect for that group, and other changes from Equation 10.1 are obvious. Subjects labeled i may usefully be numbered consecutively across groups, making a total of 24 in our hypothetical example of six sequences and four subjects per sequence group. Standard distributional assumptions are made here as well.

Method C: Analyzing Data From This Design

Obviously, these modifications of design and model will require a program with an increase in the number of lines of input compared to the program of Table 10.3 for an unreplicated design. As in Method C of chapter 9, it will be convenient to include a SEQ (for sequence) column in the INPUT statement and each line of data typed into the program. Here is part of the new program, with the first data point from the old Subject 1 now being the data point for Group 1, Subject 1, Stage 1 and a series of dots indicating sets of missing lines (Table 10.6).

TABLE 10.6
Sample Lines for a Revision of the Program in Table 10.3
for Use With a Replicated Design
(See Table 9.6 for a related program.)

```
* Program MULTBREV.SAS—6 sequences of a 3-stage dual-balanced design;
DATA MULTBREV; INPUT SEQ SUBJ STAGE TREAT $ CARRY $ Y
@@; CARDS;
1 1 1 A 0 20.46      1 1 2 A A 19.97      1 1 3 A A 19.28
. . . . . . . . . .
PROC GLM; CLASS SUBJ STAGE TREAT CARRY;
MODEL Y = SUBJ STAGE TREAT CARRY/E2 SOLUTION;
RANDOM SUBJ; RUN;
```

Table 10.6 is used to assess the effects of familiar variables in this book: subjects, stages, treatments, and carryovers. If the sample size for one or more treatment sequences is large enough, we can assess sphericity by employing the "REPEATED" option in analyses similar to those of Method C in chapter 9. Especially if there is evidence of nonsphericity, we may wish to consider an alternate analysis method employing contrasts like those found in Methods B and D of chapter 8. Method B, for example involved a four-stage two-sequence dual design, whereas we now have a three-stage six-sequence dual design a bit different from the four- and six-sequence dual designs also discussed by Jones and Kenward (1989).

Longer Series of Experimental Treatments

One way to increase the length of an experimental series is to systematically vary the number of stages prior to any treatment change. For example, having two or four stages before such a change, or six stages without a change, would yield the following (Table 10.7).

TABLE 10.7

A Possible 6 Stage Dual-Balanced Multiple–Baseline Design

	Stage 1	Stage 2	Stage 3	Stage 4	Stage 5	Stage 6
Subject 1	A	A	B	B	B	B
Subject 2	A	A	A	A	B	B
Subject 3	A	A	A	A	A	A
Subject 4	B	B	A	A	A	A
Subject 5	B	B	B	B	A	A
Subject 6	B	B	B	B	B	B

The model for this experiment is again Equation 10.1, and the only required change in the program of Table 10.3 is to delete the old data entries and include the 36 new data points obtained with the proposed experiment, plus values for associated descriptors such as SUBJ and STAGE.

New Stages Plus New Sequences of Treatments

It is possible to use a new design, such as that just given, and add more subjects, each with a new treatment sequence. For example, we could add:

	Stage 1	Stage 2	Stage 3	Stage 4	Stage 5	Stage 6
Subject 1A	A	B	B	B	B	B
Subject 2A	A	A	A	B	B	B
Subject 3A	A	A	A	A	A	B

to that design. Now we are comparing subjects whose first experience with B is on Stage 2, 3, 4, 5, 6, or never, depending on which of the six subjects we are studying. Another three subjects with comparable new sequences beginning with B could be added. Again our original model,

Equation 10.1, can be applied to the new design. The SAS® GLM program merely needs an added line for each new data point. The contents of each new line will be very similar to existing lines in the program.

FINAL THOUGHTS

This chapter is an example of tying an experimental design and a data analysis to an empirical phenomenon in a way that has theoretical implications. First we increased the complexity of our experimental designs, compared to multiple-baseline designs in chapter 9. Then we increased the complexity of the carryover effects modeled for the current designs. These two changes enabled us to show that specific differences in first-order carryover effects in the present setting correspond to elation or depression effects lasting across only one observational stage. If elation or depression effects last through $k > 1$ stages, new models with carryover effects for first through k-th order could be used to describe such effects. If necessary, even more complicated experimental designs could be employed in order to estimate such carryover effects.

THINGS TO REMEMBER

Major Analysis Options

1. A routine SAS® GLM program for a 6-sequence unreplicated multiple baseline design.

2. A modification of the first design to involve replication of at least one treatment-sequence can lead to an analysis program similar to that of Table 9.6 and (with large enough sample sizes in one or more treatment sequences), to follow-up analyses using the "REPEATED" option to assess sphericity.

Interpreting Results of Computational Methods Not Previously Discussed

1. Appropriate selection of carryovers to compare permits identification of one such difference as an estimate of elation effect and another as an estimate of depression effect in an experiment on the effects of changing reward levels given to individual subjects.

2. If there is evidence of nonsphericity in a repeated measurements analysis from the second option shown previously, one may consider use of contrasts in a further analysis, just as was done in Methods B and D of chapter 8.

EXERCISES

1. Run the programs in this chapter, making up new data as needed for Table 10.6. Otherwise, do you obtain the same results as previously reported?

2. Can you use a model like Equation 10.1 but with one carryover $\lambda_A - \lambda_B$ and an interaction of direct and residual (carryover) effects of treatments $(\tau\lambda)_{AA} - (\tau\lambda)_{AB} - (\tau\lambda)_{BA} + (\tau\lambda)_{BB}$? Try to develop appropriate computer programs for assessing the effects assumed in this model and for evaluating the efficiency values of this design with the new model. How do the new efficiencies compare to those of Table 10.5?

11

Block-Randomization Experiments With Multiple Treatments, Each Once Per Block of Stages

INTRODUCTION

Sometimes psychologists want to perform an experiment with more than one block of observations of each subject and with each block having as many stages as there are treatments to compare (McBurney, 1983; Shaughnessy & Zechmeister, 1990). Then each treatment is given once in each block for each subject. This approach is attractive because it ensures that each subject has the same amount of experience with each treatment in each block, possibly minimizing contamination of estimates of treatment effects by time-related effects. It is tempting to find a mean for each treatment for each subject and treat these means as raw data for analyzing treatment effects. One might also find a mean for each stage of the experiment and examine those means for evidence of practice effects. Cotton (1994) has warned, however, that failure to do a full analysis of data from this design may cause distortions in the conclusions one draws from those data.

METHOD A: DATA ANALYSIS ASSUMING CLASSICAL CARRYOVER EFFECTS

Orientation and Representative Design

We illustrate an analysis method for data from block-randomized experiments with the following example. For three blocks and six subjects, a specific random selection of permutations of four treatments yields the design in Table 11.1. Note that the number of stages per subject is equal to 12, the number of blocks times the number of treatments.

TABLE 11.1

A Block-Randomized Design for Comparing Four Treatments
in Three Blocks

	Block 1				Block 2				Block 3			
Stage	1	2	3	4	5	6	7	8	9	10	11	12
Subject 1	D	C	B	A	D	A	B	C	C	B	D	A
Subject 2	B	D	A	C	B	C	A	D	D	B	A	C
Subject 3	C	B	A	D	A	B	C	D	B	C	A	D
Subject 4	A	D	C	B	C	D	B	A	C	A	B	D
Subject 5	B	C	D	A	A	C	D	B	B	D	C	A
Subject 6	C	A	B	D	B	C	A	D	A	C	D	B

This design is nicely balanced for each subject and even for each subject in each block. Each subject in this design has three blocks with each block containing each treatment exactly once. However, some stages are quite unbalanced. For example, in Stage 6, A, B, and D occur once each and C appears three times. Each line of this design has some similarity to what could be called a systematic design with blocking of replicates (Cox, 1951), often a source of efficiency. However, there is more randomization and less system here than in Cox's examples.

For completely balanced designs, the reader may want to use the Latin square design of chapter 8 or the Berenblut designs discussed in Jones and Kenward (1989). Lack of balance in a design may reduce the probability of finding a true effect of a certain kind and size (statistical power) as well as reducing its efficiency for estimating such effects. However, unless the SAS® GLM output for a specific design and its associated statistical model fails to show reasonable expected mean squares and estimability information, we can proceed with confidence in an experiment based on such a design.

Hypothetical Data for This Block-Randomization Experiment

A possible set of data for this design appears in Table 11.2. The means in this table show an irregular trend toward higher scores for later stages of the experiment. They also show that mean performance is highest on Treatment D and lowest on Treatment C.

TABLE 11.2
Hypothetical Data for a Three Block, Four Treatment Design With Six Subjects

Block 1			Block 2				Block 3			
Stage 2	Stage 3	Stage 4	Stage 5	Stage 6	Stage 7	Stage 8	Stage 9	Stage 10	Stage 11	S
66.5	74.5	57.4	81.5	153.9	85.9	47.6	53.2	81.0	136.3	
(C)	(B)	(A)	(D)	(A)	(B)	(C)	(C)	(B)	(D)	
160.0	142.9	104.4	166.8	119.0	129.8	168.9	228.3	192.4	153.4	1
(D)	(A)	(C)	(B)	(C)	(A)	(D)	(D)	(B)	(A)	
65.2	74.9	125.8	77.0	115.3	110.2	143.0	172.8	158.7	111.9	
(B)	(A)	(D)	(A)	(B)	(C)	(D)	(B)	(C)	(A)	
155.9	146.5	102.5	150.5	149.7	192.7	151.2	111.0	192.7	217.9	1
(D)	(C)	(B)	(C)	(D)	(B)	(A)	(C)	(A)	(B)	
134.4	118.3	193.2	142.1	162.0	165.5	204.4	203.7	227.8	162.4	1
(C)	(D)	(A)	(A)	(C)	(D)	(B)	(B)	(D)	(C)	
66.6	131.7	193.8	166.2	118.5	119.1	149.6	140.2	125.9	221.9	1
(A)	(B)	(D)	(B)	(C)	(A)	(D)	(A)	(C)	(D)	
108.10	114.80	129.52	130.68	136.40	133.87	144.12	151.53	163.08	167.30	1
s	123.93 (A)		140.82 (B)		106.82 (C)		148.08 (D)			

What Should We Try to Learn From Data Obtained With This Design?

1. Are there any significant differences in performance for different subjects of this experiment?

2. Is there a change in performance as subjects gain more practice with this task? If so, we want to look for effects of the 12 stages.

3. Are there different effects of Treatments A, B, C, and D?

4. Is there a change in performance as a function of what treatment occurred on the previous stage (i.e., a carryover effect of previous treatments)?

A Model for Data From This Experiment

These questions can be answered by an appropriate analysis based on the following model:

$$Y_{ijk} = \mu + s_i + \pi_j + \tau_k + \lambda_{k'} + e_{ijk} \qquad (11.1)$$

where s_i is the random subject effect for Subject i, π_j is the effect for Stage j, τ_k is the effect of Treatment k, $\lambda_{k'}$ is the carryover from Treatment k' on the previous stage, and e_{ijk} is random error for Subject i on Stage j with Treatment k. As usual, we assume each subject has errors that are normal with a mean of zero and a Type H covariance structure, that subject effects are i.i.d. $N(0, \sigma_s^2)$, and that error and subject effects are independent. This implies multisample sphericity of the observations.

Analysis of Data

An Appropriate SAS® GLM Program

Here is a SAS® GLM program for analyzing the data for this experiment (Table 11.3).

TABLE 11.3

A Program for Analyzing Results From a Three Block, Four Treatment
Design With Six Subjects, Using Hypothetical Data From Table 11.2

---

* PROGRAM NAME IS BLOCRAN.SAS;
DATA BLOCRAN; INPUT SUBJ STAGE TREAT $ CARRY $ Y @@;
CARDS;

1	1	D	0	49.1	1	2	C	D	66.5	1	3	B	C	74.5
1	4	A	B	57.4	1	5	D	A	81.5	1	6	A	D	153.9
1	7	B	A	85.9	1	8	C	B	47.6	1	9	C	C	53.2
1	10	B	C	81.0	1	11	D	B	136.3	1	12	A	D	98.3
2	1	B	0	119.2	2	2	D	B	160.0	2	3	A	D	142.9
2	4	C	A	104.4	2	5	B	C	166.8	2	6	C	B	119.0
2	7	A	C	129.8	2	8	D	A	168.9	2	9	D	D	228.3
2	10	B	D	192.4	2	11	A	B	153.4	2	12	C	A	132.1
3	1	C	0	13.9	3	2	B	C	65.2	3	3	A	B	74.9
3	4	D	A	125.8	3	5	A	D	77.0	3	6	B	A	115.3
3	7	C	B	110.2	3	8	D	C	143.0	3	9	B	D	172.8
3	10	C	B	158.7	3	11	A	C	111.9	3	12	D	A	55.1
4	1	A	0	81.4	4	2	D	A	155.9	4	3	C	D	146.5
4	4	B	C	102.5	4	5	C	B	150.5	4	6	D	C	149.7
4	7	B	D	192.7	4	8	A	B	151.2	4	9	C	A	111.0
4	10	A	C	192.7	4	11	B	A	217.9	4	12	D	B	135.0
5	1	B	0	75.6	5	2	C	B	134.4	5	3	D	C	118.3
5	4	A	D	193.2	5	5	A	A	142.1	5	6	C	A	162.0
5	7	D	C	165.5	5	8	B	D	204.4	5	9	B	B	203.7
5	10	D	B	227.8	5	11	C	D	162.4	5	12	A	C	144.7
6	1	C	0	6.0	6	2	A	C	66.6	6	3	B	A	131.7
6	4	D	B	193.8	6	5	B	D	166.2	6	6	C	B	118.5
6	7	A	C	119.1	6	8	D	A	149.6	6	9	A	D	140.2
6	10	C	A	125.9	6	11	D	C	221.9	6	12	B	D	166.9

RUN; PROC GLM; CLASS SUBJ STAGE TREAT CARRY;
MODEL Y = SUBJ STAGE TREAT CARRY/SS1 E2 SS3 SS4 SOLUTION;
RANDOM SUBJ; MEANS SUBJ; MEANS STAGE; MEANS TREAT;
ESTIMATE 'STAGE 2 – STAGE 12' STAGE 0 1 0 0 0 0 0 0 0 0 0 –1;
ESTIMATE 'STAGE 3 – STAGE 12' STAGE 0 0 1 0 0 0 0 0 0 0 0 –1;
ESTIMATE 'STAGE 4 – STAGE 12' STAGE 0 0 0 1 0 0 0 0 0 0 0 –1;
ESTIMATE 'STAGE 5 – STAGE 12' STAGE 0 0 0 0 1 0 0 0 0 0 0 –1;
ESTIMATE 'STAGE 6 – STAGE 12' STAGE 0 0 0 0 0 1 0 0 0 0 0 –1;
ESTIMATE 'STAGE 7 – STAGE 12' STAGE 0 0 0 0 0 0 1 0 0 0 0 –1;
ESTIMATE 'STAGE 8 – STAGE 12' STAGE 0 0 0 0 0 0 0 1 0 0 0 –1;
ESTIMATE 'STAGE 9 – STAGE 12' STAGE 0 0 0 0 0 0 0 0 1 0 0 –1;
ESTIMATE 'STAGE 10 – STAGE 12' STAGE 0 0 0 0 0 0 0 0 0 1 0 –1;
ESTIMATE 'STAGE 11 – STAGE 12' STAGE 0 0 0 0 0 0 0 0 0 0 1 –1;
ESTIMATE 'TREAT A – TREAT D' TREAT 1 0 0 –1;
ESTIMATE 'TREAT B – TREAT D' TREAT 0 1 0 –1;

(Continued)

TABLE 11.3
(Continued)

ESTIMATE 'TREAT C – TREAT D' TREAT 0 0 1 –1;
ESTIMATE 'CARRY A – CARRY D' CARRY 0 1 0 0 –1;
ESTIMATE 'CARRY B – CARRY D' CARRY 0 0 1 0 –1;
ESTIMATE 'CARRY C – CARRY D' CARRY 0 0 0 1 –1;
TITLE 'BLOCK RANDOMIZATION WITH 4 TREATMENTS, 3 BLOCKS.
BLOCRAN.SAS.'; RUN ;

Results of Data Analysis

ANOVA. Table 11.4 summarizes the Type SAS® GLM II analysis of variance performed with the program just shown.

TABLE 11.4
Type II ANOVA Table Resulting from Table 11.3 Program

Source	Sum of Squares	df	Mean Square	F
Subjects	57,848.24	5	11,569.65	16.98****
Treatments	22,074.86	3	7,358.29	10.80****
Stages 2:12	22,464.69	10	2,246.47	3.30**
Carryovers	14,923.68	3	4,974.56	7.30***
Error	33,396.54	49	681.56	—

Note ** $p < 0.01$. *** $p < 0.001$. **** $p < 0.0001$.

This table indicates that all effects tested are significant at the 0.01 level or better.

Estimation of Effects. Results generated by the SOLUTION option in our MODEL statement and the ESTIMATE commands agree in implying that TREAT A – TREAT D = –32.23, TREAT B – TREAT D = –11.83, and TREAT C – TREAT D = –47.57 are unbiased estimates of the treatment effects: $\tau_A - \tau_D$, $\tau_B - \tau_D$, and $\tau_C - \tau_D$, respectively. However, only the two largest estimates were associated with significant t-values. Similarly, our SOLUTION and ESTIMATE computer output both imply the following unbiased values of carryover estimates: CARRY A – CARRY D = –34.33, CARRY B – CARRY D = –20.62, and CARRY C – CARRY D = –42.07 as estimates of $\lambda_A - \lambda_D$, $\lambda_B - \lambda_D$, and $\lambda_C - \lambda_D$, respectively, each being significant at the 0.05 level or better.

The estimation of stage effects is more complicated. As is often true, the E2 output regarding estimability (not shown) shows that no function of the STAGE 1 effect (π_1) effect and other stage effects but not involving carryover effects can be estimated.   Accordingly, the SOLUTION output for STAGE 1 is not very useful to us; we can only estimate 10 stage effect differences. This is why there are only 10 degrees of freedom for stages in Table 11.4 instead of the 11 degrees of freedom we would expect for 12 stages. Results generated by the SOLUTION option in our MODEL statement and the ESTIMATE commands agree in implying the following:

STAGE   2 – STAGE 12 = –6.63,   STAGE 3 – STAGE 12 = –3.95,
STAGE   4 – STAGE 12 = 10.94,   STAGE 5 – STAGE 12 = 10.64,
STAGE   6 – STAGE 12 = 28.30,   STAGE 7 – STAGE 12 = 22.12,
STAGE   8 – STAGE 12 = 20.17,   STAGE 9 – STAGE 12 = 28.32,
STAGE 10 – STAGE 12 = 50.32, and STAGE 11 – STAGE 12 = 50.01

as unbiased estimators of each respective π value for a certain stage minus π_{12}. For example, $\pi_{10} - \pi_{12}$ is estimated by the STAGE 10 – STAGE 12 estimate: 50.32. The only significant t-tests for stage effects are for STAGE 10 – STAGE 12 and STAGE 11 – STAGE 12.

Because we actually assumed subject effects to be random, the SAS® estimates of fixed subject effects are not useful to examine here.   We know From chapter 4 we know how to find expected mean squares for subjects and for error. If the former does not contain contribution from factors other than those two, chapter 4 also tells us how to compute an estimate of σ_s^2, the variance of subject effects. Behavior scientists usually find such random effect estimates of less interest than fixed effect estimates, however.

Computing Efficiencies and Dimensionless Variances of Estimators for Parameter Differences in This Example. Using standard methods allows us to find efficiencies and variances (in multiples of $\frac{\sigma^2}{n}$) for the estimators of parameter differences modeled in (11.1) for this design (Table 11.5).

TABLE 11.5

Efficiencies and Dimensionless Variances of Estimators for Parameter Differences of the Block Randomization Design and Model Investigated in Table 11.4

	$\sum \sum a_{gj}^2 =$ Estimator Variance In multiples of $\dfrac{\sigma^2}{n}$	Efficiency = E
Stage 2 – Stage 12	0.3453	96.53
Stage 3 – Stage 12	0.3405	97.90
Stage 4 – Stage 12	0.3374	98.79
Stage 5 – Stage 12	0.3369	98.94
Stage 6 – Stage 12	0.3467	96.14
Stage 7 – Stage 12	0.3490	95.51
Stage 8 – Stage 12	0.3395	98.18
Stage 9 – Stage 12	0.3446	96.73
Stage 10 – Stage 12	0.3500	95.24
Stage 11 – Stage 12	0.3409	97.78
Treat A – Treat D	0.1270	87.49
Treat B – Treat D	0.1275	87.15
Treat C – Treat D	0.1245	89.25
Carry A – Carry D	0.1472	75.48
Carry B – Carry D	0.1447	76.79
Carry C – Carry D	0.1362	81.58

This specific block randomization design is somewhat more sensitive to stage effects than to treatment and carryover effects. The values of these variances generally appear small, and the efficiencies large, compared to other designs we have considered. This suggests that the present design is quite a useful one. However, note that its sensitivity to treatment and carryover effect differences stems in part from the use of three four-stage blocks and, thus, three replications of each treatment for each subject. This is good because it is often more convenient to use a within-subjects design to make repeated measurements on a small number of subjects than to use a between-subjects design with a larger number of subjects to get the same efficiency of design. Note that these efficiencies, like those for the randomized block designs of chapter 3, are conditional upon selection of the specific stimulus sequences employed in a given experiment rather than averaging across all possible experiments of a given basic design, model, numbers of treatments, and stages, as well as of randomly selected sequences.

METHOD B1: DATA ANALYSIS ASSUMING TRANSITIONAL CARRYOVER EFFECTS

Orientation

Instead of the classical carryover effects, λ_A, λ_B, λ_C, and λ_D included in Equation 11.1, we might want to model 16 different carryovers such as λ_{AA}, λ_{AB}, λ_{AC}, and λ_{AD} (for carryovers from A, the first subscript, on one stage to another treatment, the second subscript, on the next stage). An analysis based on this approach would be an expansion for a four-treatment design of the use of a model in chapter 10 with λ_{AA}, λ_{AB}, λ_{BA}, and λ_{BB} with a two-treatment counterbalanced design.

A Transitional Carryover Model for This Kind of Experiment

One difficulty with such an analysis here is that carryovers from a treatment to the same treatment can only occur at the end of one block and the beginning of the next block. This is because no treatment is allowed to appear more than once in a block. With random selection of blocks, some or all of these matched cases such as λ_{AA} will apply, but more rarely than for most specific pairs of different treatments. This causes poorer estimation of functions of so-called standpat carryovers (λ_{AA}, λ_{BB}, λ_{CC}, and λ_{DD}) than of others, the so-called switching carryovers. Nonetheless, we have analyzed data for the following model:

$$Y_{ijk} = \mu + s_i + \pi_j + \tau_k + \lambda_{k'k} + e_{ijk} \qquad (11.2)$$

where all terms have the same definitions and distributional properties as with Equation 11.1 except that we include $\lambda_{k'k}$ as the carryover from Treatment k' on the previous stage to Treatment k on the present stage.

Re-Analysis of Hypothetical Data From a Block-Randomized Experiment

An Appropriate Data Analysis Program

For use with Equation 11.2, the Table 11.3 program is modified so that when an AA pattern appears, the CARRY column entry reads AA; when AB appears, it reads AB; and so on through patterns beginning with Bs and with Cs and on to DA, DB, DC, and DD patterns. Table 11.6 presents the revised CARRY labels in six rows for the six subjects rather than as a single column of 72 entries for the actual program.

TABLE 11.6

Revised CARRY Labels for the Program of Table 11.3 With Equation 11.2

(Row 1 for Subject 1, Row 2 for Subject 2, and so on.)

0	DC	CB	BA	AD	DA	AB	BC	CC	CB	BD	DA
0	BD	DA	AC	CB	BC	CA	AD	DD	DB	BA	AC
0	CB	BA	AD	DA	AB	BC	CD	DB	BC	CA	AD
0	AD	DC	CB	BC	CD	DB	BA	AC	CA	AB	BD
0	BC	CD	DA	AA	AC	CD	DB	BB	BD	DC	CA
0	CA	AB	BD	DB	BC	CA	AD	DA	AC	CD	DB

Results of Data Analysis

ANOVA. Table 11.7 summarizes the Type SAS® GLM II analysis of variance performed with the modifications just recommended.

TABLE 11.7

Type II ANOVA Table Resulting From the Table 11.3 Program
Modified to Include Material From Table 11.6

Source	Sum of Squares	df	Mean Square	F
Subjects	35,369.47	5	7,073.89	9.10****
Treatments	4,450.23	3	1,483.41	1.91
Stages 2:12	18,704.65	10	1,870.46	2.41*
Carryovers	19,558.42	15	1,303.89	1.68
Error	28,761.80	37	777.35	—

Note. $* p < 0.05.-**** p < 0.0001.$

As with Table 11.4, subject and stage effects are statistically significant. However, there is difficulty with other previously significant effects: Treatments now do not approach significance ($p = 0.1452$), and carryover effects are only slightly closer to significance ($p = 0.0999$).

Estimation of Effects. Because of inconsistencies in the results of analyses for the models in (11.1) and (11.2), we do not present parameter estimates for the latter, transitional carryover model, analysis. Rather we turn to a supplementary method, Method B2.

METHOD B2: FINDING DIRECT
PLUS TRANSITIONAL CARRYOVER EFFECTS

Introduction

An approach not previously considered in this book is to assess something like cumulative effects of treatments (i. e., the sum of treatment effects and of carryovers of those treatments; Kershner & Federer, 1981). There a cumulative effect was defined in terms of the current treatment effect plus the carryover from a prior treatment, with a model like that of (11.1). But something more interesting might be a total effect of the current treatment and carryover to that treatment. Thus $\tau_A + \lambda_{AA}$ would apply on a stage receiving Treatment A after Treatment A, and $\tau_A + \lambda_{BA}$ would apply on a stage receiving Treatment A after Treatment B. Averaging across prior treatments would yield a total Treatment k effect, τ_k^*, like this: $\tau_k^* = \tau_k + \overline{\lambda}_{.k}$. We perform this averaging using equal weights with each relevant carryover. For example, this implies that $\overline{\lambda}_{.A} = .25(\lambda_{AA} + \lambda_{BA} + \lambda_{CA} + \lambda_{DA})$.

What Should We Try to Learn About Total Treatment Effects?

The total treatment effects of a single treatment will not ordinarily be estimable. However, because E2 estimability information implies that $\tau_k - \tau_D$ and $\lambda_{k'k} - \lambda_{Dk}$ for any current treatment k and prior treatment k', we are always able to estimate $\tau_k^* - \tau_D^*$, the difference between the total treatment effects for a certain treatment and for the final treatment. We would like to test such a difference for statistical significance. Finally, we would like an overall test comparing such differences.

Programming the Supplementary Analysis

The SAS® GLM program based on Tables 11.3 and 11.6 simply needs the addition of appropriate ESTIMATE and CONTRAST commands to satisfy the goals just established. Table 11.8 presents those commands, to precede the TITLE statements in the program used previously.

Results of the Supplementary Analysis

The test of combined total effects of treatments and carryovers has $MS_{TR\&CARRY} = 4,932.60$ which, with the mean square for error from Table 11.7, yields $F(3,37) = 6.35$, $p = 0.0014$. Separate analyses yield $\hat{\tau}_A^* - \hat{\tau}_D^* = -38.23$, $t(37) = -2.80$, $p = 0.0080$, $\hat{\tau}_B^* - \hat{\tau}_D^* = -10.01$, $t(37)$ $= -0.77$, $p = 0.4436$, and $\hat{\tau}_C^* - \hat{\tau}_D^* = -49.41$, $t(37) = -3.75$, $p = 0.0006$. These estimates are fairly close in value and significance to the estimates of -32.23, -11.83, and -47.57, respectively, associated with Method A and presented just after Table 11.4.

Note that a comparison of total effects for treatments and transitional carryovers with the current design is much like a comparison of main effects plus average carryovers in the within-subjects factorial design of chapter 5.

FINAL THOUGHTS

Obviously, the use here of six subjects, four treatments and three blocks, with each treatment occurring exactly once per block, is just one possibility. Another design option is to use this same type of design with modified numbers of subjects, treatments, and blocks. For greater sensitivity of research in studies with few observations per subject, we recommend use of the Latin square and Berenblut designs mentioned earlier in this chapter. Another possibility with many observations per subject is to have each block contain several examples of each treatment (Schneider & Fisk, 1984) or even weight the frequency of each treat-

TABLE 11.8

ESTIMATE and CONTRAST Commands to Be Added to the Program Combining Tables 11.3 and
in Order to Assess Total Treatment Effects

U_A* – TAU_D*'	TREAT 1 0 0 –1 CARRY 0 .25 0 0 –.25 .25 0 0 –.25 .25 0 0 –.25
U_B* – TAU_D*	TREAT 0 1 0 –1 CARRY 0 0 .25 0 –.25 0 .25 0 –.25 0 .25 0 –.25
U_C* – TAU_D*'	TREAT 0 0 1 –1 CARRY 0 0 0 .25 –.25 0 0 .25 –.25 0 0 .25 –.25
COMB TR & CARRY'	TREAT 1 0 0 –1 CARRY 0 .25 0 0 –.25 .25 0 0 –.25 .25 0 0 –.25 .2
	TREAT 0 1 0 –1 CARRY 0 0 .25 0 –.25 0 .25 0 –.25 0 .25 0 –.25 0
	TREAT 0 0 1 –1 CARRY 0 0 0 .25 –.25 0 0 .25 –.25 0 0 .25 –.25 0

ment by the number of possibilities in its category (Carlson & Schneider, 1989).

THINGS TO REMEMBER

Major Analysis Options

1. Analyzing data from a block-randomized experiment with SAS® GLM when the model equation involves an intercept, a random subject effect and random error plus fixed stage, treatment, and carryover effects from immediately prior treatments.

2. Analyzing data from a block-randomized experiment with SAS® GLM when the model equation involves an intercept, a random subject effect and random error plus fixed stage, treatment, and transitional carryover effects. The latter (e.g., $\lambda_{AA}, \lambda_{AB}, \lambda_{AC},$ or λ_{AD}) depend both on the immediately prior treatment and on the current treatment.

Interpreting Results of Computational Methods
Not Previously Discussed

1. From printed output you obtain by re-running the program associated with Table 11.6 in Exercise 1 (next), you can estimate $\lambda_{AA} - \lambda_{DA}$. Its value tells you how differently you respond to an A following an A than to an A following a D. In general, you may wish to pay attention to two kinds of such carryovers, standpat carryovers reflecting no change in treatment from one stage to the next ($\lambda_{AA}, \lambda_{BB}, \lambda_{CC},$ and λ_{DD}) and switching carryovers (e.g., $\lambda_{BA}, \lambda_{CA}, \lambda_{DA},$ and λ_{AB}).

EXERCISES

1. Run the programs based on Tables 11.3, 11.6, and 11.8 to verify the results shown in this chapter.

2. Using output from the Table 11.6 and 11.8 programs, compute the dimensionless variances and efficiencies of estimating parameters of in-

terest with the current experimental design for the model of Equation 11.2.

3. Can you make up an example of a three-subject, three-block, three-treatment design block randomized design? What must you check to be sure it meets the definition of such a design? How different would the alternate models' programs for this design be from the ones you see in Tables 11.3 and 11.6?

4. (a) Could you make the example in Exercise 2 be such that every subject in the design had its nine scores forming a 3 × 3 Latin square with blocks as a row variable and stages as a column variable? (b) If so, how many different Latin squares would be needed? Why? (c) Would it be better to analyze data from this design with the techniques of this chapter or with techniques suited for Latin square model? Explain.

5. Suppose that we changed the design of our first example so that it would look like Table 11.9 (next), with hypothetical data as in Table 11.2 but tied to different arrangements of treatments. What difficulties of estimation arise with this specific design when the transitional carryover model of (11.2) is employed here? Explain what you think is the source of difficulty in the design.

TABLE 11.9
Hypothetical Data for a Three Block, Four Treatment Design With Six Subjects

Block 1				Block 2				Block 3	
Stage 2	Stage 3	Stage 4	Stage 5	Stage 6	Stage 7	Stage 8	Stage 9	Stage 10	Stage 11
66.5	74.5	57.4	81.5	153.9	85.9	47.6	53.2	81.0	136.3
(C)	(B)	(A)	(B)	(D)	(C)	(A)	(C)	(B)	(D)
160.0	142.9	104.4	166.8	119.0	129.8	168.9	228.3	192.4	153.4
(D)	(A)	(C)	(B)	(C)	(A)	(D)	(D)	(B)	(C)
65.2	74.9	125.8	77.0	115.3	110.2	143.0	172.8	158.7	111.9
(B)	(A)	(D)	(A)	(B)	(C)	(D)	(B)	(D)	(C)
155.9	146.5	102.5	150.5	149.7	192.7	151.2	111.0	192.7	217.9
(D)	(C)	(A)	(B)	(C)	(D)	(A)	(C)	(D)	(B)
134.4	118.3	193.2	142.1	162.0	165.5	204.4	203.7	227.8	162.4
(C)	(B)	(A)	(A)	(C)	(D)	(B)	(B)	(D)	(C)
66.6	131.7	193.8	166.2	118.5	119.1	149.6	140.2	125.9	221.9
(A)	(B)	(D)	(B)	(C)	(A)	(D)	(A)	(B)	(D)
108.10	114.80	129.52	130.68	136.40	133.87	144.12	151.53	163.08	167.30

is   111.65 (A)   137.15 (B)   109.77 (C)   161.08 (D)

12

Analyzing Data From an ABBA Versus BAAB Counterbalanced Design

INTRODUCTION

Orientation

A replicated ABBA design is a well-known psychological design in which the average stage number is constant for two treatments, A and B. For example, with four stages, the A condition in a ABBA sequence has $\frac{(1+4)}{2} = 2.5$ as an average stage number; the B condition has $\frac{(2+3)}{2} = 2.5$ as well. The original purpose of such designs was to give an equal average amount of practice effect at each treatment when performance under it was tested. If one could assume that practice effects were linear and carryover effects did not distort treatment mean differences, then the difference between average performance under A and average performance under B would be the difference between effects of Treatments A and B, uncontaminated by differences in practice effects.

To analyze data from dual-balanced experiments with replicated ABBA and BAAB sequences, we let our units of analysis be secondary data called contrasts like those of chapter 8, for example. Relying on an earlier source (Cotton & Kenward, 1991), we now use such contrasts as we analyze hypothetical data from such an experiment. These contrasts form the input to t-tests of possible effects. For readers who have progressed this far in the study of crossover designs, it seems appropriate to show how the GAUSS mathematical programming package (Aptech Systems, 1993) can be used to generate these contrasts, rather than using SAS® GLM in the indirect fashion discussed in chapter 8.

Historical Example of This Design in Use

An example of a variant of the ABBA design in psychology is the $A^{24}B^{24} \; B^{24}A^{24}$ design (or should we infer that it was balanced to have an $A^{24}B^{24}B^{24}A^{24}$ versus $B^{24}A^{24} \; A^{24}B^{24}$ structure?) in MacArthur and Sekuler's (1982) third task (direction uncertainty) in a study of the effects of drinking alcohol on motion perception. Each of nine male subjects pressed a button as soon as he saw a dot moving on a cathode ray tube screen, with reaction time being the primary response measure. In the A condition there were blocks of 24 trials in which movement was always to the right; in the B condition the blocks included 12 trials each randomly assigned to left and 12 trials each to right movement. Mean reaction time increased in the B (direction uncertainty) condition but was unaffected by presence or absence of alcohol of various dosages or by the time since that dose.

A full analysis of a crossover design experiment of this complexity is beyond the scope of this chapter. However, we will simulate data and analyze them to reflect processes that might have been observed by MacArthur and Sekuler. Each subject will be measured in an ABBA condition or a BAAB condition, not an $A^{24}B^{24}B^{24}A^{24}$ or $B^{24}A^{24}A^{24}B^{24}$ condition; no variation in alcohol dosage or time since drinking will be involved. In a trial with Condition A, each subject is told to expect the dot to move to the right. In a trial with Condition B each subject is told to expect the dot to move to the right with probability one-half and to the left with probability one-half. On the average, one-fourth of the subjects will see left–right, one-fourth will see right–left, one-fourth will see left–left, and one-fourth will see right–right movements on their B trials.

Now we turn to a model for data from this hypothetical experiment, with reaction time being assumed to be a linear function of stage number and an unrestricted function of treatments (Conditions A and B) and of prior treatments forming a carryover effect. As usual, random subject effects will be assumed to be present. For convenience, reaction times (RT values) will be assumed normally distributed, a most unlikely event. Normality assumptions do often fail in real experiments (Micceri, 1989) and the reader may wish to make the basic datum for analysis be log RT as used by MacArthur and Sekuler or some other transformation of RT.

METHOD A: DATA ANALYSIS ASSUMING LINEAR STAGE EFFECTS

A Model for an ABBA Versus BAAB Replicated Design With Linear Trend

Suppose that we let i be the sequence number $i = 1$ for ABBA and $i = 2$ for BAAB. Also let j be the stage number, k be the subject number, m be the current treatment, and m' be the treatment on the preceding stage. If our earlier analysis of variance methods were to be employed here, a natural model for behavior observed with this design might be:

$$Y_{ijkm} = \mu + s_{ik} + j\,\beta_1 + \tau_m + \lambda_{m'm} + e_{ijkm} \tag{12.1}$$

where Y_{ijkm} is the observation, μ is an additive constant, the s_{ik} are random subject effects for Subject k of Treatment Sequence i and are i.i.d. $N(0, \sigma_s^2)$, β_1 is the slope constant for a linear practice effect, τ_m is a treatment effect, $\lambda_{m'm}$ is the carryover effect from Treatment m' on the immediately preceding stage to Treatment m on the present stage, and e_{ijkm} is the random error component on Stage j of Subject k in Sequence i with Treatment m. The error component vectors for different subjects are normally distributed with a zero mean and a Type H covariance structure across stages. Error components e_{ijk} and subject effects $s_{i'k'}$ are independent regardless of whether $[i,k] = [i',k']$. So, multisample sphericity holds under this model.

For the analyses in the present chapter, however, we relax the foregoing distributional assumptions to require only that contrasts for individual samples be drawn randomly from normal distributions for populations applicable to each sequence group. If population variance are equal for a given type of contrast, the t-distribution applies when the hypothesis of equal means is true. So a conventional t-test can be used to test that hypothesis or, with evidence of unequal population variances, one applies a so-called Satterthwaite correction.

Hypothetical Data for a Replicated ABBA Versus BAAB Design

Table 12.1 shows hypothetical data for the present design with six subjects receiving ABBA and six receiving BAAB treatment.

TABLE 12.1

Data for a Hypothetical Motion Perception Experiment
Using ABBA and BAAB Sequences for Six Subjects Each
(A = Directional Certainty, B = Directional Uncertainty, Responses in ms)

Stage	Stage and Treatment				Mean
	1	2	3	4	
Subject	(A)	(B)	(B)	(A)	
S1	244.9	255.6	238.0	209.7	237.05
S2	276.3	283.6	274.6	235.5	267.50
S3	255.8	275.6	256.6	213.7	250.42
S4	270.4	289.6	275.2	229.8	266.25
S5	273.2	288.4	271.5	226.0	264.78
S6	263.8	269.2	268.5	233.8	258.82
Mean	264.07	277.00	264.07	224.75	257.47
Subject	(B)	(A)	(A)	(B)	
S7	299.3	248.3	220.7	227.1	248.85
S8	287.7	237.5	213.9	239.5	244.65
S9	294.8	240.6	225.1	237.6	249.52
S10	298.1	240.0	230.4	248.5	254.25
S11	299.0	254.1	225.5	248.3	256.72
S12	289.0	250.9	234.4	252.3	256.65
Mean	294.65	245.23	225.00	242.22	251.78
Overall Mean	279.36	261.12	244.53	233.48	254.62
Treatment Mean	239.76 (A)		269.48 (B)		

Analysis of Data

An Appropriate SAS® Program

Table 12.2 presents a SAS® program for analyzing these data. Note that it uses "proc ttest", not "proc GLM". Saying "class seq;" says to do t-tests comparing mean contrast scores for the ABBA and BAAB sequences. As in earlier examples, because we want each t-test to compare a certain pair of sums of contrasts for the ABBA and BAAB sequences, the BAAB sequence contrasts are temporarily defined incorrectly as the negative of their real value. There are six such t-test comparisons, one for each of six new measures called "var" in the program, "slope" for linear trend in stages,"tau_AB" for the difference between treatment effects for Conditions A and B, and "lam_AA", "lam_AB", "lam_BA", and "lam_BB" for carryovers from the treatment on the immediately prior stage to that on the current stage.

TABLE 12.2

A Program for Analyzing Data From an ABBA Versus BAAB Design
If Stage Effects Are Linear

```
/*  Program name is abbalin.sas, a program for finding and using summary
contrast scores for a linear trend model using an ABBA vs. BAAB design
with 6 subjects per sequence.  Testing for 4 carryovers.            */
data abba; input y1 y2 y3 y4 seq subject @@; mult = 2 - seq;
slope = .25*(mult*(-y2+y4)+(1-mult)*(y2-y4));
tauA_B = .5*mult*(2*y1-y2-y4)+.5*(1-mult)*(2*y1-y2-y4);
lam_AA = mult*(-y1+y2)+(1-mult)*(-y3+y4);
lam_AB= .75*mult*(y2-y4)+(1-mult)*(y1-.75*y2-.25*y4);
lam_BA = mult*(-y1+.75*y2+.25*y4)+.75*(1-mult)*(-y2+y4);
lam_BB = mult*(y3-y4)+(1-mult)*(y1-y2); cards;
244.9 255.6 238.0 209.7 1   1     276.3 283.6 274.6 235.5 1   2
255.8 275.6 256.6 213.7 1   3     270.4 289.6 275.2 229.8 1   4
273.2 288.4 271.5 226.0 1   5     263.8 269.2 268.5 233.8 1   6
299.3 248.3 220.7 227.1 2   7     287.7 237.5 213.9 239.5 2   8
294.8 240.6 225.1 237.6 2   9     298.1 240.0 230.4 248.5 2  10
299.0 254.1 225.5 248.3 2  11     289.0 250.9 234.4 252.3 2  12
run; proc means; proc ttest; class seq;  var slope tauA_B lam_AA
lam_AB lam_BA lam_BB; proc print; data abba;
title 'BEWARE: Sequence 2 estimates are the negative of true ones.';
title2 'This permits automatic calculation of t values.'; run;
```

Further Interpretation of What This SAS® Program Has to Say. Like similar programs (e.g., chapter 8, this volume), the *t*-test program in Table 12.2 has its data step include not only input but also the definitions of new variables: One is called "mult" and is equal to 2 minus the sequence number, making it 1 for the ABBA sequence and 0 for the BAAB sequence. The other six definitions form summary scores, called contrasts, of the four basic observations for each subject. For example, *lam_BB* for a given subject, is equal to: [a constant, *mult*, times ($y_3 - y_4$) for that subject] plus [($1 - mult$) times ($y_1 - y_2$) for that subject]. Combining *lam_BB* contrasts properly leads to an estimate of λ_{BB} even though no individual contrast score is an unbiased estimate of that carryover. Justification for the definitions of specific contrast scores is deferred to Appendix 2 because it requires discussion of the GAUSS™ computer language (Aptech Systems, 1993).

Results of Data Analysis

When the program of Table 12.2 is run, the following contrast scores and t-tests in Table 12.3 result.

TABLE 12.3
Contrast Scores[1] and Their Analysis, for the Data of Table 12.1

Subject	Treat Contr	AA Contr	AB Contr	BA Contr	BB Contr	Slope Contr
S1	12.2	10.7	34.4	−0.8	28.3	−11.5
S2	16.8	7.3	36.1	−4.7	39.1	−12.0
S3	11.2	19.8	46.4	4.3	42.9	−15.5
S4	10.7	19.2	44.8	4.2	45.4	−15.0
S5	16.0	15.2	46.8	−0.4	45.5	−15.6
S6	12.3	5.4	26.6	−3.4	34.7	−8.8
Mean 1	13.19	12.93	39.19	−0.13	39.32	−13.06
s	2.55	6.08	8.18	3.79	6.79	2.73
S7	61.6	6.4	56.3	−15.9	51.0	5.3
S8	49.2	25.6	49.7	1.5	50.2	−0.5
S9	55.7	12.5	55.0	−2.2	54.2	0.8
S10	53.8	18.1	56.0	6.4	58.1	−2.1
S11	47.8	22.8	46.4	-4.4	44.9	1.4
S12	37.4	17.9	37.8	1.0	38.1	-0.4
Mean 2	50.92	17.22	50.17	−2.26	49.42	0.75
s	8.26	6.96	7.26	7.62	7.07	2.54
Comb. Est.[2]	−37.73	−4.29	−10.98	2.13	−10.10	−13.81
t	−10.69 ****	−1.14	−2.46*	0.61	−2.52*	−9.08 ****
df	5.9	10	10	10	10	10

Note. * $p < 0.05$. **** $p < 0.0001$. [1]Scores for S7 through S12 are negatives of true contrasts; combined estimates and t's use Mean 1 − Mean 2 from above. [2]Hand computed as Mean 1 − Mean 2 before rounding of other computer output.

As indicated earlier, a great advantage of using contrasts here is that even regardless of whether a multigroup sphericity property holds for the observations, a t-test of some form comparing mean contrasts is legitimate. Ordinarily one assumes that variances for the two sequences are equal. There are two ways to assess this equality: (a) On the basis of theory, we know that, if the covariance structures for observations from different sequences are identical, having the same basic definition (except possibly for algebraic sign) of a contrast for one sequence (ABBA) and of another (BAAB) implies equal variances for their contrasts. (b) We can be more empirical and simply perform an F-test of the assumption of homogeneity of variances for contrasts from the two sequences.

Consider the first option: In the symbols of our program of Table 12.2, we estimate the slope, b, with the following contrasts for either ABBA or BAAB sequences: $.25(-y_2 + y_4)$ provided that we correct the sign changes mentioned in Table 12.2. In the more detailed terms of (12.1), the slope contrast for an ABBA subject is $.25 (-y_2 + y_4) = .25(-Y_{12kB} + Y_{14kA})$ and the corrected slope contrast for a BAAB subject is $-.25(y_2 - y_4) = .25(-Y_{22kA} + Y_{24kB})$. Clearly, slope has an identical basic definition in each sequence group. For treatment effect differences $(\tau_A - \tau_B)$, the contrast for an ABBA subject is $.5(2y_1 - y_2 + y_4)$, and the corrected contrast for a BAAB subject is its negative, $-.5(2y_1 - y_2 + y_4)$. Except for this change of sign, the definitions of the two kinds of contrasts for treatment effect differences are the same. So the assumptions of homogeneity of variances of the two kinds of slope contrasts and of the two kinds of treatment difference contrasts are justified if the further assumption of equal covariance structures of the Y_{ijkm} values for the two treatment sequences holds. Identity of basic definitions does not occur for any of the other contrast types computed with the program of Table 12.2.

Now consider the second option: SAS® PROC TTEST routinely does an F-test of the hypothesis of homogeneity of variances of its data entries. Because the assumption of equal covariance structures for original observations from the two sequence groups might fail in any example, we choose to be guided by information from Option b in all cases. Therefore, whenever a test for unequal variances shown in SAS® output just below a t-test is significant, we report the so-called Satterthwaite correction, yielding the same t as otherwise but with a reduced degree of freedom value.

For example, despite the identity of basic contrast definitions noted earlier, the t-test for treatment contrasts in Table 12.3 uses a fractional number of degrees of freedom, 5.9, rather than the 10 expected with two independent groups of six subjects each. A corrected value (the "Unequal Variances" result) is reported by SAS® for every t-test, together with the traditional value (the "Equal Variances" result).

Table 12.3 exhibits significant ($p < 0.05$) effects for λ_{AB} and λ_{BB} plus highly significant ($p < 0.0001$ or better) effects of slope and treatment effects. The combined estimate of slope suggests a decreased reaction time of almost 14 ms for each new stage, after taking out other estimates of effects. The combined estimate of Treat_Contr, -37.73, suggests a lower population mean reaction time for Treatment A (decision certainty) than for Treatment B (decision uncertainty), all other things being equal.

The present analysis based on a linear trend model follows the spirit of psychological experimentation using within-subject counterbalancing of treatments. That approach, even with only an ABBA or a BAAB sequence, assumes linear trend in order to imply equal average performance on Stages 1 and 4 compared to Stages 2 and 3 in the absence of differences in treatment effects and of differences in carryover effects. In addition to equalizing practice effects under each treatment for each subject in each treatment sequence, use of the present model with the ABBA versus BAAB counterbalanced design permits assessment of more carryover effect differences than were considered in classical carryover models (Kershner & Federer, 1981). There surely are many experimental situations, however, in which an assumption of a linear trend with stages would seem a poor approximation to reality.

For example, it is common to assume an exponential learning curve in a repeated measurements design in which the same treatment is given on every trial. If we can measure four equally spaced and (if the growth rate is large) very closely-spaced points on an exponential curve, the learning curve will be approximately linear. Even an ABBA or a BAAB design might then be a reasonable substitute for the repeated measurements design, and Equation 12.1 might be a reasonable model on which to base a data analysis even though the learning curve is really exponential. But, if such close and equal spacing is impossible, we should not assume linear trend at all nor expect to find an experimental means of equalizing practice effects for each treatment with a single treatment sequence (McBurney, 1983). If there are no differential effects of treatments nor of prior treatments (no differential carryover), use of dual-balanced designs like ABBA versus BAAB can nonetheless equalize means for Treatments A and B in the absence of linearity, however. To face this problem, the next section of this chapter presents an alternative model and associated data analysis.

Determining Efficiencies and Dimensionless Variances of Estimates of Effects From This Design and Linear Trend Model

We describe, but do not illustrate, computational techniques needed in order to obtain variances of estimates of effects in $\frac{\sigma^2}{n}$ units in this chapter as well as their associated efficiencies. First, consider the current design when modeled with Equation 12.1, assuming a linear stage effect and four transitional carryover effects. A standard SAS® GLM program was run with raw scores, not contrasts, as the data for analysis. The MODEL statement involved three class variables (subjects, treatments, and carryovers) as predictors plus one quantitative predictor (stages). ESTIMATE commands were of the forms:

```
ESTIMATE 'STAGE' STAGE 1;
ESTIMATE 'TREAT A – TREAT B' TREAT 1 –1;
ESTIMATE 'CARRY AA – CARRY 0' CARRY –1 1 0 0 0;
```

As suggested in the third of those ESTIMATE commands, a difficulty reflected in estimating carryover effects is that, with this design and model, SAS® GLM has to estimate the difference between each carryover and CARRY 0. The results, however, do apply to a comparable model without CARRY 0 and not analyzed with SAS® GLM. For example, programming with the model of (12.1) and the GAUSS™ computer language (Aptech Systems, 1993) mentioned earlier yields appropriate results here.

Finally, the methods of chapter 5 were employed to determine the dimensionless variances of each type of estimator. Linear trend is much better assessed than treatment effects and carryover effects, with dimensionless variance for slope (b) being 0.2500 ($E = 100.0$), for the treatment effect difference ($\tau_A - \tau_B$) being 3.000 ($E = 16.67$), for Carryover AA or Carryover BB (λ_{AA} or λ_{BB}) both being 4.000 ($E = 25.00$), and for Carryover AB or Carryover BA (λ_{AB} or λ_{BA}) both being 2.7500 ($E = 36.36$).

METHOD B: DATA WITH POSSIBLY NONLINEAR STAGE EFFECTS

A Model Involving Unrestricted Stage Effects

Once more, we model behavior under the present design, but now with stage effects being unrestricted rather than linear:

$$Y_{ijkm} = \mu + s_{ik} + \pi_j + \tau_m + \lambda_{m'm} + e_{ijkm} \qquad (12.2)$$

Again s_{ik} is a random subject effect for Subject k of Treatment Sequence i, τ_m is a treatment effect, $\lambda_{m'm}$ is the carryover effect from Treatment m' on the immediately preceding stage to Treatment m on the present stage, and e_{ijkm} is the random error component on Stage j of Subject k in Sequence i with Treatment m. The new term, π_j, is an effect for Stage j. For an analysis of variance approach rather than a contrast analysis, distributional assumptions about subject effects and error would be as given for Equation 12.1. However, t-tests using contrast analysis methods will be employed because of their advantages of requiring less stringent distributional assumptions than analysis of variance. It will turn out that only two carryover differences, rather than four separate carryovers, are estimable with the current model and experimental design.

Analysis of Data

An Appropriate SAS® Program

We need a further program which can be used to analyze data where non-linear stage effects may be present. Table 12.4 presents such a SAS® program for use with Equation 12.2 and the example data presented already. We are looking for any estimable stage, treatment, and carryover effect differences. However, we will not estimate nor test significance of the subject effects modeled in (12.2)—use of contrast analysis has the minor disadvantage of precluding such analyses.

TABLE 12.4

A Program for Analyzing Data From an ABBA Versus BAAB Design
Even If Stage Effects Are Not Linear

/* Program name is abbanl.sas, for finding and using summary contrast scores
for an arbitrary trend model using an ABBA versus BAAB design with 6 sub-
subjects per sequence. Testing 2 carry diffs. A = directional certainty, B =
uncertainty.   */

```
data abba; input y1 y2 y3 y4 seq subject @@; mult = 2 - seq;
tauA_B = .5*mult*(2*y1-y2-y4)+.5*(1-mult)*(2*y1-y2-y4);
IAB_BA = mult*(y1-y4)+(1-mult)*(y1-y4);
IAA_BB= mult*(-y1+y2-y3+y4)+(1-mult)*(-y1+y2-y3+y4);
pi2_4 = .5*mult*(y2-y4)-.5*(1-mult)*(y2-y4); cards;
244.9 255.6 238.0 209.7 1  1      276.3 283.6 274.6 235.5 1  2
255.8 275.6 256.6 213.7 1  3      270.4 289.6 275.2 229.8 1  4
273.2 288.4 271.5 226.0 1  5      263.8 269.2 268.5 233.8 1  6
299.3 248.3 220.7 227.1 2  7      287.7 237.5 213.9 239.5 2  8
294.8 240.6 225.1 237.6 2  9      298.1 240.0 230.4 248.5 2 10
299.0 254.1 225.5 248.3 2 11      289.0 250.9 234.4 252.3 2 12
run; proc means; proc ttest; class seq; var IAB_BA IAA_BB
tauA_B pi2_4; proc print; data abba2;
title 'BEWARE: Sequence 2 estimates are the negative of true ones.';
title2 'This permits automatic calculation of t values.';
proc glm data = abba; class seq; model y1-y4=seq/nouni;
repeated stage polynomial/short summary printe;
title 'ABBAnl.sas program for unrestricted stage effects.'; run;
```

Testing Individual Effects With t-Tests. Again, justification for the
definitions of specific contrasts is presented in Appendix 2. Table 12.4
allows us to test for treatment effects, two kinds of carryover effect differences, and the difference between stage effects for the second and
fourth stages only. See Equations 12.3 through 12.4a for model changes
that could permit comparison of all four stage effects in the current design unless we change the model based on Equation 12.2 slightly in
order to make the GLM portion of the previous program legitimate.

Results of New Data Analysis

Table 12.5 summarizes the contrasts and t-tests computed with the
program of Table 12.4.

TABLE 12.5

Contrast Scores[1] and Their Analysis for the Data of Table 12.1,
Under an Arbitrary Stage Effect Model Involving Two Carryover Differences

Subject	Treat_Contr	AB–BA Contr	AA–BB Contr	Stage2–4 Contr
S1	12.2	35.2	–17.6	23.0
S2	16.8	40.8	–31.8	24.0
S3	11.2	42.1	–23.1	31.0
S4	10.7	40.6	–26.2	29.9
S5	16.0	47.2	–30.3	31.2
S6	12.3	30.0	–29.3	17.7
Mean 1	13.19	39.32	–26.38	26.12
s	2.55	5.96	5.31	5.45
S7	61.6	72.2	–44.6	–10.6
S8	49.2	48.2	–24.6	1.0
S9	55.7	57.2	–41.7	–1.5
S10	53.8	49.6	–40.0	4.2
S11	47.8	50.7	–22.1	–2.9
S12	37.4	36.7	-20.2	0.7
Mean 2	50.92	52.43	–32.20	–1.51
s	8.26	11.75	11.03	5.08
Comb. Est.[2]	–37.73	–13.11	5.82	27.63
t	–10.69****	–2.44*	1.16	9.08****
df	5.9	10	10	10

Note. $* \ p < 0.05.$ $**** \ p < 0.0001.$ [1]Scores for S7 through S12 are negatives of true contrasts; combined estimates and t's use Mean 1 – Mean 2 from above. 2 Hand computed as Mean 1 – Mean 2 before rounding of computer output.

This table shows a significant ($p < 0.05$) difference between estimates of switching carryovers, $\lambda_{AB} - \lambda_{BA}$ with the latter appearing to be 13.11 ms larger than the former. There are highly significant ($p < 0.0001$ or better) differences between estimated treatment effects (exactly the same as in the analysis based on Equation 12.1) and also between estimated values of π_2 and π_4, with almost a 28 ms higher value for Stage 2 than for Stage 4.

Testing for Differences Among Stage Means. The "proc glm" section in Table 12.4 analyzes raw scores rather than contrasts, leading to various tests of the following hypothesis:

$$H: [\bar{\mu}_{.1} - \bar{\mu}_{.4}, \bar{\mu}_{.2} - \bar{\mu}_{.4}, \bar{\mu}_{.3} - \bar{\mu}_{.4})] = [0,0,0] \tag{12.3}$$

which says that each difference between a stage population mean and the Stage 4 population mean is zero—that the plot of stage population means against stages is flat. It is easy to show algebraically from Equation 12.2 and its average values for different stages that Equation 12.3 implies:

$$H: [\pi_1 - \pi_4 - .5(\lambda_{AB} + \lambda_{BA}), \pi_2 - \pi_4, \pi_3 - \pi_4 +$$

$$.5(\lambda_{AA} - \lambda_{AB} - \lambda_{BA} + \lambda_{BB})] = [0, 0, 0] \tag{12.4}$$

However, we have implicitly rejected this hypothesis in our t-test for differences between Stage 2 and 4 effects. So we need not report either the univariate test (requiring a multisample sphericity property) or multivariate test of stage effects related to the Hs. On the other hand, if this t-test had not been significant, we still might wish to test the H of (12.3) and (12.4).

Constraining Carryover Effects to Permit Checking for Nonlinearity of Stage Effects. Suppose that we assume $\lambda_{AB} + \lambda_{BA} = 0$ and $\lambda_{AA} + \lambda_{BB} = 0$ in Equation 12.2. Then (12.4) becomes:

$$H^*: [\pi_1 - \pi_4, \pi_2 - \pi_4, \pi_3 - \pi_4] = [0, 0, 0] \tag{12.4a}$$

Each stage effect difference from Stage Effect 4 is equal to zero. Under appropriate assumptions, the univariate and multivariate tests of H just mentioned would now test H^*. However, once again H^* is implicitly rejected because of our earlier significant t-test for differences between Stage 2 and 4 effects.

Also, under a multisample sphericity condition, the univariate polynomial function tests of the current program would be tests of linear, quadratic, and cubic components of stage means. For the present data the $F(1,10)$ for linear trend is 277.96 ($p < 0.001$), and the $F(1,10)$ for quadratic trend is 5.82 ($p < 0.05$), but the $F(1,10) = 0.49$ for cubic trend does not approach significance. However, unless good reason can be found to assume $\lambda_{AB} + \lambda_{BA} = 0$ and $\lambda_{AA} + \lambda_{BB} = 0$, it is better to interpret these Fs (labeled as having a source = Mean in the computer output) as implying significant linear and quadratic components for stage means, not for stage effects. Multivariate tests are reported with SAS® GLM for repeated measurements and can be invoked here if multisample sphericity seems doubtful.

Despite our inability to develop a convincing set of assumptions justifying a test of nonlinearity of stage effects, we advocate the use of (12.2) rather than (12.1) as the model for data from the ABBA versus BAAB design. The test of treatment effects is the same for each model, and the tests of Stage 2 minus Stage 4 effects and carryover effects are easier to justify with (12.2) because linearity of stage effects is not required.

Efficiencies (E) and Variances of Parameter Function Estimates (in $\frac{\sigma^2}{n}$ units) With This Design When Nonlinear Stage Effects May Exist

No new techniques need to be illustrated in order to report dimensionless variances (variances in $\frac{\sigma^2}{n}$ units) of parameter difference estimates for the current design when modeled with Equation 12.2, and assuming arbitrary stage effects in a new SAS® GLM program. Except for stage effects, with estimates of Stage 2 − Stage 4 effects ($\pi_2 - \pi_4$) having a dimensionless variance of 1.0000, the results are disappointing, however: the Treatment A − Treatment B effect difference ($\tau_A - \tau_B$) is estimated with a comparable variance of 3.0000, just as for the linear trend model. Also Carryover AA − Carryover BB ($\lambda_{AA} - \lambda_{BB}$) and Carryover AB − Carryover BA ($\lambda_{AB} - \lambda_{BA}$) are estimated with variances of 8.0000 and 4.0000, respectively, higher on average than with the prior model with four estimable carryovers. Correspondingly, most of the E values (100.00 for $\pi_2 - \pi_4$, 16.67 for $\tau_A - \tau_B$, 12.50 for $\lambda_{AA} - \lambda_{BB}$, and 25.00 for $\lambda_{AB} - \lambda_{BA}$) also show low sensitivity of this design.

One could say that our problem is that, in both the cases just examined, we are paying a price for a more sophisticated model that may indeed match reality better than simpler models. Here is what happens

with a variation of (12.2) having only one degree of freedom for carryover effects:

$$Y_{ijkm} = \mu + s_{ik} + \pi_j + \tau_m + \lambda_{m'} + e_{ijkm} \tag{12.5}$$

Now we have a single classical carryover depending on the immediately prior treatment, and we will estimate $\lambda_A - \lambda_B$. Standard
methods tell us that, for this simpler model, $\pi_2 - \pi_4$ and $\pi_3 - \pi_4$ are
estimated with the dimensionless variance of 1.000 for $\pi_2 - \pi_4$ before,
but $\tau_A - \tau_B$ and $\lambda_A - \lambda_B$ have dimensionless variances of 0.5500 and
0.8000, much more satisfactory values than with the 2-estimable car-
ryover model, with corresponding E values of 100.00, 90.91, and 62.50.
Obviously (12.5) is an attractive model from an estimation point of view
and should be preferred to (12.1) or (12.2) if it is psychologically tenable.

FINAL THOUGHTS

Similar logic may be used to test for treatment, stage, and carryover
effects in more complicated counterbalanced designs such as one using
ABCCBA, BCAACB, and CABBAC sequences in different groups of
subjects. One may also wish to examine Cox's (1951) discussion of an
ABCCBAABCCBA experimental design for a single subject with cubic
trend and treatment effects but no carryover effects.

THINGS TO REMEMBER

Major Analysis Options

1. Under a model assuming linear trend as a function of stages, it is
possible to compute a contrast for each subject for representative 1-df
functions of parameters. Then a t-test can be computed to test a hypothesis about each such function. Sphericity is not required for such tests.

2. Under a model allowing arbitrary trend, it is also possible to compute a contrast for each subject for representative 1-df functions of parameters. Then a t-test can be computed to test a hypothesis about each
such function regardless of whether sphericity holds. That property may
be required for univariate F-tests of hypotheses about more than two

parameter values. Alternatively, multivariate tests can be used in order to minimize assumptions about covariance structures.

Interpreting Results of Computational Methods
Not Previously Discussed

1. Often formulas for contrasts to be employed in SAS® programs must be computed. This can be done once one learns some GAUSS™ programming and a bit of estimation theory given in Appendix 2.

2. It is necessary to decide for each t-test performed with the SAS® PROC TTEST whether to use the conventional degree of freedom value and associated significance level or the correct values applicable when an assumption of equality of variances in the two treatment-sequence groups is untenable.

3. In the case of possibly nonlinear trend, appropriate assessment of stage effects may be quite limited. Once any acceptable t-tests have been performed and any adjustments in assumptions have been made, it may be necessary to decide between follow-up univariate and multivariate tests. This decision will be related to one's judgment about the plausibility of a sphericity assumption.

EXERCISES

1. Redo the programs of this chapter to verify that they yield the previously reported results.

2. It has been argued that a carryover effect, as a delayed treatment effect, should be no larger than the treatment effect itself, sometimes called a direct treatment effect. So $\tau_m - \tau_{m*} \geq \lambda_{m'} - \lambda_{m*'}$ when the carryover is classical, depending only on the previous treatment. For the case of transitional and standpat carryovers, it is not so clear what might make sense. Indicate which of the following four constraints seem plausible to you and give your reasons for these choices.

(a) $\tau_A - \tau_B \geq \lambda_{AB} - \lambda_{BA}$

(b) $\tau_A - \tau_B \geq \lambda_{AA} - \lambda_{BB}$

(c) $\tau_A - \tau_B \geq \lambda_{AB} - \lambda_{BB}$

(d) $\tau_A - \tau_B \geq \lambda_{BA} - \lambda_{BB}$

13

Should "Optimal Designs" Be Preferred in Behavior Science Crossover Experiments?

INTRODUCTION

We now know a good deal about many crossover designs of interest to behavioral scientists. But, we have ignored many designs used in other fields of research. Furthermore, we have not really asked what makes a good design. From a psychological perspective, we care that we are studying an important problem, such as factors that control retrieval from short-term memory. We care most that the design is clean—that we are not completely confounding variables by manipulating two independent variables in paralllel when we think we are manipulating just one.

As experimenters, we also are aware of statistical demands for our experimental design: We want to meet the assumptions of the model underlying our statistical analysis, so that we can be confident of the parameter estimates and significance test levels that we report. We know that we would like estimability: interesting parameters or differences between parameters should be ones we can assess by standard statistical techniques. (In part, this is a statistical counterpart of the requirement of a clean design in which complete confounding does not occur.) We also would like the power for our most important statistical tests to be relatively high, possibly 0.70 or better against reasonable alternative hypotheses. From our discussions of variances of estimates of parameter differences (in $\frac{\sigma^2}{n}$ units where n is the number of subjects per treatment sequence), we know that we would like to have small dimensionless variances and large efficiencies for our parameter estimates. But we have little idea yet about how to get designs with the smallest dimensionless variances or other properties that could be used to define optimal designs. That is what this chapter is intended to consider.

First, we define an optimal design for an experiment. Because some kinds of balancing of experimental treatments can produce optimal designs, we also define a variety of forms of such balancing. We also provide examples of optimal designs and information about what is required to produce optimality. Optimality is not treated as a certain indication that a design is useful, however. Accordingly, other indications of good designs receive attention here. Because of differences in their controlling features, the case of two treatments is separated from that of three or more treatments.

Next we mention other ways that investigators in agriculture, biology, medicine, and statistics have used to select experimental designs or to obtain desirable designs. We will consider such matters as *washout observations* (observations without special treatment, included to prevent carryover from previous treatments to apply on subsequent stages of an experiment), and extra stages at the end of an experiment, and other devices intended to increase sensitivity through balancing the designs. Finally, it seems appropriate to further organize and interpret some of the information in chapters 1 through 12 concerning the efficiencies of different designs in estimating parameters or differences between parameters.

OPTIMAL DESIGN FOR TWO-TREATMENT EXPERIMENTS

Preliminary Definitions Related to Optimality

We would like to employ an experimental design that finds existing effects as well as possible, considering the effort given to the experiment. It is tempting to say that the best design of a given type is what is called *optimal* here. Let us not be unrealistic—what is best has to depend on what we are expecting in our experimental results. So, we must specify a model to be tested and establish what effects can be assessed with a certain kind of experiment (check for estimability) before we can obtain an optimal design. Then we may look for further information to tell us if we have the best design for our research problem. At first, we use standard definitions of these ideas, after which we consider questions of practical optimality and discuss some objections raised against certain designs that have been found optimal under them.

For the most part, we restrict our discussion to the case of models assuming symmetric covariance structure and random subject effects. Note also that we discuss only the simple case where n is a constant number of individuals for each treatment-sequence group. See Jones and Kenward (1989) for more general analyses.

For the moment, the best design is taken to be the design of a certain type that has minimum variance for estimating treatment and carryover effects. The type of design is identified by its numbers of treatments (T), stages (p), and treatment sequences (s), but we may not find an optimal sequence for every combination of these three numbers. Given this language, a quotation from Jones and Kenward (1989) follows, "For two treatments the criterion usually adopted in the literature is that a cross-over design is optimal if it provides minimum-variance unbiased estimators of [treatment and classical carryover effect parameters]". Here the bracketed section is our substitute for symbols at the end of their sentence.[1] We add that there may be one or more optimal designs for each different number of stages.

We emphasize that this definition of optimality does not guarantee desirability of a specific design. Even if most features of the design and associated model seem reasonable, an optimal design may have too large a variance for a parameter estimate to be satisfactory; also its efficiency values may be too small compared to those of designs of other types appropriate to a given experimental problem. For example, although the two-period, two-treatment Balaam design is optimal under a standard model with only one estimable carryover difference (Laska & Meisner, 1985), we found in chapter 7 that it has efficiencies of only 25.00 for Treatment A – Treatment B effects and 12.50 for Carryover A – Carryover B effects. In addition, stage effects are not estimable at all with this design. Accordingly, the two-period two-treatment optimal design is quite unsatisfactory compared to comparable designs with larger numbers of treatments. Clearly we must compare different designs by more than one criterion in order to select the appropriate one to use in a given situation.

---

[1]Adapted from Jones, B., & Kenward, M. G. (1989). *Design and analysis of cross-over trials.* London: Chapman and Hall, p. 142, with the permnission of the authors and publisher.

There is a large theoretical literature concerning optimal design for crossover experiments, some of which is discussed, for two-treatment cases, in Kershner and Federer (1981) and elsewhere. A variety of references in this chapter deal with the case of three or more treatments. We provide a bare minimum of information about that research; interested readers should use this chapter simply as a point of entry to the topic as a whole.

Balanced Designs

Balance in General

By *balance* in a crossover design, we mean something more than an apparent symmetry of design. For example, a two-group repeated measurements design with different treatments for different groups but constant treatments on successive stages within subjects has some symmetry but would not be called balanced here. Instead, we will be interested, for example, in the total number of times each treatment appears in each treatment-sequence group, the frequency with which different treatments appear on a given stage for different subjects, the frequency of patterns such as AB or AA on successive stages for different subjects, and the frequency with which opposite patterns such as AB and BA appear for different subjects.

We now use almost the same words as in a definition by Jones and Kenward (1989), ". . . in a balanced design, every treatment occurs once with each subject. In addition, for the entire design each treatment appears the same number of times on each stage, and every possible pattern of two successive different treatments such as AB or BA occurs the same number of times."[2] Examples of such designs are the balanced Williams Latin squares already mentioned and minimal balanced designs (i.e., balanced designs that use the smallest possible number of subjects to assess a set of T treatments). We will also say that an otherwise balanced design in which every treatment occurs exactly k times $(k > 1)$ with each subject is a balanced design.

Dual-Balanced Designs

A dual-balanced design has dual sequences, with one sequence such

---

[2]Adapted from Jones, B., & Kenward, M. G. (1989). *Design and analysis of cross-over trials.* London: Chapman and Hall, p. 195, with the permnission of the authors and publisher.

as ABB being matched by its mirror image (i.e., a design with the previous letters for treatments interchanged). Thus, the dual sequence of ABB is BAA. For a design to be dual-balanced, it must both have dual sequences and have equal numbers of subjects in each sequence.

It is possible to have more than one pair of dual sequences. For example, the Balaam design of chapter 7 has two such pairs: AA and BB accompanied by AB and BA. Also a further design in the same chapter has the pairs A^3A^3 and B^3B^3 as well as A^3B^3 and B^3A^3. Chapter 8 has one dual pair, ABAB and BABA, to be compared with a similar pair ABBA and BAAB in chapter 12. Chapter 10 has AAA and BBB, as well as AAB and BBA, and (finally) ABB and BAA as dual-balanced pairs. We have seen in earlier chapters that a data analysis method using contrasts is convenient to use with dual-balanced designs. A second reason to be interested in them is that Laska and Meisner (1985) and Matthews (1987) have proven that, with two treatments in an experiment, there will always be a dual-balanced optimal design; other optimal designs of the same size may also appear.

Completely Balanced Designs

Definition. A *completely balanced design* (sometimes also called a *strongly balanced design*) is an otherwise balanced design in which every treatment follows every other treatment (including itself) an equal number of times, making one treatment have more occurrences than each other one for any given subject. Some completely balanced designs such as the so-called Quenouille design for three treatments (Jones and Kenward, 1989) have the number of stages be an exact multiple of the number of treatments.

Completely balanced designs often prove to be optimal designs though not necessarily designs with efficiency of 100 for a given type of effect (Jones & Kenward, 1989). A later section is related to this issue.

Extra-Period Completely Balanced Designs. There is also a form of completely balanced designs called *completely balanced extra-period designs* in which there are $T+1$ stages for each subject and the last treatment for each subject is the same as its immediate predecessor. An example from Jones and Kenward (1989) is built on a 4×4 Williams Latin square, with the result that the efficiency E for estimating treatment effect differences increases from 90.91 to 96.00 and the E for estimating carryover effect differences increases from 62.50 to 80.00.

Balanced Designs With Fewer Stages Than Treatments

If there are fewer stages than treatments, no subject can receive each treatment once. However, it is possible to satisfy the other conditions of balance: For the entire design each treatment can appear the same number of times on each stage, and every possible pattern of two successive different treatments can occur the same number of times.

Various Kinds of Uniform Designs

A *uniform crossover design* is one in which every subject receives each treatment an equal number of times and each stage involves the same number of cases of each treatment. For example, the following Latin square from Jones and Kenward (1989) is uniform:

	Stage			
	1	2	3	4
Subject 1	A	B	C	D
Subject 2	B	C	D	A
Subject 3	C	D	A	B
Subject 4	D	A	B	C

However, because this design falls far short of having every possible pair of different treatments appear equally often (e.g., AB occurs three times, but AC and AD are never present), this is not a balanced design; Jones and Kenward (1989) reported its efficiencies for each treatment effect difference in the presence of carryover and for each carryover effect difference as 18.18 and 12.50, respectively. Corresponding efficiencies for all estimable stage effect differences are all 100, as in many other crossover designs.

On the other hand, all designs meeting the general definition of balanced designs are also *uniform balanced designs*. There are also *completely balanced uniform designs (strongly balanced uniform designs)* such as the three-treatment Quenouille design previously mentioned.

In this book we also speak of a partially uniform design, one that has each treatment for every subject, for example. Such a design would be called *uniform across subjects*. A design with every treatment on each stage would be called *uniform across stages*, and one with every treatment in each block for each subject would be called *uniform across blocks for subjects.*

Two-Treatment Optimal Designs: Examples and Further Theory

Earlier chapters discuss only one two-treatment design that is now seen to be optimal in the previous sense, having minimal variances for its estimates of treatment and carryover effects: the Balaam design of chapter 7 just mentioned. Jones and Kenward (1989) also display a three-stage design (ABB vs. BAA), a four-stage design (AABB, BBAA, ABBA, and BAAB), and two six-stage designs with different numbers of sequences as optimal. Laska and Meisner's (1985) three-part Theorem 1 for (a) p an even number greater than two, (b) p an odd number, and (c) $p = 2$, respectively, justifies all these examples.

Each of these designs employs one or more pairs of dual sequences. More importantly, each design is completely balanced, which we know implies optimality as well. The four-stage design just described is one example of what is called a two-treatment Quenouille design.

Comparing Attractiveness of Some Two-Treatment Designs

Table 13.1 compares the optimal two-treatment Quenouille design to a design consisting of two of its treatment sequences, the ABBA versus BAAB counterbalanced design of chapter 12. Models for the latter design involving either one or two estimable carryover effects are compared to the standard Quenouille design modeled with only one such effect.

Although the ABBA versus BAAB counterbalanced design is not optimal under an unrestricted stage effects assumption, we can see in Table 13.1 that its model with one estimable carryover is almost as good with respect to efficiency as the optimal design and leads to substantially smaller dimensionless variances and larger efficiencies for estimates of treatment and carryover effects than the switching design with ABAB and BABA as its treatment sequences. The corresponding model with two estimable carryovers is competitive with the latter design and has the advantage of providing more information about carryovers, but at the price of inability to estimate the difference between Stage 3 and Stage 4 effects. Optimal two-treatment designs under linear trend may not yet be known.

TABLE 13.1

Variances of Estimators (in $\frac{\sigma^2}{n}$ Units) and Efficiencies for Various

Two-Treatment Designs and Models Allowing Nonlinear Stage Effects

ABBA versus BAAB versus AABB versus BBAA Design (Quenouille design, 1 estimable carry-over diff.)	ADBA versus BAAB Design (1 estimable carryover diff.)	ABBA versus BAAB Design (2 estimable carryover diffs.)	ABAB versus BABA Design (1 estimable carryover diff.)
No Previous Chapter	Chapter 12		Chapter 8
$\pi_2 - \pi_4$ or $\pi_3 - \pi_4$: 0.5000 (E = 100.00)	$\pi_2 - \pi_4$ or $\pi_3 - \pi_4$: 1.0000 (E = 100.00)	$\pi_2 - \pi_4$: 1.0000 (E = 100.00)	$\pi_2 - \pi_4$ or $\pi_3 - \pi_4$: 1.0000 (E = 100.00)
$\tau_A - \tau_B$: 0.2500 (E = 100.00)	$\tau_A - \tau_B$: 0.5500 (E = 90.91)	$\tau_A - \tau_B$: 3.0000 (E = 16.67)	$\tau_A - \tau_B$: 2.7500 (E = 18.18)
$\lambda_A - \lambda_B$: 0.3636 (E = 68.75)	$\lambda_A - \lambda_B$: 0.8000 (E = 62.50)	$\lambda_{AA} - \lambda_{BB}$: 8.000 (E = 12.50) $\lambda_{AB} - \lambda_{AB}$: 4.0000 (E = 25.00)	$\lambda_A - \lambda_B$: 4.0000 (E = 12.50)

For the case of $m > 1$ identical treatments in a row, could alternating or switching designs, such as the $A^m A^m$ versus $A^m B^m$ versus $B^m A^m$ versus $B^m B^m$ designs of chapter 7, be optimal? Note that this set of designs has $p = 2m$ stages. We can apply Laska and Meisner's (1985) Theorem 1, Part 1, for a symmetric covariance carryover model identical to the one assumed in this book for such designs and an even number of stages. First, however, we need to define the quantity whose variance is estimated in that theorem.

Theorem 1 actually provides variances for the best linear unbiased estimators of $\tau_A - \tau_B$ and not the variances of the best linear unbiased estimators of $\tau = \dfrac{\tau_A - \tau_B}{2}$ as might be supposed from the sentence just above their Equation (3.1). This is because their constraint Equation (3.4) applies to only half of the sequences in the dual balanced design. Therefore, they obtain unbiased estimators of $2\tau = (\tau_A - \tau_B)$ (Laska and Meisner, Personal Communication, August 17, 1995). Accordingly, Theorem 1, Part 1 implies that a completely balanced (and uniform on the periods) design with constant number of subjects per sequence has a minimum variance of $4\dfrac{\sigma^2}{nps}$ for estimates of $\tau_A - \tau_B$. Note that both complete balance and uniformity on the periods is required. In $\dfrac{\sigma^2}{n}$ units, the variance of $\tau_A - \tau_B$ would therefore be $\dfrac{4}{ps}$ = 0.25 for a four-sequence ($s = 4$), four-period ($p = 4$) design. This confirms our report in Table 13.1 of a dimensionless variance of 0.25 for the estimator of $\tau_A - \tau_B$ in the Quenouille design of Table 13.1, as implied by Kershner and Federer (1981).

How does this result compare to the sensitivity of the A^3A^3 versus A^3B^3 versus B^3A^3 versus B^3B^3 design of chapter 7? Laska and Meisner's Theorem 1, Part 2 tells us that an optimal $s = 4$ and $p = 6$ design yields a minimum variance for estimating $\tau_A - \tau_B$ of $4\dfrac{\sigma^2}{nps} = \dfrac{4\sigma^2}{24n}$, which is 0.16667 in dimensionless terms. This may be compared to a dimensionless variance value of 1.3426 obtained for this chapter 7 design. The latter variance is discouragingly larger than the optimal value. Laska and Meisner (1985) give examples of two six-stage, four-sequence optimal designs and one six-stage, eight-sequence optimal design: "(a) ABBAAB, AABBBA, and their duals; (b) ABBBAA, ABBAAB, and their duals; and (c) ABBAAB, AABBBA, ABBBAA, ABBAAB, and their duals."

The A^3A^3 versus A^3B^3 versus B^3A^3 versus B^3B^3 design has some advantages, such as convenience of experimental procedures or opportunity to check for failures of the statistical model when the same treatment appears in three or more stages. However, because of its frequent high standard errors of estimate and low efficiencies, we see good reason to consider using a completely balanced design in place of this chapter 7 option, thereby preferring to make each treatment value follow each other treatment value (including itself) an equal number of times or, alternatively, to choose some other optimal design such as those of Laska and Meisner previously mentioned. Laska and Meisner also report that the conditions for their Theorem 1, Part 1, imply optimality for estimation of classical carryover effects, as well. No values for minimal variances in this case are provided.

Optimality Issues for Two-Way Factorial Designs
With Two Levels Each

Jones and Kenward (1989) noted the potential importance of crossover designs with four within-subject treatments having a 2×2 factorial structure as in the main computational example of our chapter 5. They point out that in some cases primary interest may lie in assessing interaction. Although they mention one class of designs that could be helpful, they do not discuss the question of optimizing the search for a certain kind of effects in this situation.

OPTIMAL DESIGN WITH MORE THAN TWO
TREATMENTS

Variance Balance in Designs With More Than Two
Treatments

The same kinds of balance mentioned earlier can be identified when there are more than two treatments. But, because the case of three or more treatments allows two or more covariances between estimates of differences in treatment effects, we can also speak of balance among the relevant variances (Jones & Kenward, 1989): Variance balance means that the model and experimental design are such that the difference in estimates between any two treatment effects has a constant variance. With a classical carryover model, the (Williams) balanced Latin squares mentioned in our chapters 5 and 6 are variance balanced designs. Completely balanced designs are also variance balanced (Jones & Kenward, 1989).

The Definition of Optimality When $T > 2$

Jones and Kenward (1989) wrote that any Latin square without carryover effects is optimal because of its minimum variance estimation of treatment effect differences. For more generality in this case of more than two treatments ($T > 2$), Jones and Kenward (1989 discuss work organized by Kiefer (1975) into the concept of universal optimality, simultaneously incorporating three other kinds of optimality, each being defined in terms of the covariance matrix V of a set of orthogonal, normalized contrasts among treatment effects: (a) minimizing the determinant of V, (b) minimizing the average variance of the orthonormal contrasts, and (c) minimizing the maximum variance of the orthonormal contrasts.

Ways to Produce Optimality When $T > 2$

Jones and Kenward (1989) relied heavily on a review by Matthews (1988) of theoretical work stating such facts as that a strongly balanced uniform crossover design is universally optimal for the estimation of treatment effects and carryover effects. Furthermore, such designs have the same optimality property for designs including treatment times carryover interaction parameters in their model.

Examples of Variance-Balanced Designs With $T > 2$

Ratkowsky, Evans, and Alldredge (1993) listed 98 variance-balanced designs with T taking on values from 3 to 16 but omitting 8, 9, 12, 14, and 15 as impossible, reporting their key design properties plus efficiency measures. These designs were all originally studied by Patterson and Lucas (1962). Jones and Kenward (1989) provide a smaller list of variance-balanced designs as well as their key design properties plus efficiency measures. They also include several variance-balanced designs not examined by Patterson and Lucas.

Examples of Optimal or Near-Optimal Designs With $T > 2$

Quenouille (1953) also showed how to generate designs with efficiencies of 100 for estimating treatment effect differences when there are three or more treatments. An example given by Jones and Kenward (1989) for the $T = 3$ case requires 6 stages and 18 sequences and, thus, a minimum of 18 subjects, making a total of 108 observations. For this case, it attains $E = 100.00$ for treatments and $E = 80.56$ for carryovers. Berenblut (1964, 1967) has shown how to reduce the number of observations in an optimal design for T treatments: He is able to generate such designs with $2T$ stages and T^2 sequences, making a minimum of $2T^3 = 54$ observations when $T = 3$.

Although Namboodiri (1972) has described Berenblut designs in a psychological journal and shown a relatively easy way to generate them, they seem not to have been used as widely in behavioral research as their efficiency properties would warrant. A more popular approach in psychology is the use of block randomization designs like the one in chapter 11. The example given there employed 6 treatment sequences of one subject, each with 3 blocks of 4 treatments (making 12 stages and 72 total observations, almost as many as for the four-treatment Berenblut design). However, the efficiency values for treatment effects ranged from 87.15 to 89.25 rather than attaining the ideal 100.00 value. Block randomization designs nearly satisfy the definition of a uniform design and may also approximate balance or even complete balance. Psychologists may want to consider modifying block randomization designs to complete balance or to replace them by Berenblut or Quenouille designs. More importantly, perhaps, they need to match their data analysis methods to the experimental designs they employ.

POSSIBLE DIFFICULTIES WITH SOME OPTIMAL DESIGNS

Omission of Relevant Effects or Inclusion of Absent Effects, Causing Selection of the Wrong Design or Inaccurate Estimation of Parameters

A design selected as optimal under one model may be quite unsatisfactory if a different model is applicable. We have seen an illustration of this problem in our discussion of a uniform 4×4 Latin square design with a cyclically shifted sequence, making it far from balanced (because Treatment B always follows Treatment A, and so on). Under a traditional model without carryover effects, this design yields $E = 100.00$ for estimating treatment effect differences and thereby optimality as well for them. However, when carryover effects are included in the model, we saw that E drops to 18.18 for treatment effect differences, and the design is not optimal. Even an optimal 4×4 Williams Latin square design for this model yields only $E = 90.91$ for estimating treatment effect differences and $E = 62.50$ for estimating carryover effect differences (Jones & Kenward, 1989); as before, $E = 100$ for each estimable stage effect difference.

The converse problem is the inclusion of too many parameters. In such situations, computed efficiency values based on the unnecessarily complicated model are correct for that model. However, an investigator using a correct, smaller model will typically find equal or larger efficiencies for estimating effects in the smaller model.

From an accuracy of estimation standpoint rather than an efficiency standpoint, each of these problems may be called misspecification of the model. This can produce biased estimators in addition to the problems just mentioned. Because one seldom is certain what model is consistent with the underlying population of data, one risks poor conclusions whenever one is arbitrary in model formulation. Such difficulties are reduced by use of so-called *nonparametric regression methods*. Although detailed discussion of such methods is beyond the scope of this book, we mention that two of their forms, generalized additive models and software (Almudevar & Tibshirani, 1990; Chambers & Hastie, 1992; Hastie & Tibshirani, 1990) and generalized regression trees (Chaudhuri, Lo, Loh, & Yang, 1995) are possible options for the reader.

Existence of Optimal Designs With Low Efficiency Values

It is certainly conceivable that a "bad" experimental design might sometimes be judged universally optimal (if $T > 2$) or optimal by the criterion of having minimal variance of its treatment and carryover estimates ($T = 2$.) Ratkowsky, Evans, and Alldredge (1993) mention some such possibilities. For example, the optimal two-stage, two-treatment Balaam design previously discussed is unsatisfactory to them because there is an 0.707 correlation between its estimates of treatment and carryover effects. This may be taken as one explanation for the low efficiency values possessed by this design ($E = 25.00$ for differences between treatment effects and $E = 12.50$ for differences between carryover effects).

Gill and Shukla (1987) have proposed a six-stage optimal design with its three sequences of ABCABC, CABCAB, and BCABCA, respectively. However, we calculate efficiency values of only 13.79 for any treatment effect difference and 11.11 for any carryover effect difference Obviously, this design has the difficulty that, after Stage 1, any A is always preceded by C, any B is always preceded by A, and any C is always preceded by B, making it difficult to separate the effects of the current treatment from the effects of the immediately prior treatment (carryover). This is clearly another example of an optimal design with little practical usefulness.

What is a reasonable strategy when the optimal design for a given situation (e.g., the Balaam design with AA versus AB versus BA versus BB conditions) has low efficiency for estimating treatment effects? The best thing to do seems to be to change the number of stages and treatment sequences in such a way as to yield a design with a large efficiency for estimating each treatment difference of interest regardless of whether the new design is also optimal.

Optimality Issues When Nonclassical Carryovers Are Assumed

We know from chapter 12 that the efficiency of estimating treatment effects for an ABBA versus BAAB design may be greatly reduced by including such complicated carryovers as λ_{AA}, λ_{AB}, λ_{BA}, and λ_{BB} in the model to be assessed. Furthermore, the efficiency of estimating carryover effects may also be low with such carryovers. It remains to be seen whether optimal designs for use with two treatments and complicated carryovers exist and whether their efficiency is reasonably high as well.

Finessing the Problem: Achieving Practical Optimality

or Eliminating Undesired Effects in Order to Make Efficient

Designs Easier to Obtain

Achieving Practical Optimality

Jones and Kenward (1989) used practical optimality to mean that one takes into account other issues than efficiency or average variance of estimators of a given effect. They mention substantive issues (likelihood of dropouts or missing data when the number of stages is large, experimental practicality of running the design if it is too complicated, and the difficulty investigators might have in interpreting a complex design). Also we would emphasize that a non-optimal design may have its efficiencies large enough to be useful, suggesting practical optimality there as well. From a previous section it appears that the specific block randomization design displayed in chapter 11 has practical optimality.

Minimizing Undesired Effects With Washout Observations

Much medical research with crossover designs involves the comparison of effectiveness of different prescription drugs or other treatments. Here carryover effects are a distraction to be avoided if possible. One does not want side-effects from an earlier drug to appear at a stage where some other drug is being evaluated. Therefore, it may be useful to stop treatment with one drug for a period of days or weeks (washout stage) before introducing the next drug whose effects are to be assessed.

Let us assume only one observation during the washout stage, taken toward its end. Although one might simply assume from theory or prior experience that the effects of the immediately preceding drug have disappeared by the end of the washout stage, it is more useful to test this assumption with a model measuring changes from the prior treatment phase to the current washout stage and on to the next observation on a treatment stage. It is customary to assume no treatment effect whatsoever on a washout observation, attributing behavior changes from the previous stage to the new stage effect plus a first-order carryover effect (carryover from the immediately preceding observation).

On the next observation, under a treatment, the model will include a stage effect, a treatment effect, and a second-order carryover effect (carryover from the second preceding observation, one made under the prior treatment; Jones & Kenward, 1989). If the second-order carryover is not significant, the statistician will conclude that the washout stage served its purpose fully. Otherwise, second-order carryovers may be expected to be smaller than the first-order effect that otherwise might have been involved in performance on the new treatment observation.

Statisticians sometimes model observations without treatments introduced yet on early stages (often only one such stage) of an experiment by including stage effects but no treatment effects or carryover effects in the model for those baseline stages. Our discussion of multiple baseline designs includes both stage effects and baseline treatment effects on each baseline stage as well as carryover effects in the model for each baseline observation except the first.

FINAL THOUGHTS: COMPARISON OF EFFICIENCIES
OF DIFFERENT CLASSES
OF POSSIBLE PSYCHOLOGICAL DESIGNS

Now it is time to summarize what we know about the efficiency of estimating different kinds of effects with some experimental designs and associated statistical models discussed in this book. Table 13.2 is, in some ways, a reprise of Table 1.1, our first introduction to variations in within-subject designs. Fortunately, we now have a technical vocabulary available for use in a new classification of the designs in question. This table dichotomizes and, thus, simplifies the efficiency results shown in this book, reporting only whether each combination of experimental design and statistical model (where specially relevant) leads to an efficiency for estimating stage effects (for example) of greater than 50.00 or not. In so doing, we are implicitly saying that we will call each given example with efficiency greater than 50 a "good" design-model combination for estimating its category of effect.

TABLE 13.2

Comparative Adequacy of Some Illustrated Experimental Designs
for Estimating Various Classes of Effects*

	Stage Effects?	Treatment Effects?	Carryover Effects?
(a) Uniform across Subjects:			
Randomized Blocks wo/ Time-Related Effects	nr	$E = 100$ not reported elsewhere in this book	nr
Randomized Blocks w/ Time-Related Effects (chap. 3)	Yes	Yes	Yes

(Continued)

TABLE 13.2
(Continued)

	Stage Effects?	Treatment Effects?	Carryover Effects?
2 × 2 Factorial Within-S (Orthog. Lat. Sqs.) (chap. 5)	Yes	Yes**	Yes
(b) Uniform Designs (chap. 13):			
Latin Square, Cyclically Shifted Sequence	Yes	No	No
Balanced Latin Square (Williams)	Yes	Yes	Yes
(c) Pretest– Posttest Control Group Designs (chap. 6):			
AA versus AB	Not Relevant to Between-S Analysis	Yes	Not Relevant to Between-S Analysis
A^3A^3 versus A^3B^3	Yes	No	No
(d) Switching Treatments in Blocks (chap. 7):			
AA versus AB versus BA versus BB (Balaam)	Not estimable	No	No
A^3A^3 versus A^3B^3 versus B^3A^3 versus B^3B^3	Yes	No	No

(Continued)

TABLE 13.2
(Continued)

	Stage Effects?	Treatment Effects?	
(e) Uniform across Subjects in Blocks:			
ABAB versus BABA Alternation chap. 8)	Yes	No	No
$A^4B^4A^4B^4$ versus $B^4A^4B^4A^4$ Alternation (chap. 8)	Yes	No	No
Block Randomization (chap. 11)	Yes	Yes	Yes
(e†) ABBA versus BAAB Counterbalanced :			
Linear Stage Effects, 4 Carryovers (chap. 12)	Yes	No	No
Unconstrained Stage Effects, 1 Estimable Carryover (chap. 13)	Yes	Yes	Yes
Unconstrained Stage Effects, 2 Estimable Carryovers (chap. 12)	Yes	No	No
(f) Multiple Baseline:			
AAA versus AAB versus ABB (chap. 9)	Yes	No	No

(Continued)

TABLE 13.2
(Continued)

	Stage Effects?	Treatment Effects	Carryover Effects?
AAA versus AAB versus ABB versus BBB versus BBA versus BAA, Classical Carryovers (chap. 10)	Yes	Yes	No
AAA versus AAB versus ABB versus BBB versus BBA versus BAA, Transitional Carryovers (chap. 10)	Yes	No	No

Note. * If most E values are greater than 50.00, "Yes" is recorded; otherwise "No." *nr* means *not relevant*. Chapter locations of efficiency information are also listed. ** Not true unless an appropriate ESTIMATE command is used for estimation rather than output from the SOLUTION option of the SAS MODEL command.

A second concern about Table 13.2 is that it applies to very specific designs, often to two-treatment designs and ones with specific treatment sequences such as those employed in our randomized block example of chapter 3. A final concern is that efficiency measures for a crossover design do not tell us the net effect of possible reduction in MS error and in efficiency when such a design is employed. Therefore, power calculations with certain kinds of data may suggest that specific inefficient designs are nonetheless attractive.

THINGS TO REMEMBER

Theory of Optimal Design

1. An optimal two-treatment design for a given number of stages is one that yields minimum-variance unbiased estimators both of treatment

effect and carryover effect differences. However, efficiency (E) values for these aspects of optimal designs are not necessarily 100.

2. In a balanced design, each treatment occurs the same number of times with each subject. It also occurs the same number of times on each stage, and every possible pattern of two successive different treatments occurs the same number of times.

3. A completely balanced design is an otherwise balanced design in which every possible pair of two successive treatments (even the same one) occurs an equal number of times, making one treatment have more occurrences than each other one for any given subject. One method of construction is to begin with a balanced design and repeat the last treatment for each subject on one extra stage, making a so-called extra-period design that is completely balanced.

4. A uniform crossover design is one in which every subject receives each treatment an equal number of times and each stage involves the same number of cases of each treatment. A completely balanced uniform design is also optimal. Given the usual covariance assumptions of our models, any completely balanced uniform two-treament design with a constant number of subjects per sequence is an optimal design.

5. A variance-balanced design ($T > 2$) is one in which there is a constant variance for the estimates of parameters or of the difference between pairs of parameters. All completely balanced designs are variance-balanced, and all completely balanced uniform designs are optimal for the estimation of treatment effects and carryover effects.

Statistically and Nonstatistically Oriented Ways to Improve Experimental Design

1. Seek optimal or near-optimal designs for the treatments compared and the desired number of stages, but also demand that relevant efficiencies be high.

2. Consider the use of extra-period designs as a means of increasing efficiency.

3. Consider the use of washout observations as a means of minimizing unwanted carryover effects in psychological experiments.

4. Consider psychological factors and other practical issues such as dropouts from a lengthy experiment in seeking practical optimality.

EXERCISES

1. (a) Do you know enough to add a row of Table 13.2 for the Quenouille two-treatment design discussed earlier? What can you say about it there?

(b) Do you know enough to add a row of Table 13.2 for the Berenblut four-treatment design discussed earlier? What can you say about it there?

A1

Appendix 1: A Little About Matrices and Vectors

INTRODUCTION

A *matrix* is a rectangular or a square array of numbers or letters. For example, $\begin{pmatrix} a\,c \\ b\,d \end{pmatrix}$ $\begin{pmatrix} 1\,2 \\ 3\,7 \end{pmatrix}$ and $\begin{pmatrix} 1\,0\,0 \\ 0\,1\,0 \end{pmatrix}$ are all matrices. A matrix can also have only one row but two columns, as with (2 3), or only one column with 3 columns, as with $\begin{pmatrix} 1 \\ 1 \\ 0 \end{pmatrix}$. A matrix with only one row is also called a *row vector*. A matrix with only one column is called a *column vector*. If someone speaks simply of a vector, that might mean either a row or a column vector. Usually, however, saying a vector is taken to mean a column vector. Matrices and vectors are implicit in the SAS® computer programs that we display in this book. However, much of the time a behavioral science SAS® user ignores the mathematical properties of matrices and vectors, letting the statisticians and programmers who developed SAS® do the serious mathematical work underlying the calculational results needed by the user. This is why the current information can safely be relegated to an appendix. Interested readers may supplement this information by examining more extensive discussions of matrix algebra in other statistics texts or in books primarily focused on matrix theory (e.g., Searle, 1982).

SOME MATRIX OPERATIONS AND PROPERTIES

Ordinary numbers (so-called *scalar* quantities) have several arithmetic operations available for manipulating them: addition, subtraction, multiplication, and division, for example. Matrices have related operations that are considered next.

Matrix Addition and Subtraction

Two or more matrices can be added together, provided that each has the same number of rows as the others and also has the same number of columns as the others. The method of addition is to add corresponding elements of each matrix. Consider $\mathbf{A} = \begin{pmatrix} 6 & 2 & 6 \\ 3 & 8 & 5 \end{pmatrix}$ and $\mathbf{B} = \begin{pmatrix} 1 & 2 & 0 \\ 3 & 4 & 1 \end{pmatrix}$. Because each of these matrices has two rows and three columns, we know they can be added.

The first row, first column entries in the two matrices are 6 and 1, respectively. Therefore, their sum is 7. Similar calculations for each position in each matrix yields

$$\mathbf{A} + \mathbf{B} = \begin{pmatrix} 6 & 2 & 6 \\ 3 & 8 & 5 \end{pmatrix} + \begin{pmatrix} 1 & 2 & 0 \\ 3 & 4 & 1 \end{pmatrix} = \begin{pmatrix} 7 & 4 & 6 \\ 6 & 12 & 6 \end{pmatrix}$$

Matrix subtraction is like matrix addition except that finding $\mathbf{A} - \mathbf{B}$ requires subtracting elements of $\mathbf{B}$ from corresponding elements of $\mathbf{A}$.

Matrix Multiplication

Consider the multiplication of a row vector by a column vector following it: $(8\ 5)$ times $\begin{pmatrix} 1 \\ 2 \end{pmatrix} = (8\ 5)\begin{pmatrix} 1 \\ 2 \end{pmatrix}$. Can they be multiplied? A natural possibility to consider is that the first element of the row vector (8) should be multiplied by the first element of the column vector (1), yielding 8. Also the second element of the row vector (5) should be multiplied by the second element of the column vector (2), yielding 10. Finally, the two products should be added together, yielding $8 + 10 = 18$. This is indeed the set of rules required for this multiplication. Let us use more symbols now, saying $\mathbf{u} = (8\ 5)$ and $\mathbf{v} = \begin{pmatrix} 1 \\ 2 \end{pmatrix}$. Then our multiplication rule may be summarized by writing $\mathbf{uv} = (8\ 5)$ times $\begin{pmatrix} 1 \\ 2 \end{pmatrix}$ $= 18$ or $\mathbf{uv} = (8\ 5) \times \begin{pmatrix} 1 \\ 2 \end{pmatrix} = 18$ or even $\mathbf{uv} = (8\ 5)\begin{pmatrix} 1 \\ 2 \end{pmatrix} = 18$.

We are accustomed to the fact that 2×3 is equal to 3×2 or 6. Could it be that the value of $\mathbf{uv}$ is the same as that of $\mathbf{vu} = \begin{pmatrix} 1 \\ 2 \end{pmatrix} \times$

$(8\ 5) = \begin{pmatrix} 1 \\ 2 \end{pmatrix}(8\ 5)$ for $\mathbf{u} = (8\ 5)$ and $\mathbf{v} = \begin{pmatrix} 1 \\ 2 \end{pmatrix}$? Notice that $\mathbf{vu} = \begin{pmatrix} 1 \\ 2 \end{pmatrix} \times$ $(8\ 5)$ looks quite different from $\mathbf{uv} = (8\ 5) \times \begin{pmatrix} 1 \\ 2 \end{pmatrix}$ suggesting that its value might be quite different. This is indeed true:

To find $\mathbf{vu} = \begin{pmatrix} 1 \\ 2 \end{pmatrix} \times (8\ 5)$, we first multiply the first element of $\mathbf{v}$ by the first element of $\mathbf{u}$, obtaining $1 \times 8 = 8$. Then we multiply the first element of $\mathbf{v}$ by the second element of $\mathbf{u}$, obtaining $1 \times 5 = 5$. Instead of adding products, we say that this yields a first row for a new matrix: 8 5.

Next we multiply the second element of $\mathbf{v}$ by the first element of $\mathbf{u}$, obtaining $2 \times 8 = 16$. Then we multiply the second element of $\mathbf{v}$ by the second element of $\mathbf{u}$, obtaining $2 \times 5 = 10$. Now we have the second row of our new matrix: 16 10.

Combining the two rows of the $\mathbf{vu}$ product yields $\mathbf{vu} = \begin{pmatrix} 8 & 5 \\ 16 & 10 \end{pmatrix}$, a very different answer from $\mathbf{uv} = 18$.

One way to understand the differences in form and answer between this pair of products, $\mathbf{uv}$ and $\mathbf{vu}$ is to note that each has the same number of rows in its answer as the number of rows in the first vector or matrix on the left. Each also has the same number of columns in its answer as the number of columns in the second matrix to be multiplied. This will be true for any pair of matrices to be multiplied. So $\mathbf{uv}$ has to have one row and one column, and $\mathbf{vu}$ has to have two rows and two columns. Notice also that the number of columns in the first matrix on the left must equal the number of rows in the next matrix if there is to be a natural way to form a product.

The next example shows how to multiply a matrix with more than one row and column by a vector of appropriate size. Because Greek letters are often needed in the rest of this book, we will spice up this example by including some of them in our vector. Let $\mathbf{X} = \begin{pmatrix} 1 & 1 & 0 \\ 1 & 0 & 1 \end{pmatrix}$ and $\beta = \begin{pmatrix} \mu \\ \alpha_1 \\ \alpha_2 \end{pmatrix}$. Then we can find $\mathbf{X}\beta$ by first multiplying the first row of $\mathbf{X}$

by β, obtaining $\mu + \alpha_1 + 0\alpha_2 = \mu + \alpha_1$, and then multiplying the second row of **X** by β, obtaining $\mu + 0\alpha_1 + \alpha_2 = \mu + \alpha_2$. Because we know that this product must have two rows from **X** and one column from β, we combine our first and second subproducts in the form $X\beta = \begin{pmatrix} \mu + \alpha_1 \\ \mu + \alpha_2 \end{pmatrix}$

Here is an example showing how to multiply a matrix with more than one row and column by a matrix that also is not a vector. Let $A = \begin{pmatrix} 1 & 1 & 0 \\ 1 & 0 & 1 \end{pmatrix}$ and $B = \begin{pmatrix} 1 & 1 \\ 1 & 3 \\ 2 & 1 \end{pmatrix}$. We find the first row of **AB** by multiplying A's first row by the first column of **B**, obtaining $(1 \times 1) + (1 \times 1) + (0 \times 2) = 2$ and then multiplying the first row of **A** by the second column of **B**, obtaining $(1 \times 1) + (1 \times 3) + (0 \times 1) = 4$. This makes the first row 2 4.

Next we find the second row of **AB** by first multiplying the second row of **A** by the first column of **B**, obtaining $(1 \times 1) + (0 \times 1) + (1 \times 2) = 3$ and then multiplying the second row of **A** by the second column of **B**, obtaining $(1 \times 1) + (0 \times 3) + (1 \times 1) = 2$. This makes the second row 3 2. When we combine these two rows, we obtain: $AB = \begin{pmatrix} 2 & 4 \\ 3 & 2 \end{pmatrix}$

Occasionally you will need to do a hand calculation to find a product of two vectors, of a matrix times a vector, or even of two matrices that are not also vectors, as in the **AB** example just given. However, we believe that the computer will do most matrix multiplications that you need.

Transposition

Transposed matrices have the same elements as the original matrices, but what were originally rows are now columns and vice versa. We usually use an apostrophe or a superscript T to indicate transposition. Therefore, if $X = \begin{pmatrix} 1 & 2 & 0 \\ 1 & 0 & 4 \end{pmatrix}$ we can write $X' = X^T = \begin{pmatrix} 1 & 1 \\ 2 & 0 \\ 0 & 4 \end{pmatrix}$.

Terminology for the Size of a Matrix and the Label for a Cell Entry

Sometimes we say that a matrix with two rows and three columns is a 2 row by 3 column matrix or simply a 2 by 3 matrix. Occasionally we may say also that it is a 2 × 3 matrix (even though this could be confusing because × is also used here to represent multiplication). Another notation for the 2 by 3 matrix X is to place appropriate subscripts on its name, calling it X_{23}.

Sometimes we want to label an individual entry in a matrix such as X. It is customary then to use a lower case letter with two subscripts, the first for the row and the second for the column. So x_{11} is the entry in Row 1, Column 1 of X. If we know its value is 3, for example, we can write $x_{11} = 3$. Similary, if the element of X in Row 1, Column 2 is –5, we can write $x_{12} = -5$.

Determinants of Small-Sized Square Matrices

The determinant of a square matrix A is labeled $|A|$. It is the sum of a certain set of products of its elements. Consider first the 2 row × 2 column matrix: $A = \begin{pmatrix} 1 & 3 \\ 2 & 1 \end{pmatrix}$. The value of $|A|$ is the product of the two numbers on the diagonal from top left to bottom right, 1×1, minus the product of the two numbers on the opposite diagonal from lower left to upper right, 2×3. This makes its value $|A| = 1 - 6 = -5$.

Now we look for the determinant of $B = \begin{pmatrix} -1 & 1 & 1 \\ 1 & 4 & 0 \\ 2 & 2 & 1 \end{pmatrix}$. In a 3 × 3 matrix like this one there are six products to combine. First we look at the main diagonal from upper left to lower right: That diagonal involves a product of the parenthesized entries here: $B = \begin{pmatrix} (-1) & 1 & 1 \\ 1 & (4) & 0 \\ 2 & 2 & (1) \end{pmatrix}$, yielding –4.

Next we need a product of two entries in a smaller diagonal and one entry in a corner: $\begin{pmatrix} -1 & (1) & 1 \\ 1 & 4 & (0) \\ (2) & 2 & 1 \end{pmatrix}$ yielding a product of 0 for the parenthesized entries. The third product is analogously based on parenthesized entries here: $\begin{pmatrix} -1 & 1 & (1) \\ (1) & 4 & 0 \\ 2 & (2) & 1 \end{pmatrix}$, yielding a product of 2. These three products -4, 0, and $+2$ sum to a total of -2.

Now we must find three products whose sum will be subtracted from our earlier sum to yield the deteminant of **B**. Our fourth product uses $\begin{pmatrix} -1 & 1 & (1) \\ 1 & (4) & 0 \\ (2) & 2 & 1 \end{pmatrix}$ and yields $+8$. Our fifth product uses $\begin{pmatrix} -1 & (1) & 1) \\ (1) & 4 & 0 \\ 2 & 2 & (1) \end{pmatrix}$ and yields $+1$. Our final product uses $\begin{pmatrix} (-1) & 1 & 1 \\ 1 & 4 & (0) \\ 2 & (2) & 1 \end{pmatrix}$ and yields 0. So the sum of these three products is $+9$. To get the determinant we must take the first total minus the second total: $|\mathbf{B}| = -2 - 9 = -11$.

Minors

A minor of an element in a square matrix is the determinant of the remaining matrix once the row and column containing that element are deleted. In $\mathbf{B} = \begin{pmatrix} -1 & 1 & 1 \\ 1 & 4 & 0 \\ 2 & 2 & 1 \end{pmatrix}$ there can be a minor for each of the nine elements. As in a previous éxample, we name our elements with lower case letters corresponding to the capital letters naming our matrices. Let us also use two subscripts for each element, with the first one indicating the row number and starting with 1 at the top of the matrix. Similarly, the second subscript indicates the column number and starts from the left of the matrix. Then b_{11} is the entry for the first row and first column of **B** and has the value -1. If we want the minor of the Row 1 Column 1 element $b_{11} = -1$, parenthesized here: $\begin{pmatrix} (-1) & 1 & 1 \\ 1 & 4 & 0 \\ 2 & 2 & 1 \end{pmatrix}$, we will delete the first row and first column, yielding $\begin{pmatrix} - & - & - \\ - & 4 & 0 \\ - & 2 & 1 \end{pmatrix}$ or more conventionally $\begin{pmatrix} 4 & 0 \\ 2 & 1 \end{pmatrix}$, with a determinant $\begin{vmatrix} 4 & 0 \\ 2 & 1 \end{vmatrix} = 4$. So 4 is the minor of the first row, first column element of the original matrix.

Consider the calculation of another minor from **B**, a minor for which the third row, second column entry $b_{32} = 2$ is parenthesized as being of interest:

$$\begin{pmatrix} -1 & 1 & 1 \\ 1 & 4 & 0 \\ 2 & (2) & 1 \end{pmatrix}$$ Now we will delete the third row and second column,

yielding $\begin{pmatrix} -1 & — & 1 \\ 1 & — & 0 \\ \hline \end{pmatrix}$. Or write more conventionally $\begin{pmatrix} -1 & 1 \\ 1 & 0 \end{pmatrix}$, with a de

terminant $\begin{vmatrix} -1 & 1 \\ 1 & 0 \end{vmatrix} = -1$. So -1 is the minor of the third row, second column element $b_{32} = 2$ of **B**. We state without further demonstration that the matrix of minors for **B** is $\begin{pmatrix} 4 & 1 & -6 \\ -1 & -3 & -4 \\ -4 & -1 & -5 \end{pmatrix}$.

Cofactors and Matrices of Cofactors

A cofactor is a minor with a $+1$ or -1 multiplier reflecting the position of the element having that minor. These multipliers form an alternating pattern beginning with $+1$ in Row 1, Column 1. Thus for a 3 by 3 matrix, the pattern (or pattern matrix) is: $\begin{pmatrix} +1 & -1 & +1 \\ -1 & +1 & -1 \\ +1 & -1 & +1 \end{pmatrix}$. The same rule can be used to form a matrix pattern for a matrix of any number of rows and columns.

We know that the minor for $b_{11} = -1$ parenthesized in the matrix $\begin{pmatrix} (-1) & 1 & 1 \\ 1 & 4 & 0 \\ 2 & 2 & 1 \end{pmatrix}$ is 4. Because the corresponding multiplier for that cell is $+1$, the cofactor of b_{11} is also 4. But for $b_{32} = 2$ parenthesized in the same matrix $\begin{pmatrix} -1 & 1 & 1 \\ 1 & 4 & 0 \\ 2 & (2) & 1 \end{pmatrix}$, the minor is -1. The corresponding multiplier in the matrix of patterns is -1. Therefore, we know the cofactor is $-1 \times -1 = 1$.

A matrix of cofactors is simply the matrix formed by finding every minor in an original matrix and then multiplying each element by +1 or −1, depending on what the pattern matrix says for that element. It is obvious from the previous matrix of minors and the pattern matrix that the matrix of cofactors for **B** is $\begin{pmatrix} 4 & -1 & -6 \\ 1 & -3 & 4 \\ -4 & 1 & -5 \end{pmatrix}$.

Adjoint Matrices

An adjoint matrix is simply the tranpose of a matrix of cofactors. Therefore, the adjoint matrix for **B** is $\begin{pmatrix} 4 & 1 & -4 \\ -1 & -3 & 1 \\ -6 & 4 & -5 \end{pmatrix}$.

Identity Matrices

A square matrix with 1s in a top left to bottom right pattern and 0s everywhere else is called an identity matrix **I**. For example, $\mathbf{I} = \mathbf{I}_{22} = \begin{pmatrix} 1 & 0 \\ 0 & 1 \end{pmatrix}$ is an identity matrix with two rows and two columns. Also $\mathbf{I} = \mathbf{I}_{33} = \begin{pmatrix} 1 & 0 & 0 \\ 0 & 1 & 0 \\ 0 & 0 & 1 \end{pmatrix}$ is an identity matrix with three rows and three columns.

Matrix Inverses

A square matrix **X** may have a unique inverse $\mathbf{X}^{-1}$, satisfying the rule $\mathbf{XX}^{-1} = \mathbf{X}^{-1}\mathbf{X} = \mathbf{I}$, with both orders of matrix multiplication yielding the same result. This constancy of result is called commutativity: **X** and $\mathbf{X}^{-1}$ commute in the sense that either order of multiplication yields the same result. Notice that an inverse is like a reciprocal and an identity matrix is like a one in ordinary arithmetic. Similarly, scalar numbers and their inverses commute in arithmetic. For example, we know that 3 times $\left(\dfrac{1}{3}\right) = \left(\dfrac{1}{3}\right)$ times 3 = 1. If $\mathbf{X} = \begin{pmatrix} 1 & 0 \\ 2 & 1 \end{pmatrix}$, then it can be shown that $\mathbf{X}^{-1} = \begin{pmatrix} 1 & 0 \\ -2 & 1 \end{pmatrix}$ You can test your skills at matrix multiplication by checking whether this new matrix $\mathbf{X}^{-1}$ is indeed the inverse of $\mathbf{X}$.

Many statistical computer packages can do some matrix operations, either on specific demand or as part of a larger routine. Because the INVERSE command in a SAS® GLM program can compute the inverse of a certain important class of matrices, we do not show how to calculate inverses of large matrices by hand. However, you may need to compute inverses of small matrices. From the section on determinants, we know that for $\mathbf{A} = \begin{pmatrix} 1 & 3 \\ 2 & 1 \end{pmatrix}$ the determinant $|\mathbf{A}| = -5$. Also for $\mathbf{B} = \begin{pmatrix} -1 & 1 & 1 \\ 1 & 4 & 0 \\ 2 & 2 & 1 \end{pmatrix}$, we know that $|\mathbf{B}| = -11$.

Any square matrix whose determinant is not zero has an inverse. Because $|\mathbf{A}|$ is not zero, it has an inverse. Because $|\mathbf{B}|$ is not zero, it also has an inverse. Now we learn how to compute those inverses and thus to compute the inverse of any 2×2 or 3×3 matrix. For $\mathbf{A} = \begin{pmatrix} 1 & 3 \\ 2 & 1 \end{pmatrix}$ we must produce its adjoint matrix $\begin{pmatrix} 1 & -3 \\ -2 & 1 \end{pmatrix}$ and divide it by the determinant $|\mathbf{A}|$: $\mathbf{A}^{-1} = \begin{pmatrix} 1 & 3 \\ 2 & 1 \end{pmatrix}^{-1} = \begin{pmatrix} 1 & -3 \\ -2 & 1 \end{pmatrix} / (-5) = \begin{pmatrix} -.2 & .6 \\ .4 & -.2 \end{pmatrix}$ The adjoint matrix could have been obtained by the previous methods. However, for a 2 by 2 matrix, it is equivalent to switch upper left and lower right entries (no change because each was 1) and then reverse the signs of the other entries.

For $\mathbf{B} = \begin{pmatrix} -1 & 1 & 1 \\ 1 & 4 & 0 \\ 2 & 2 & 1 \end{pmatrix}$ we have already computed the adjoint matrix: $\begin{pmatrix} 4 & 1 & -4 \\ -1 & -3 & 1 \\ -6 & 4 & -5 \end{pmatrix}$ We must simply divide that adjoint matrix by the determinant $|\mathbf{B}| = -11$:

$$\mathbf{B}^{-1} = \begin{pmatrix} -1 & 1 & 1 \\ 1 & 4 & 0 \\ 2 & 2 & 1 \end{pmatrix}^{-1} = \begin{pmatrix} 4 & 1 & -4 \\ -1 & -3 & 1 \\ -6 & 4 & -5 \end{pmatrix} \div -11 = \begin{pmatrix} -\frac{4}{11} & -\frac{1}{11} & \frac{4}{11} \\ \frac{1}{11} & \frac{3}{11} & -\frac{1}{11} \\ \frac{6}{11} & -\frac{4}{11} & \frac{5}{11} \end{pmatrix}$$

Rank of a Matrix

The rank of a matrix is the number of rows (= number of columns) in the largest square submatrix that has a nonzero determinant. So, if a 3 by 3 matrix has a nonzero determinant, the rank of that matrix is 3. Such a matrix is called a *matrix of full rank*. If it does not have a nonzero determinant, but a submatrix of size 2 by 2 does have a nonzero determinant, the rank of the original matrix is 2. In this case the 3 by 3 matrix is said to be of less than full rank or not of full rank.

Generalized Inverses

All matrices $\mathbf{A}$, whether square or not, have generalized inverses $\mathbf{G}$ satisfying the equation $\mathbf{AGA} = \mathbf{A}$. Except for cases in which $\mathbf{A}$ has an inverse, most such matrices have non-unique generalized inverses. Any square matrix with a zero determinant does not have an inverse. Here is a case of a square matrix, $\mathbf{A} = \begin{pmatrix} 1 & 0 \\ 0 & 0 \end{pmatrix}$ without an inverse but with a generalized inverse, $\mathbf{G} = \begin{pmatrix} 1 & 0 \\ 0 & 1 \end{pmatrix}$, that may be unique. Can you verify that $\mathbf{G}$ is indeed a generalized inverse of $\mathbf{A}$?

The inverse of the design matrix when existent (i.e., when the relevant matrix is of full rank) or a generalized inverse for any design matrix not of full rank can be produced by using the "INVERSE" option after "/" in the "MODEL" command. This book does not use this option very often, but something similar appears in the GAUSS programs of Appendix 2.

Determinants of Larger Square Matrices

We need a general rule for computing the determinant of a square matrix even if it is larger than 3 by 3. Suppose that the n by n matrix $\mathbf{A}$ has elements $\begin{pmatrix} a_{11} & a_{12} & \dots & a_{1n} \\ a_{21} & a_{22} & \dots & a_{2n} \\ \dots & \dots & \dots & \dots \\ a_{n1} & a_{n2} & \dots & a_{nn} \end{pmatrix}$ and a cofactor matrix C with elements

$\begin{pmatrix} c_{11} & c_{12} & \dots & c_{1n} \\ c_{21} & c_{22} & \dots & c_{2n} \\ \dots & \dots & \dots & \dots \\ c_{n1} & c_{n2} & \dots & c_{nn} \end{pmatrix}$. Then the determinant, $|A|$ can be computed in several

different ways.   Depending on such things as whether a given row or column includes some zeroes, one picks a certain row or column of A and does what is called expanding along that row or column. Suppose we want to expand along Row 2: Then we must find products of second row elements from A and C and sum them up: $|A| = a_{21} c_{21} + a_{22} c_{22} + \dots + a_{2n} c_{2n}$.

A2

Appendix 2: Using the GAUSS Matrix Programming Language

The GAUSS™ language (Aptech Systems, 1993) is a matrix algebra language often used in statistical applications. We introduce it now by presenting two GAUSS programs needed to develop some results presented in chapter 12.

A GAUSS™ PROGRAM FOR ESTIMATING

PARAMETERS FOR ABBA VERSUS BAAB DESIGN

DATA WITH LINEAR SLOPE

The Program Itself

Table A2.1 is a variant of a GAUSS program to generate contrasts used in Table 12.2 with a model assuming linear slope as a function of stage of practice. It would apply exactly if the ABBA and BAAB sequence groups of the associated data set had two subjects each.

TABLE A2.1

A GAUSS Program to Facilitate Finding Appropriate Contrasts for an
an ABBA vs. BAAB Design Model Assuming Linear Practice Effects

---

```
new; output file=temp.out reset; @ User can choose filename with a certain
drive and directory if desired.@ output reset; date;
/* ABBA2S.EST program for finding estimation matrix for a 2-group (ABBA
versus BAAB) 2-S per group  4-stage design with a linear trend plus 4
carryovers. */   let x[16,10] =
1 0 1 1 0 0 0 0 1 0
1 0 2 0 0 1 0 0 1 0
1 0 3 0 0 0 0 1 1 0
```

(Continued)

TABLE A2.1
(Continued)

```
1 0 4 1 0 0 1 0 1 0
1 0 1 1 0 0 0 0 0 0
1 0 2 0 0 1 0 0 0 0
1 0 3 0 0 0 0 1 0 0
1 0 4 1 0 0 1 0 0 0
0 1 1 0 0 0 0 0 0 1
0 1 2 1 0 0 1 0 0 1
0 1 3 1 1 0 0 0 0 1
0 1 4 0 0 1 0 0 0 1
0 1 1 0 0 0 0 0 0 0
0 1 2 1 0 0 1 0 0 0
0 1 3 1 1 0 0 0 0 0
0 1 4 0 0 1 0 0 0 0;
```

@ Each row is for 1 subject of a certain sequence on a certain stage. Columns
are for parameters for seq1=mu+tau_B+subj1n, seq2=mu+tau_B+subj2n, b,
tau_A-tau_B, lambda_AA, lambda_AB, lambda_BA, lambda_BB,
subj11-subj1n, and subj21-subj2n. @
x_prod = x'x; prod_inv = inv(x_prod); fndn = prod_inv*x';
"Estimation matrix (foundation for parameter estimation) = "; fndn;
output off; end;

Some Rules About Symbols Used in a GAUSS Program

As in SAS® each GAUSS command ends with a semicolon. A matrix
such as x above has a certain number of rows and a possibly different
number of columns. One way to tell the GAUSS system how many
rows and columns appear in a matrix is to say something like "let
x[16,10] =" indicating that there are to be 16 rows and 10 columns in
the x matrix. This implies that there are 160 elements in the matrix.
Without further specification of format requirements, they must be numbers separated by spaces or line breaks. First the numbers in the first
row are given, then the numbers in the second row, and so on. However, we need not display exactly one row of a matrix in each line. In
order to save space, more than one row or even several rows plus part of
another row can appear on one line so long as everything appears in the

correct order. When the data are all entered, the final line (not the next line as in SAS®) contains a semicolon.

GAUSS has no boldfacing for any symbols, including matrices. When a matrix label such as "x" ends with an apostrophe, making it x', the transpose of the matrix is defined. Multiplication is indicated by "x*y" or "x'y", depending on whether x or x' is the first matrix in the product. The expression "inv(x)" defines the inverse of x if it exists.

The command "new;" clears GAUSS so that no old computations will be used in the current program. The "output file = ..." tells the output filename selected and, if desired, in what drive and directory the output from the current program will be stored. The expression "reset;" at its end destroys any old output file by the same name, creates the new output file, and causes GAUSS to store all output in the output file. Also "@" signs around parts or wholes of one or more lines form comments to help the user remember what a certain part of a GAUSS program does. A sequence beginning "/" and ending with "*/" does the same. Quoted material is printed as shown, but a command such as: "fndn;" or equivalently, "print fndn;" (each without quotes) says to print the value of the quoted concept. The expression "output off;" closes the current output file. The command "end;" stops all program execution.

Additional General Linear Model Theory Needed Here

We know from chapter 1 that $Y = X\beta + E$, making the expected value of the observation vector $E(Y) = X\beta$, where X is the design matrix and β is the parameter vector. When $X'X$ is not of full rank, it has no inverse and we cannot estimate the parameter value uniquely. Because there will be a multiplicity of generalized inverses, $(X'X)^-$ quantities, a multiplicity of solutions is available using the equation $\hat{\beta}^0 = (X'X)^- X'Y$. We find a unique solution based on a set-to-zero reparametrization of this theory of the form $Y = x\beta^* + E$, with the property that $x'x$ is of full rank, implying that $x'x$ has a true inverse. (By a set-to-zero reparameterization, we mean that the estimated value of the last parameter in each family such as τ_A and τ_B, is set to zero. This lets us say, $\hat{\tau}_B = 0$, for example, in which case it is possible to use this information in estimating $\hat{\tau}_A - \hat{\tau}_B$ uniquely; see chapter 6 for more details.)

Now we know that we can estimate the modified parameter vector with the following equation:

$$\hat{\beta}^* = (x'x)^{-1}x'Y \qquad (A2.1)$$

The GAUSS command in Table A2.1, "fndn = prod_inv*x';" calculates a portion of the right hand side of (A2.1):

$$fndn = (x'x)^{-1}x' \qquad (A2.2)$$

where *fndn* is shorthand for *foundation*.

Interpreting What This GAUSS Program Has to Say

The comment following the definition of x[16,10] tells us that successive rows refer to Stages 1 through 4 for Sequence 1, Subject 1, to Stages 1 through 4 for Sequence 1, Subject 2, and then on to Stages 1 through 4 for each subject of Sequence 2. Similarly columns refer to parameters or parameter combinations. A specific row of x is like a predictive equation for a subject in a certain sequence on a certain stage. Vector multiplication of such a row by the column vector for parameters (column headings of x) yields a prediction for the observation. For example, Row 1 for Subject 1 in Sequence 1, Stage 1 and the codings of the columns of the columns of x imply a predicted value equal to the estimated value of $(\hat{\mu} + \hat{\tau}_B + \hat{s}_{1_a})\cdot \hat{b} + (\hat{\tau}_A - \hat{\tau}_B) + (\hat{s}_{11} - \hat{s}_{1n}) = \hat{\mu} + \hat{b} + \hat{\tau}_A + \hat{s}_{11}$.

The command "x_prod = x'x;" says to multiply x' by x; "prod_inv = inv(x_prod);" says to find the inverse of x_prod. The command "fndn = prod_inv*x';" says to multiply prod_inv times the transpose of x, forming what is called the estimation matrix and printed out for use in later programs. Table A2.2 gives that output matrix with entries rounded to three digits after the decimal place, except that numbers in scientific notation and simplifying to zero are shortened further. Some authors also define a so-called "hat matrix" equal here to x*fndn. The name follows from the property that the "hat matrix" postmultiplied by the observation vector y is equal to the predicted vector of observations, $\hat{y}$.

TABLE A2.2

Realigned Estimation Matrix (*fndn*) for an ABBA Versus BAAB Design
With *n* = 2 per Sequence Group, Based on the Linear Trend Model of (12.1)

−0.125	0.250	−0.125	−1e−16	0.125	0.500	0.125	0.250
0.500	−0.125	−1e−16	−0.375	0.500	−0.125	−1e−16	−0.375
−2e−16	0.125	−2e−16	−0.125	−2e−16	0.125	−2e−16	−0.125
0.375	−1e−16	−0.125	−0.250	0.625	0.250	0.125	−2e−16
0.000	−0.125	0.000	0.125	0.000	−0.125	0.000	0.125
0.000	−0.125	6e−17	0.125	0.000	−0.125	6e−7	0.125
0.500	−0.250	2e−16	−0.250	0.500	−0.250	2e−16	−0.250
−0.500	0.250	−2e−16	0.250	−0.500	0.250	−2e−16	0.250
−0.500	0.500	0.000	−7e−16	−0.500	0.500	0.000	−7e−16
0.000	7e−16	0.500	−0.500	0.000	7e−16	0.500	−0.500
−1e−16	0.375	0.000	−0.375	−1e−16	0.375	0.000	−0.375
−0.500	0.375	−4e−16	0.125	−0.500	0.375	−4e−16	0.125
−0.500	0.375	0.000	0.125	−0.500	0.375	0.000	0.125
0.000	0.375	−2e−16	−0.375	0.000	0.375	−2e−16	−0.375
−1e−16	7e−16	0.500	−0.500	−1e−16	7e−16	0.500	−0.500
−0.500	0.500	−4e−16	−4e−16	−0.500	0.500	−4−e16	−4e−16
0.250	0.250	0.250	0.250	−0.250	−0.250	−0.250	−0.250
0.000	0.000	0.000	0.000	0.000	0.000	0.000	0.000
0.000	0.000	0.000	0.000	0.000	0.000	0.000	0.000
0.250	0.250	0.250	0.250	−0.250	−0.250	−0.250	−0.250

We know that in scientific notation e−16 is $10^{-16} \approx 0$. So all the entries involving e−16 or a similar term have values that may be replaced by zero. Because Table A2.2 applies only with two subjects per sequence group, we examine it only briefly. First, notice that *fndn* from (A2.2) should have 10 rows for different parameters and 4(2n) = 16 columns for different observations. This means that it takes two rows of Table A2.2 to represent 1 row of *fndn*, which is why it is called a realigned matrix. Also the observation vector, *Y*, should have 4(2n) = 16 rows and 1 column. This means that postmultiplication of the first row of *fndn by Y* yields an estimate of the first parameter of β^* from (A2.1), and so on, yielding 10 rows and 1 column.

The relatively uninteresting rows 1 through 4 of Table A2.2 are for estimating $seq_1 = \mu + \tau_B + s_{1n}$ and $seq_2 = \mu + \tau_B + s_{2n}$, respectively, with $n = 2$ in this case. Let us move on to the 16 entries from rows 5 and 6 for estimating the next parameter estimate, $\hat{b}$:

| 0 | −0.125 | 0 | 0.125 | 0 | −0.125 | 0 | 0.125 |
| 0 | −0.125 | 0 | 0.125 | 0 | −0.125 | 0 | 0.125 |

after replacing e−16 or similar terms by zero. The first four entries apply to Subject 1 in the ABBA sequence group, the second four to Subject 2 in that group and the last eight to the first and second subjects in the BAAB sequence group. These 16 entries combine to represent the fifth and sixth rows of *fndn* from (A2.2). For sequence *g*, subject *i*, and stage *j*, we can use the symbol Y_{gij}. Then the vector multiplication just recommended means that each entry of this third row is multiplied by the corresponding observed score in a sequence such as Y_{1i1}, Y_{1i2}, Y_{1i3}, and Y_{1i4} for the *i*-th subject in the ABBA sequence group. This yields:

$$\hat{b} = (-.125Y_{112[B]} + .125Y_{114[A]}) + (-.125Y_{122[B]} + .125Y_{124[A]})$$

$$+ (-.125Y_{212[A]} + .125Y_{214[B]}) + (-.125Y_{222[A]} + .125Y_{224[B]})$$

After reading further we will be able to see that, for any specific number, *n*, of subjects per sequence group, the multipliers in the previous equation will be $\frac{.25}{n}$ and there will be *n* parenthesized terms per sequence group (one for each subject), corresponding to the two parenthesized terms per sequence group in that equation. Even though no one of the four parenthesized quantities in this $\hat{b}$ equation is itself an unbiased estimator of the slope *b*, or even of $\frac{b}{4}$, each is a contrast helping to define the estimated slope. So we choose to write:

$$\hat{b} = Slope\_Contr_{ABBA} \text{ for } Subject_{11} + Slope\_Contr_{ABBA} \text{ for } Subject_{12} +$$

Slope_Contr_BAAB for *Subject$_{21}$* + *Slope_Contr$_{BAAB}$* for *Subject$_{22}$*

where the slope contrasts are as used in chapter 12.

A GAUSS™ PROGRAM FOR FINDING CONTRASTS
FOR ABBA VERSUS BAAB DESIGN DATA
WITH LINEAR SLOPE

Table A2.1 is intended to facilitate computation of parameter estimates for combined data from several subjects in each sequence group. However, for the t-tests of chapter 12, we need individual contrasts related to each parameter for each separate subject. Therefore, we use Table A2.3 to obtain estimates for all parameters except those involving μ and subjects effects s_{ij} with a simpler GAUSS™ program for $n = 1$ per sequence group. Comparison to results from Table A2.4 will permit us to use the present program to find all needed contrasts for the present design and model, regardless of the sample sizes used with each treatment group.

TABLE A2.3

A GAUSS™ Program to Facilitate Finding Individual Subjects' Contrasts
for an ABBA Versus BAA Design Model Assuming Linear Practice Effects

---

```
new;  output file = temp.out reset; date;
/* ABBA4C.EST program for a 2-group (ABBA vs. BAAB sequence),
4-period
design with a linear trend plus 4 carryovers. Estimation matrix provided for
all effects but subject effects. Works for arbitrary sample size, n.          */
let x[8,8] =
1 0 1 1 0 0 0 0   1 0 2 0 0 1 0 0   1 0 3 0 0 0 0 1   1 0 4 1 0 0 1 0
0 1 1 0 0 0 0 0   0 1 2 1 0 0 1 0   0 1 3 1 1 0 0 0   0 1 4 0 0 1 0 0;
@ Columns for seq1 = mu + subj1n + tau_B, seq2 = mu + subj2n + tau_B, b,
tau_A – tau_B, lambda_AA, lambda_AB, lambda_BA, and lambda_BB,
respectively.  4 sets of columns for 4 stages of a single sequence group.  @
x_prod = x'x; prod_inv = inv(x_prod);
fndn = prod_inv*x'; "Estimation matrix = "; fndn;
output off; end;
```

This program leads to the next estimation matrix, with zeroes replacing scientific notation quantities having that approximate value (Table A2.4).

TABLE A2.4

Estimation Matrix (*fndn*) for an ABBA Versus BAAB Design
With Sample Size $n = 1$ per Sequence Group,
Based on the Linear Trend Model of (12.1)

0	0.750	0	0.250	1.000	−0.250	0	−0.750
0	0.250	0	−0.250	1.000	0.250	0	−0.250
0	−0.250	0	0.250	0	−0.250	0	0.250
1.000	−0.500	0	−0.500	−1.000	0.500	0	0.500
−1.000	1.000	0	0	0	0	1.000	−1.000
0	0.750	0	−0.750	−1.000	0.750	0	0.250
−1.000	0.750	0	0.250	0	0.750	0	−0.750
0	0	1.000	−1.000	−1.000	1.000	0	0

Now, *fndn* from (A2.2) should have eight rows for its parameters and eight columns, one for each stage for each sequence group. Again we ignore the vector products using the first two rows of our output. So our vector postmultiplication of the second row of *fndn* by Y for one member of each sequence group yields: $\hat{b} = -.25Y_{112[B]} + .25Y_{114[A]} -.25Y_{212[A]} + .25Y_{214[B]}$. In terms of contrasts, we can write:

$\hat{b} = Slope\_Contr_{ABBA}$ for $Subject_{11} + Slope\_Contr_{BAAB}$ for $Subject_{21}$,

where $Slope\_Contr_{ABBA}$ for $Subject_{11} = -.25Y_{112[B]} + .25Y_{114[A]}$

and $Slope\_Contr_{BAAB}$ for $Subject_{21} = (-.25Y_{212[A]} + .25Y_{214[B]}.)$

RELATION TO SAS® DEFINITIONS OF CONTRASTS BASED ON TABLE 12.2

For a subject in the ABBA group, the mult of Table 12.2 = 1, and the two entries for $Slope\_Contr_{ABBA}$ for $Subject_{11}$ correspond to "slope =

.25*(mult*(−y2 + y4) + (1 − mult)*(y2 − y4));" or .25*(−y2 + y4)" in the SAS® definition of that table. Similarly, for a subject in the BAAB group, mult = 0, and the two entries for− $Slope\_Contr_{BAAB}$ for $Subject_{21}$ correspond to "slope = .25*(mult*(−y2 + y4) + (1 − mult)*(y2 − y4)) = .25*(y2 - y4)", just as implied by Table A2.4. This SAS® coding leads to a separate contrast for slope for each subject in each treatment group.

Next let us think about combining the slope contrasts for all subjects in this kind of experiment. We need the average of all such contrasts for the ABBA subjects plus the average of all such contrasts for the BAAB subjects. Calling the first average $\overline{Slope\_Contr}_{ABBA}$ and the second average $\overline{Slope\_Contr}_{BAAB}$, we can say that we need to compute $\hat{b} = \overline{Slope\_Contr}_{ABBA} + \overline{Slope\_Contr}_{BAAB}$. This is what our GAUSS program output from Table A2.2 tells us to do in estimating the slope constant b for this data set; it is also what is done when SAS® performs the t-test for slope effects using the program of Table 12.2.

In general $Slope\_Contr_{BAAB} = 0Y_{2i1} - .25Y_{2i2} + 0Y_{1i3} + .25Y_{2i4}$

$$= -.25Y_{2i2} + .25Y2i4.$$

Now with the BAAB sequence present, mult = 0, making this new equation activate the second part of the SAS® slope definition). But with the ABBA sequence present, mult = 1, making the original equations for $\hat{b}$ above activate the first part of the SAS® definition in our earlier Table 12.2.

Remember the issue in chapters 8 and 12 about negatives of true contrasts being invoked in our t-test computations? We now expand our explanation of that process to point out that we want to compute $t = \dfrac{\overline{Slope\_Contr}_{ABBA} + \overline{Slope\_Contr}_{BAAB}}{s_{\overline{Slope\_Contr}_{ABBA} + \overline{Slope\_Contr}_{BAAB}}}$ with the SAS® PROC TTEST program. But SAS® and we as well are more accustomed to computing quantities like $t = \dfrac{\overline{X}_{ABBA} - \overline{X}_{BAAB}}{s_{\overline{X}_{ABBA} - \overline{X}_{BAAB}}}$. Also, for independent groups, the standard errors of the sums and differences are identical: $s_{\overline{X}_{ABBA} + \overline{X}_{BAAB}} = s_{\overline{X}_{ABBA} - \overline{X}_{BAAB}}$. So we trick the computer program by feeding into it correct contrasts for the ABBA subjects but negative contrasts, $-$Slope_Contr$_{BAAB}$, for the BAAB subjects.   Does this make sense to you?

We do not present or describe the use of the remainder of the estimation matrix we have been discussing. The principles of its use for estimating other parameter values are exactly the same as for estimating the previous slope.

FINDING CONTRASTS FOR DATA WITHOUT LINEAR SLOPE

The Program Itself

For a model permitting nonlinear stage effects, Table A2.5 shows an analogue to the GAUSS™ program of Table A2.3. It is used to develop the contrast score formulas in Table 12.4 for our model permitting nonlinear stage effects. As before, a set-to-zero recoding has been invoked to permit unique parameter estimation (Table A2.5).

TABLE A2.5
A GAUSS™ Program to Facilitate Finding Individual Subjects' Contrasts
for an ABBA Versus BAAB Design Model Not Assuming
Linear Practice Effects

```
new; output file= temp.out reset; date;
/* COUNSET0.EST program to find estimation matrix for a 2-group 4-period
design with 2 carryover parameters with n = 1 per group.*/
let x[8,8] =
1 0 1 0 0 1  0  0
1 0 0 1 0 0 .5  0
1 0 0 0 1 0  0 -.5
1 0 0 0 0 1 -.5  0
0 1 1 0 0 0  0  0
0 1 0 1 0 1 -.5  0
0 1 0 0 1 1  0 .5
0 1 0 0 0 0 .5  0;
```

(Continued)

TABLE A2.5

(Continued)

@ Columns for seq1 = mu + subj1n + pi_4 + tau_B + .5(lam_AB + lam_BA),
seq2 = mu + subj2n + pi_4 + tau_B + .5(lam_AB + lam_BA), pi_1 – pi_4 –
.5 (lam_AB + lam_BA, pi_2 – pi_4, pi_3 – pi_4 + .5(lam_AA – lam_AB –
lam_BA + lam_BB), tau_A – tau_B, lam_AB – lam_BA, and lam_AA –
lam_BB. @ x_prod = x'x; prod_inv = inv(x_prod); fndn = prod_inv*x';
"Estimation matrix = " ; fndn; output off; end;

Interpreting What This GAUSS™ Program Has to Say

The logic on which this new table is based is similar to that for Table
A2.3 for a model with linear trend. Notice that the three functions of
stages represented earlier in Equation 12.4, $\pi_1 - \pi_4 - .5(\lambda_{AB} + \lambda_{BA})$,
$\pi_2 - \pi_4$, and $\pi_3 - \pi_4 + .5(\lambda_{AA} - \lambda_{AB} - \lambda_{BA} + \lambda_{BB})$ are assigned to Columns 3 through 5. However, only $\pi_2 - \pi_4$ was interesting enough to be
included in the SAS® program of Table 12.4. Output from this table is
used to produce contrasts for different parameters and subjects and to do
t-tests in a manner comparable to that associated with Table A2.3.

USE OF GAUSS™ IN EFFICIENCY ESTIMATION

Most efficiency calculations for this book were performed twice, once
with SAS® and once with GAUSS™, yielding results consistent within
reasonable limits of rounding effects. We do not show extensions of
GAUSS™ programs such as those of Tables A2.3 and A2.5, noting simply that Equation 5.15, for example, is easy to apply in that language.

GAUSS™ IS JUST ONE OPTION

There are other possibilities than GAUSS™ for use in performing matrix
computations and supplementing the work of conventional statistical
procedures such as SAS® GLM. Two popular options are Mathematica
(Wolfram, 1991) and SAS®/IML (SAS Institute Inc., 1989a).

References

Adair, J. G. (1984). The Hawthorne effect: A reconsideration of the methodological artifact. *Journal of Applied Psychology, 69*, 334–345.

Almudevar, T., & Tibshirani, R. (1990). *GAIM. Version 1.0.* Toronto: S. N. Tibshirani Enterprises, Inc.

Anscombe, F., & Tukey, J. W. (1963). The examination and analysis of residuals. *Biometrics, 5*, 141–160.

Aptech Systems. (1993). *GAUSS 3.1.12.* Maple Valley, WA: Aptech Systems.

Baalam, L. N. (1968). A two-period design with t^2 experimental units. *Biometrics, 24*, 61–73.

Barlow, D. H., & Hersen, M. (1984). *Single case experimental designs. Strategies for studying behavior changes* (2nd ed.). New York: Pergamon Press.

Berenblut, I. I. (1964). Change-over designs with complete balance for first residual effects. *Biometrics, 20*, 707–712.

Berenblut, I. I. (1967). The analysis of change-over designs with complete balance for first residual effects. *Biometrics, 23*, 578–580.

Bethell-Fox, C. E., & Shepard, R. N. (1988). Mental rotation: Effects of stimulus complexity and familiarity. *Journal of Experimental Psychology: Human Perception and Performance, 14*, 12–23.

Boik, R. J. (1981). A priori effects in repeated measures designs: Effects of non-sphericity. *Psychometrika, 46*, 241–255.

Campbell, D. T., & Stanley, J. C. (1966). *Experimental and quasi-experimental designs for research.* Chicago: Rand McNally.

Carlson, R. A., & Schneider, W. (1989). Acquisition context and the use of causal rules. *Memory & Cognition, 17,* 240–248.

Chambers, J. M., & Hastie, T. J. (Eds.) (1992). *Statistical methods in S.* Pacific Grove, CA: Wadsworth & Brooks/Cole Advanced Books & Software.

Chatfield, C. (1989). *The analysis of time series. An introduction* (4th ed.). London: Chapman and Hall.

Chaudhuri, P., Lo, W-D., Loh, W-Y., & Yang, C-C. (1995). Generalized regression trees: Function estimation via recursive partitioning and maximum likelihood. *Statistica Sinica, 5,* 641–666.

Cochran, W. G., & Cox, G. M. (1957). *Experimental designs* (2nd ed.). New York: Wiley.

Collier, R. O., Jr., Baker, F. B., & Mandeville, G. K. (1967). Tests of hypotheses in a repeated measures design from a permutation viewpoint. *Psychometrika, 32,* 15–24.

Cook, R. D., & Weisberg, S. (1982). *Residuals and influence in regression.* NewYork: Chapman and Hall.

Cook, T. D., & Campbell, D. T. (1983). The design and conduct of quasi-experiments and true experiments in field settings. In M. D. Dunnette (Ed.), *Handbook of industrial and organizational psychology* (pp. 223–326). New York: Wiley.

Cornell, J. E., Young, D. M., Seaman, S. L., & Kirk, R. E. (1992). Power comparisons of eight tests for sphericity in repeated measurements designs, *Journal of Educational Statistics, 17,* 233-249.

Cotton, J. W. (1989). Interpreting data from 2–period crossover designs. (Also termed the replicated 2 by 2 Latin square design.) *Psychological Bulletin, 106,* 503–515.

Cotton, J. W. (1993). Latin square designs. In L. K. Edwards (Ed.), *Applied analysis of variance in behavioral science.* New York: Marcel Dekker.

Cotton, J. W. (1994). Effects of collapsing data from crossover designs. In G. H. Fischer & D. Laming (Eds.), *Contributions to mathematical psychology, psychometrics, and methodology.* New York: Springer-Verlag.

Cotton, J. W., & Kenward, M. G. (1991, June). *Data analysis for 2-treatment within-subject designs with few observations per subject.* Paper presented at joint meeting of the Psychometric Society and the

Classification Society of North America, New Brunswick, NJ.

Cox, D. R. (1951). Some systematic experimental designs. *Biometrika*, *38*, 312–323.

Crespi, L. P. (1942). Quantitative variation of incentive and performance in the white rat. *American Journal of Psychology*, *55*, 467–517.

Crespi, L. P. (1944). Amount of reinforcement and level of performance. *Psychological Review*, *51*, 341–357.

Crowder, M. J., & Hand, D. J. (1990). *Analysis of repeated measures.* London: Chapman and Hall.

De Carlo, L. T. (1994). A dynamic theory of proportional judgment: Context and judgment of length, heaviness, and roughness. *Journal of Experimental Psychology: Human Perception and Performance*, *20*, 372–381.

Dixon, W. J., Brown, M. B., Engelman, L., Hill, M. A., & Jennrich, R. I. (1990). *BMDP statistical software manual.* Berkeley, CA: University of California Press.

Draper, N. R., & Joiner, B. L. (1984). Residuals with one degree of freedom. *American Statistician*, *38*, 55–57.

Draper, N. R., & Smith, H. (1981). *Applied regression analysis* (2nd ed.). New York: Wiley.

Edgington, E. S. (1995). *Randomization tests* (3rd ed.). New York: Marcel Dekker.

Edwards, L. K., & Bland, P. C. (1993). Some computer programs for selected ANOVA programs. In L. K. Edwards (Ed.), *Applied analysis of variance in behavioral science.* New York: Marcel Dekker.

Elashoff, J. (1997). *NQuery Advisor®.* Boston: Statistical Solutions.

Fulenwider, D. O. (1989). Using the GLM procedure and the CONTRAST statement: A very basic approach. In *Proceedings of the Fourteenth Annual SAS Users Group International Conference* (pp. 152–162). Cary, NC: SAS Institute Inc.

Geisser, S., & Greenhouse, S. W. (1958). An extension of Box's results on the use of the *F*-distribution in multivariate analysis. *Annals of Mathematical Statistics*, *29*, 885–891.

Gentile, J. R., Roden, A. H., & Klein, R. (1972). An analysis-of-variance model for the intrasubject replication design. *Journal of Applied Behavior Analysis*, *5*, 193–198.

Gentleman, J. F., & Wilk, M. B. (1975). Detecting outliers in a two-way table: I. Statistical behavior of residuals. *Technometrics*, *17*,

1–14.

Gill, P. S., & Shukla, G. K. (1987). Optimal change-over designs for correlated observations. *Communications in Statisics—Theory and Methods, 16*, 2243–2261.

Girden, E. R. (1992). *ANOVA Repeated measures. Quantitative applications in the social sciences, paper 84.* Newbury Park, CA: Sage.

Gottsdanker, R. (1978). *Experimenting in psychology.* Englewood Cliffs, NJ: Prentice-Hall.

Hall, J. F. (1966). *The psychology of learning.* Philadelphia: J. B. Lippincott.

Hartmann, D. P. (1974). Forcing square pegs into round holes: Some comments on "An analysis-of-variance model for the intrasubject replication design." *Journal of Applied Behavior Analysis, 7*, 635–638.

Hastie, T. J., & Tibshirani, R. J. (1990). *Generalized additive models.* London: Chapman and Hall.

Hays, W. L. (1994). *Statistics* (5th ed.). Fort Worth: Harcourt Brace.

Huynh, H., & Feldt, L. S. (1970). Conditions under which mean square ratios in repeated measurements designs have exact F-distributions. *Journal of the American Statistical Association, 65*, 1582–1589.

Huynh, H., & Feldt, L. S. (1976). Estimation of the Box correction for degrees of freedom from sample data in randomized block and split-plot designs. *Journal of Educational Statistics, 1*, 69–82.

Ingham, R. J., & Andrews, G. (1973). An analysis of a token economy in stuttering therapy. *Journal of Applied Behavior Analysis, 6, 219–229.*

John, S. (1971). Some optimal multivariate tests. *Biometrika, 58*, 123-127.

John, S. (1972). The distribution of a statistic used for testing sphericity of normal distributions. *Biometrika, 59*, 169-173.

Jones, B., & Kenward, M. G. (1989). *Design and analysis of cross-over trials.* London: Chapman and Hall.

Jones, R. H. (1993). *Longitudinal data with serial correlation: A state-space approach.* London: Chapman and Hall.

Kempthorne, O. (1952). *The design and analysis of experiments.* New York: Wiley.

Keppel, G. (1982). *Design and analysis. A researcher's handbook* (2nd ed.). Englewood Cliffs, NJ: Prentice-Hall.

Kershner, R. P., & Federer, W. T. (1981). Two-treatment crossover designs for estimating a variety of effects. *Journal of the American*

Statistical Association, 76, 612–619.

Kiefer, J. (1975). Construction and optimality of generalized Youden designs. In J. N. Srivastava (Ed.), *A survey of statistical design and linear models.* Amsterdam: North-Holland.

Kirk, R. E. (1982). *Experimental design: Procedures for the behavioral sciences* (2nd ed.). Belmont, CA: Brooks/Cole.

Kirk, R. E. (1995). *Experimental design: Procedures for the behavioral sciences* (3rd ed.). Belmont, CA: Brooks/Cole.

Kratochwill, T. R. (Ed.). (1978). *Single subject research: Strategies for evaluating change.* New York: Academic Press.

Kratochwill, T. R., & Levin, J. R. (Eds.). (1992). *Single-case research design and analysis: New directions for psychology and education.* Hillsdale, NJ: Lawrence Erlbaum Associates.

Laska, E. M., & Meisner, M. (1985). A variational approach to optimal two-treatment crossover designs: Application to carryover-effect models. *Journal of the American Statistical Association, 80,* 704–710.

Lorch, R. F., & Myers, J. L. (1990). Regression analyses of repeated measures data in cognitive research. *Journal of Experimental Psychology: Learning, Memory, and Cognition, 16,* 149–157.

Lunneborg, C. E. (1994). *Modeling experimental and observational data.* Belmont, CA: Duxbury Press.

MacArthur, R. D., & Sekuler, R. (1982). Alcohol and motion perception. *Perception & Psychophysics, 31,* 502–505.

Manly, B. F. J. (1991). *Randomization and Monte Carlo methods in biology.* London: Chapman and Hall.

Matthews, J. N. S. (1987). Optimal crossover designs for the comparison of two treatments in the presence of carryover effects and autocorrelated errors. *Biometrika, 74,* 311–320.

Matthews, J. N. S. (1988). Recent developments in crossover designs. *International Statistical Review, 56,* 311–320.

Mauchly, J. W. (1940). Significance test for sphericity of a normal *n*-variate distirbution. *Annals of Mathematical Statistics, 11,* 204–209.

Maxwell, S. E. (1980). Pairwise multiple comparisons in repeated measures designs. *Journal of Educational Statistics, 5,* 269–287.

Maxwell, S. E., & Delaney, H. D. (1990). *Designing experiments and analyzing data. A model comparison perspective.* Belmont, CA: Wadsworth.

McBurney, D. H. (1983). *Experimental psychology.* Belmont, CA: Wadsworth.

Micceri, T. (1989). The unicorn, the normal curve, and other improbable creatures. *Psychological Bulletin, 105,* 156–166.

Milliken, G. A., & Johnson, D. E. (1984). *Analysis of messy data. Vol. 1: Designed experiments.* Belmont, CA: Lifetime Learning Publications.

Morrison, D. F. (1990). *Multivariate statistical methods* (3rd ed.). New York: McGraw-Hill.

Myers, J. L. (1979). *Fundamentals of experimental design* (3rd ed.). Boston: Allyn and Bacon.

Namboodiri, N. K. (1972). Experimental designs in which each subject is used repeatedly. *Psychological Bulletin, 77,* 54–64.

Norusis, M. J. (1990a). *SPSS® base system user's guide.* Chicago: SPSS Inc.

Norusis, M. J. (1990b). *SPSS® advanced statistics™ user's guide.* Chicago: SPSS Inc.

O'Brien, R. G., & Muller, K. E. (1993). Unified power analysis for *t*-tests through multivariate hypotheses. In L. K. Edwards (Ed.), *Applied analysis of variance in behavioral science.* New York: Marcel Dekker.

Patel, H. I. (1986). Analysis of repeated measures designs with changing covariates in clinical trials. *Biometrika, 73,* 707–715.

Patel, H. I., & Hearne, E. M. (1980). Multivariate analysis for the two-period repeated measures crossover design with application to clinical trials. *Communications in Statistics—Theory and Methods, 9,* 1919–1929.

Patterson, H. D., & Lucas, H. L. (1962). *Change-over designs.* North Carolina Agricultural Experiment Station and U.S. Department of Agriculture, Technical Bulletin No. 147.

Quenouille, M. H. (1953). *The design and analysis of experiment.* London: Griffin.

Ratkowsky, D. A., Evans, M. A., & Alldredge, J. R. (1993). *Cross-over experiments: Design, analysis, and application.* New York: Marcel Dekker.

Roethlisberger, F. J., & Dickson, W. J. (1939). *Management and the worker: An account of a research program conducted by the Western Electric Company, Hawthorne Works.* Cambridge, MA: Harvard University Press.

Rouanet, H., & Lepine, D. (1970). Comparison between treatments in a repeated measures design: ANOVA and multivariate methods. *British Journal of Mathematical and Statistical Psychology, 23,* 147–163.

Rousseeuw, P. J. (1991). Tutorial to robust statistics. *Journal of Chemometrics, 5,* 1–20.

Rousseeuw, P. J., & Leroy, A. M. (1987). *Robust regression and outlier detection.* New York: Wiley.

SAS Institute Inc. (1985). *SAS/IML™ user's guide for personal computers. Version 6 edition.* Cary, NC: SAS Institute, Inc.

SAS Institute Inc. (1988a). *SAS® introductory guide for personal computers. Release 6.03 edition.* Cary, NC: SAS Institute Inc.

SAS Institute Inc. (1988b). *SAS/SAT® user's guide. Release 6.03 edition.* Cary, NC: SAS Institute Inc.

SAS Institute Inc. (1989a). *SAS/IML® software: Usage and reference, Version 6* (1st ed.), Cary, NC: SAS Institute Inc.

SAS Institute Inc. (1989b). *SAS® language and procedures: Usage. Version 6* (1st ed.), Cary, NC: SAS Institute Inc.

SAS Institute Inc. (1989c). *SAS/STAT user's guide, Version 6* (4th ed.). Vol. 1. Cary, NC: SAS Institute, Inc.

SAS Institute Inc. (1989d). *SAS/STAT® user's guide. Version 6 (4th ed.). Vol. 2. Cary, NC: SAS Institute Inc.*

SAS Institute Inc. (1990). *SAS® language. Reference version 6* (1st ed.). Cary, NC: SAS Institute Inc.

Scheffé, H. (1959). *The analysis of variance.* New York: Wiley.

Schneider, W., & Fisk, A. D. (1984). Automatic category search and its transfer. *Journal of Experimental Psychology: Learning, Memory, and Cognition, 10,* 1–15.

Searle, S. R. (1971). *Linear models.* New York: Wiley.

Searle, S. R. (1982). *Matrix algebra useful for statistics.* New York: Wiley.

Searle, S. R. (1987). *Linear models for unbalanced data.* New York: Wiley.

Seber, G. A. E. (1984). *Multivariate observations.* New York: Wiley.

Senn, S. (1993). *Cross-over trials in clinical research.* New York: Wiley.

Shaughnessy, J. J., & Zechmeister, E. B. (1990). *Research methods in psychology* (2nd ed.). New York: McGraw-Hill.

Shepard, R. N., & Metzler, J. (1971). Mental rotation of three-dimensional objects. *Science, 171,* 701–703.

Smith, M. D. (1996). *The design and analysis of crossover trials with many periods.* Unpublished doctoral dissertation, University of Kent at Canterbury. Canterbury, England.

Stevens, J. (1996). *Applied multivariate statistics for the social sciences* (3rd ed.). Mahwah, NJ: Lawrence Erlbaum Associates.

Wallenstein, S., & Fisher, A. C. (1977). The analysis of the two-period repeated measurements crossover design with applications to clinical trials. *Biometrics, 33,* 261–269.

Wilkinson, L. (1989). *SYSTAT™: The system for statistics.* Evanston, IL: SYSTAT Inc.

Williams, E. J. (1949). Experimental designs balanced for the estimation of residual effects of treatments. *Australian Journal of Scientific Research, A2,* 149–168.

Winer, B. J., Brown, D. R., & Michels, K. M. (1991). *Statistical principles in experimental design* (3rd ed.). New York: McGraw-Hill.

Wolfram, S. (1991). *Mathematica: A system for doing mathematics by computer* (2nd ed.). Redwood City, CA: Addison-Wesley.

Wood, C. (1978). A large sample Kolmogorov-Smirnov test for normality of experimental error in a randomized block design. *Biometrika, 65,* 673–676.

Young, A. W., Ellis, A. W., Flude, B. M., McWeeny, K. H., & Hay, D. C. (1986). Face-name interference. *Journal of Experimental Psychology: Human Perception and Performance, 12,* 466–475.

Young, A. W., McWeeny, K. H., Ellis, A. W., & Hay, D. C. (1986). Naming and categorizing faces and written names. *Quarterly Journal of Experimental Psychology, 38A,* 297–318.

Zeaman, D. (1949). Response latency as a function of the amount of reinforcement. *Journal of Experimental Psychology, 39,* 466–483.

Author Index

Subject Index